WITHDRAWN
WRIGHT STATE UNIVERSITY LIBRARIES

CARDIAC PACING AND ELECTROPHYSIOLOGY

Cardiac Pacing and Electrophysiology

A bridge to the 21st century

Edited by

A.E. AUBERT
University Hospital Gasthuisberg, Leuven, Belgium

H. ECTOR
University Hospital Gasthuisberg, Leuven, Belgium

and

R. STROOBANDT
St. Jozef Hospital, Oostende, Belgium

Kluwer Academic Publishers
Dordrecht / Boston / London

Library of Congress Cataloging-in-Publication Data

```
Cardiac pacing and electrophysiology : a bridge to the 21st century /
   edited by A.E. Aubert, H. Ector, and R. Stroobandt.
      p.   cm.
   Includes index.
   ISBN 0-7923-2627-X (hb : alk. paper)
   1. Cardiac pacing.   I. Aubert, André E., 1943-   . II. Ector,
Hugo, 1943-   .  III. Stroobandt, R. (Roland)
   [DNLM: 1. Cardiac Pacing, Artificial--trends.
2. Electrophysiology--trends.  3. Electrophysiology-
-instrumentation.  4. Pacemaker, Artificial--trends.
5. Defibrillators, Implantable--trends.   WG 168 C2633 1944]
RC684.P3C314  1994
617.4'120645--dc20
DNLM/DLC
for Library of Congress                                   93-38818
```
ISBN 0-7923-2627-X

Published by Kluwer Academic Publishers,
P.O. Box 17, 3300 AA Dordrecht, The Netherlands.

Kluwer Academic Publishers incorporates
the publishing programmes of
D. Reidel, Martinus Nijhoff, Dr W. Junk and MTP Press.

Sold and distributed in the U.S.A. and Canada
by Kluwer Academic Publishers,
101 Philip Drive, Norwell, MA 02061, U.S.A.

In all other countries, sold and distributed
by Kluwer Adademic Publishers Group,
P.O. Box 322, 3300 AH Dordrecht, The Netherlands.

Printed on acid-free paper

All Rights Reserved
© 1994 Kluwer Academic Publishers
No part of the material protected by this copyright notice may be reproduced or
utilized in any form or by any means, electronic or mechanical,
including photocopying, recording or by any information storage and
retrieval system, without written permission from the copyright owner.

Printed in the Netherlands

This book is dedicated to the memory of His Majesty King Baudouin, King of the Belgians (1930–1993)

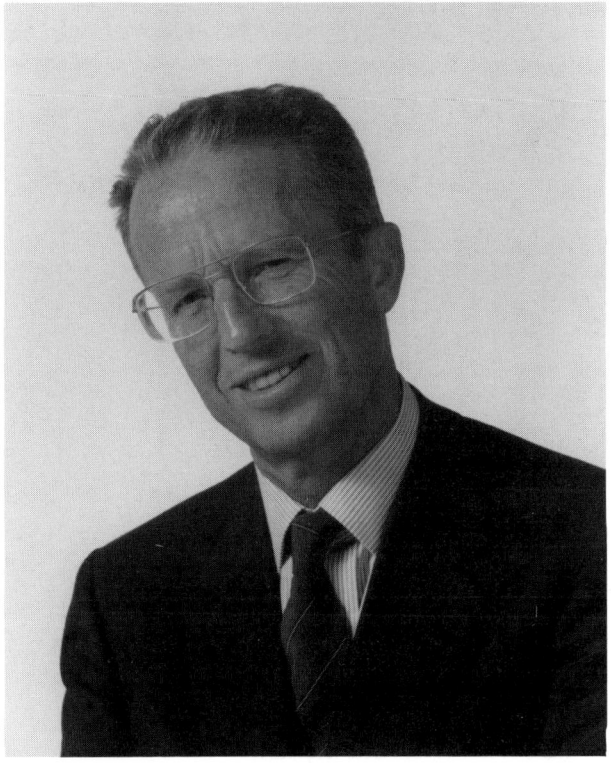

"His Majesty the King of the Belgians Patron of the 6th European Symposium on Cardiac Pacing"

F. Kuypers @ INBEL
Regentlaan 54   Bd du Régent 54
1000 Brussel   1000 Bruxelles
tel.   32-02-2171111

Contents

Foreword xiii
List of Contributors xvii

PART ONE: Electrophysiology

1. Equipment for the electrophysiology laboratory: possibilities and limitations
   Willem R.M. Dassen, Rob G.A. Mulleneers & Joep R.L.M. Smeets 3

2. Vasovagal syncope: clinical presentation, classification and management
   Richard Sutton 15

3. Classification of antiarrhythmic drugs in relation to mechanisms of arrhythmias
   Michiel J. Janse 23

4. Electrophysiological characteristics in arrhythmogenic right ventricular dysplasia and dilated cardiomyopathies
   Guy Fontaine, R. Frank, R. Tsezana, J. Tonet, E. Velasquez & G. Lascault 31

5. Classification of death in patients under antiarrhythmic treatment
   Ralph Rogers, Hugo Ector, Ann Rubens, Carl Timmermans, Hein Heidbüchel & Hilaire De Geest 41

6. Heart rate variability. Methodology and physiological basis
   Lü Fei & Marek Malik 49

7. Heart rate variability and QT interval: their relationships with the cardiac frequency
Philippe Coumel & Pierre Maison-Blanche ... 63

8. Role of dynamic QT interval in Holter tapes to stratify risk in postmyocardial infarction patients
E. Rodriguez Font, E. Homs, J. Guindo, V. Martí, X. Viñolas, A. Bayés Genís & A. Bayés de Luna ... 73

9. Heart rate variability in patients with angina pectoris
Nina Rehnqvist, Inge Björkander, Lennart Forslund, Claes Held & Paul Hjemdahl ... 79

10. Time and frequency domain analysis of heart rate variability after myocardial infarction
Federico Lombardi, Giulia Sandrone & Alberto Malliani ... 83

11. Signal averaged ECG. Technical principles, possibilities and limitations
Alfons Sinnaeve & Hugo Tassignon ... 93

12. Optimizing the predictive value of the signal-averaged ECG for serious arrhythmic events in the post-infarction period
Nabil El-Sherif ... 117

13. Signal-averaged analysis of the P wave: possible applications in different settings
M. Ali Oto ... 125

14. Late potentials during acute myocardial ischaemia
P.E. Vardas, F.J. Parthenakis & E.G. Manios ... 131

15. Radiofrequency catheter ablation in the treatment of supraventricular tachycardias
Frank Simonis, Erik Andries & Pedro Brugada ... 137

16. Anatomical versus electrophysiological approaches for ablation of the slow pathway in patients with AV nodal reentrant tachycardia
Michel Haissaguerre, Bruno Fischer, Philippe le Métayer, Pierre Jais, Philippe Egloff & Jean-François Warin ... 145

PART TWO: Pacing

17. Cardiac pacing in Europe in 1992: a new survey
    Giorgio A. Feruglio 157

18. The myocardium-electrode interface at the cellular level
    Max Schaldach 169

19. The myocardium-electrode interface at the macro level
    W. Irnich 189

20. Unipolar versus bipolar leads
    Ivo Kersschot 203

21. Single lead VDD pacing: an update
    Giovanni Enrico Antonioli, Lucia Ansani, Roberto Audoglio,
    Gabriele Guardigli, Gianfranco Percoco & Tiziano Toselli 209

22. Substantial improvement of screw-in electrodes
    Petras Stirbys 221

23. Physiological cardiac pacing: an individual objective
    J. Claude Daubert, Philippe Mabo, Daniel Gras, Christophe
    Leclercq & Thierry Lelièvre 227

24. Pacemaker syndrome during atrial-based pacing
    S. Serge Barold 251

25. Dual chamber pacemaker therapy in cardiomyopathy
    S. Serge Barold, Lukas Kappenberger, Claude Daubert & Guy
    Fontaine 269

26. DDD rate-responsive pacing: state of the art
    Massimo Santini, G. Ansalone & G. Cacciatore 281

27. Heart rate response based on changes in central venous oxygen
    saturation, minute ventilation and body activity
    Ole-Jörgen Ohm, Svein Fœrestrand & Finn Hegbom 289

28. DDDR and atrial arrhythmia
    Véronique Mahaux 303

29. Holter and pacemaker diagnostics
    Paul A. Levine 309

x *Contents*

30. Clinical relevance of histograms in the follow-up of DDDR pacemakers
    Marc M.J. Berkhof, Jozef P. Snoeck, Marnix P.N. Goethals & Marc J. Claeys   325

31. Holter and telemetry in pacemakers and ICDs: new developments
    Alain Ripart   333

32. Automatic measure of the interface capacitor and the total cardiac impedance
    Francisco Pérez Gómez, Manuel Montero, Miguel A. Pastor, Francisco Pérez-Vizcaíno, María J. Pérez-Vizcaíno & Pablo González   347

33. Critical analysis of the different algorithms designed to protect the paced patient against atrial tachyarrhythmias in dual chamber pacing
    Philippe Ritter, S. Cazeau, Y. Kojoukharov, L. Henry, H. Podeur, A. Lazarus & J. Mugica   355

34. Mode switching in DDDR pacing
    Richard Sutton   363

PART THREE: Defibrillators

35. Indication for ICD implantation and selection of patients: present and future
    Luc Jordaens   373

36. The optimum tilt for defibrillation
    W. Irnich   381

37. Cerebrovasomotor reactivity predicts tolerance to tiered therapy with implantable cardioverter-defibrillators
    Igor Singer & Harvey Edmonds, Jr.   387

38. Clinical utility of telemetered electrograms in pacemakers and ICDs
    Roland Stroobandt, Filiep Vandenbulcke, Roger Willems & Alfons Sinnaeve   399

Contents xi

39. High patient acceptance for implantable cardioverter/
defibrillator (ICD): quality of life and patient acceptance
Berndt Lüderitz, Werner Jung & Matthias Manz   411

40. Cardiac pacing and electrophysiology: how much technology do
we need?
R.W.F. Campbell   419

41. Medical technology assessment and reimbursement policy of
implantable devices in Belgium: possibilities and limitations for
the future
Rob van den Oever   423

42. Socioeconomic aspects of implantable devices: can we afford
new technology?
Konrad K. Steinbach   431

Index   439

Foreword

In 1992, clinical cardiac electrophysiology became a recognized sub-speciality of the American Board of Internal Medicine. The formal recognition of this highly specialized and technical field of medicine represents the culmination of thirty years of remarkable scientific and intellectual discovery. Beginning in the 1950s, cardiologists realized that cardiac arrhythmias were the cause of significant morbidity and the sudden death of at least 350,000 patients every year in the United States alone. At that time the only tools available for analyzing abnormal heart rhythms were the standard EKG machine and careful deductive reasoning.

During the early 1960s, cardiac pacemakers reflected the first foray in the electrical therapy of cardiac arrhythmias. Pacemakers were first implanted in order to control syncopal episodes related to bradycardic heart rhythms. Although crude and bulky devices, their utility was immediately obvious to physicians and patients alike. The recognition that electrical signals could be recorded from *inside* the heart and that the heart's rhythm could be controlled by the application of electrical energy began the era of clinical cardiac electrophysiology which was to follow.

In the late 1960s and early 1970s and at the peak of the Vietnam conflict, a group of cardiologists with special training in cardiac electrophysiology were sequestered at the US Public Health Service Hospital at Staten Island. Their sole responsibility was to develop techniques which would enable the clinical study of arrhythmias. Nearly simultaneously, at several cardiologic centers in Europe, identical clinical investigations proceeding independently were developing similar techniques with similar exciting results. Out of those preliminary and ground-breaking investigations came procedures now broadly known as Electrophysiologic Studies.

ELECTROPHYSIOLOGY

The current book as edited by Drs. A.E. Aubert, H. Ector and R. Stroobandt reflects the nearly unbelievable advances made in the field of cardiac electrophysiology over the past thirty years. In the first section a variety of techniques never imagined as recently as ten years ago are discussed. The analysis of electrocardiograms by signal averaging techniques is discussed in the chapters by Drs. El-Sherif, Oto and Vardas. This sophisticated method of signal analysis applied at both the atrial and ventricular levels has allowed analysis of the statistical probability of arrhythmia development. In the setting of coronary artery disease, the signal-averaged EKG has been an extraordinarily accurate independent predictor for the development of malignant ventricular arrhythmias and sudden death.

Heart rate variability as yet another predictor of the likelihood of arrhythmic events is similarly discussed. The physiologic basis of blunted heart rate variability as well as its relationship to ischemia, infarction and sudden death is detailed in the chapters by Drs. Fei, Coumel, Rehnqvist and Lombardi. A review of the equipment required in the modern electrophysiology laboratory as well as discussion of anti arrhythmic therapy in the current era is similarly presented.

Perhaps the most revolutionary aspect of modern clinical electrophysiology is the current ability to 'cure' specific cardiac arrhythmias by the application of ablative energy to specific areas of cardiac tissue responsible for them. The use of radio-frequency catheter ablation in the treatment of patients with reentrant supraventricular tachycardia is detailed in the articles by Simonis and Haissaguerre. It is apparent that this new field of clinical cardiac electrophysiology, still in its infancy, holds dramatic promise as the therapy of choice in a variety of cardiac arrhythmias.

PACING

The chapters dealing with cardiac pacing attest to the extraordinary developments which have occurred in a field less than forty years old. A far cry from the primitive devices of the 1960s, today's pacemakers employ not only new lead technologies (see the chapters of Drs. Schaldach, Irnich, Kersschot, Antonioli, and Stirbys) but reflect a detailed understanding of the myocardial electrode interface required for both cardiac pacing and the discriminate recognition of intracardiac signals. Physiologic pacing employing dual-chambered and rate responsive devices is also discussed. Drs. Barold, Santini and Mahaux critically review the efficacy of dual chamber rate responsive pacing devices as well as their inherent limitations. The ability of these pacemakers to sense abnormal cardiac rhythms and automatically switch to an appropriate pacing mode is outlined by Dr. Sutton.

Technologies allowing modern pacemakers to store data reflecting their function forms the basis of additional chapters in the section on cardiac pacing. Pacemaker diagnostics as discussed by Drs. Levine and Berkhof reflect the ability of current devices to analyze, store and allow subsequent retrieval of cardiac electrophysiologic data. The use of cardiac pacemakers as diagnostic devices is clearly an area which will receive additional attention during the years to come.

DEFIBRILLATION

With the rapid improvement in permanent pacemaker technology which occurred during the 1970s, the possibility of using electrical energy to treat abnormally rapid heart rhythms became a reality. Not only were implanted pacemakers used to 'stimulate' the heart and treat symptomatic bradyarrhythmias, they began to be used to terminate abnormally rapid heart rhythms using pacing algorithms just recently discovered in the electrophysiology laboratories of Europe and the United States. Shortly thereafter a new device was to revolutionize the treatment of patients at risk of sudden death.

In the 1960s, Sudden Cardiac Death (SCD) was found to be the result of a specific abnormal heart rhythm – ventricular fibrillation. This lethal arrhythmia was shown to begin with single ventricular premature depolarizations which under specific electrophysiologic circumstances demonstrated 'reentry' within abnormal areas of ventricular myocardium. Finding multiple available reentrant pathways, the resultant ventricular tachycardia degenerated into the electrical chaos which so frequently resulted in sudden death.

The recognition that a large electrical shock applied to the chest could simultaneously depolarize large areas of ventricular myocardium and restore the heart beat to normal, resulted in a small but significant survivorship of what would ordinarily have been a terminal event. In the mid 1980s the first practical *implantable* defibrillator was placed in patients in the United States and Europe. This small but incredibly complex device, changed the risk of dying suddenly as a result of ventricular fibrillation from 50% over two years, to less than 5% at the end of five.

In the section on Defibrillation, the state of the art available implantable devices (pacemaker-cardiovertor-defibrillators) are reviewed. Drs. Jordaens and Lüderitz consider the issues of appropriate patient selection as well as acceptance of this type of device therapy. Technical aspects of the defibrillation pulse are discussed in the chapter by Dr Irnich. Drs. Singer and Stroobandt review the sophisticated algorithms required by these multitasked devices as well as their necessary patient and physician interfaces. In conclusion, the socio-economic ramifications of these expensive new technologies are explored in the chapters provided by Drs. van den Oever and Steinbach.

Cardiac pacing and electrophysiology as presented in the current publication truly represents a bridge to the 21st century. As a progress report on one of the most exciting areas of medical/scientific/engineering endeavor to have emerged in the later twentieth century one can only marvel at the accomplishments thus far achieved. With a societal commitment to continued technological advancement there seems no limit to the patient benefits which will be derived.

BRUCE N. GOLDREYER, M.D. *Clinical Professor of Medicine*
University of Southern California
Director, Clinical Electrophysiology
San Pedro Peninsula Hospital
San Pedro, CA, USA

List of contributors

GIOVANNI ENRICO ANTONIOLI
  Department of Cardiology, Arcispedale S. Anna, C. So Giovecca 203, I-44100 Ferrara, Italy
  Co-authors: Lucia Ansani, Roberto Audoglio, Gabriele Guardigli, Gianfranco Percoco and Tiziano Toselli

ANDRÉ E. AUBERT
  University Hospital Gasthuisberg O/N, Herestraat 49, B-3000 Leuven, Belgium

S. SERGE BAROLD
  Division of Cardiology, Department of Medicine, The Genesee Hospital, University of Rochester, 224 Alexander Street, Rochester NY 14607, U.S.A.
  Co-authors: Lukas Kappenberger, Claude Daubert and Guy Fontaine

MARC M.J. BERKHOF
  Department of Cardiology, University Hospital Antwerp, Wilrijkstraat 10, B-2650 Edegem, Belgium
  Co-authors: Jozef P. Snoeck, Marnix P.N. Goethals and Marc J. Claeys

PEDRO BRUGADA
  Cardiovascular Centre, OLV Hospital, Moorselbaan 164, B-9300 Aalst, Belgium
  Co-authors: Frank Simonis and Erik Andries

R.W.F. CAMPBELL
  Department of Academic Cardiology, University of Newcastle upon Tyne, Framlington Place, Newcastle upon Tyne NE2 4HH, U.K.

List of contributors

PHILIPPE COUMEL
  Hôpital Lariboisière, 2, Rue Ambroise Paré, F-75010 Paris Cedex 10, France
  Co-author: Pierre Maison-Blanche

WILLEM R.M. DASSEN
  Department of Cardiology, University Hospital, University of Limburg, P. Debyelaan 25, P.O. Box 5800, NL-6202 AZ Maastricht, The Netherlands
  Co-authors: Rob G.A. Mulleneers and Joep R.L.M. Smeets

J. CLAUDE DAUBERT
  Service de Cardiologie A, Centre Hospitalier Univ/CHRU, 2 Rue de l'Hotel Dieu, F-35033 Rennes Cedex, France
  Co-authors: Philippe Mabo, Daniel Gras, Christophe Leclercq and Thierry Lelièvre

HUGO ECTOR
  Department of Cardiology, University Hospital Gasthuisberg, Herestraat 49, B-3000 Leuven, Belgium
  Co-authors: Ralph Rogers, Ann Rubens, Carl Timmermans, Hein Heidbüchel and Hilaire De Geest

NABIL EL-SHERIF
  Cardiology Division, SUNY Health Science Center, VA Medical Center, 450 Clarkson Avenue, PO Box 1199, Brooklyn, NY 11203-2098, U.S.A.

LÜ FEI
  Department of Cardiological Sciences, St. George's Hospital, Medical School, Cranmer Terrace, London SW17 ORE, U.K.
  Co-author: Marek Malik

GIORGIO A. FERUGLIO
  Cardiology Department, Regional Hospital, Piazzale S. Maria della Misericordia 15, I-33100 Udine, Italy

E. RODRIGUEZ FONT
  Department of Cardiology, Hospital De La Santa Creu i Sant Pau, Sant Antoni M. Claret 167, E-08025 Barcelona, Spain
  Co-authors: E. Homs, J. Guindo, V. Martí, X. Viñolas, A. Bayés Genís and A. Bayés de Luna

GUY FONTAINE
Department of Cardiac Pacing, Hospital Jean Rostand, 39–41 Rue Jean le Galleu, F-94200 Ivry sur Seine, France
Co-authors: R. Frank, R. Tsezana, J. Tonet, E. Velasquez and G. Lascault

BRUCE N. GOLDREYER
1360 West 6th Street/Ste 200, San Pedro, CA 90732, U.S.A.

FRANCISCO PÉREZ GÓMEZ
Department of Cardiology, University Hospital San Carlos, Ciudad Universitaria, E-28040 Madrid, Spain
Co-authors: Manuel Montero, Miguel A. Pastor, Francisco Pérez-Vizcaíno, María J. Pérez-Vizcaíno and Pablo González

MICHEL HAISSAGUERRE
Department of Cardiology, Hospital Saint–André, F-33000 Bordeaux, France
Co-authors: Bruno Fischer, Philippe le Métayer, Pierre Jais, Philippe Egloff and Jean-François Warin

W. IRNICH
Department of Medical Engineering, Justus-Liebig-University, Aulweg 123, D-35392 Giessen, Germany

MICHIEL J. JANSE
Laboratory of Experimental Cardiology, Academic Medical Center, Meibergdreef 9, NL-1105 AZ Amsterdam, The Netherlands

LUC JORDAENS
Department of Cardiology, University Hospital, De Pintelaan 185, B-9000 Gent, Belgium

IVO KERSSCHOT
Department of Cardiology, St. Vincentius Hospital, St. Vincentiusstraat 20, B-2018 Antwerp, Belgium

PAUL A. LEVINE
Siemens Pacesetter, Inc., 15900 Valley View Court, P.O. Box 9221, Sylmar, CA 91392–9221, U.S.A.

FEDERICO LOMBARDI
Internal Medicine II, Ospedale L. Sacco, University of Milan, Via GB Grassi, 74, I-20157 Milano, Italy
Co-authors: Giulia Sandrone and Alberto Malliani

BERNDT LÜDERITZ
  Department of Cardiology, Medical University Clinic, Sigmund-Freud-Strasse 25, D-5300 Bonn 1, Germany
  Co-authors: Werner Jung and Matthias Manz

VÉRONIQUE MAHAUX
  Department of Cardiology, University of Liège, CHU Sart Tilman, P.O. Box 35, B-4000 Liege, Belgium

ROB VAN DEN OEVER
  Landsbond der Christelijke Mutualiteiten, Wetstraat 121, B-1040 Brussels, Belgium

OLE-JÖRGEN OHM
  Department of Cardiology, Medical Department A, University School of Medicine, Haukeland Sykehus, N-5021 Bergen, Norway
  Co-authors: Svein Faerestrand and Finn Hegbom

M. ALI OTO
  Hacettepe University, Tip Fakültesi, Kardiyoloji Ana Bilim Dali, Sihhiye, Ankara, Turkey

NINA REHNQVIST
  Department of Medicine, Danderyd Hospital, S-182 88 Danderyd, Sweden
  Co-authors: Inge Björkander, Lennart Forslund, Claes Held and Paul Hjemdahl

ALAIN RIPART
  ELA Medical, C.A. La Boursidière, F-92357 Le Plessis Robinson Cedex, France

PHILIPPE RITTER
  Department of Cardiac Stimulation and Electrophysiology, Centre Chirurg Val d'Or, 16 Rue Pasteur, F-92211 Saint Cloud Cedex, France
  Co-authors: S. Cazeau, Y. Kojoukharov, L. Henry, H. Podeur, A. Lazarus and J. Mugica

MASSIMO SANTINI
  Via del Collegio Capranica n. 30, I-00186 Rome, Italy
  Co-authors: G. Ansalone and G. Cacciatore

MAX SCHALDACH
  Central Institute for Biomedical Technique, Friedrich-Alexander-University, Erlangen-Nürnberg, Turnstrasse 5, D-91054 Erlangen, Germany

IGOR SINGER
Cardiac Electrophysiology and Pacing, Arrhythmia Service, University of Louisville, 530 South Jackson Street, Louisville, KY 40292, U.S.A.
Co-author: Harvey Edmonds, Jr.

ALFONS SINNAEVE
Zeedijk 101, B-8400 Oostende, Belgium
Co-author: Hugo Tassignon

KONRAD K. STEINBACH
Ludwig Boltzmann Institute on Arrhythmia Research, Cardiac Department, Wilheminenspital, Montleartstrasse 37, A-1171 Vienna, Austria

PETRAS STIRBYS
Cardiac Pacing Clinic, Kaunas Medical Academy, Eiveniu Str 2, Kaunas 3007, Lithuania

ROLAND STROOBANDT
Department of Cardiology, Sint-Jozef Hospital, Nieuwpoortsesteenweg 57, B-8400 Ostend, Belgium
Co-authors: Filiep Vandenbulcke, Roger Willems and Alfons Sinnaeve

RICHARD SUTTON
Chelsea and Westminster Hospital, 369 Fulham Road, London SW10 9NH, U.K.

P.E. VARDAS
Department of Cardiology, University Hospital, University of Crete, P.O. Box 1352, Stravrakia Heraklion, Crete, Greece
Co-authors: F.J. Parthenakis and E.G. Manios

PART ONE

Electrophysiology

1. Equipment for the electrophysiology laboratory: possibilities and limitations

WILLEM R.M. DASSEN, ROB G.A. MULLENEERS & JOEP R.L.M. SMEETS

INTRODUCTION

In this chapter, an overview will be presented of the equipment required for invasive electrophysiological investigations in patients suffering from cardiac arrhythmias or conduction disturbances. In this context, the term electrophysiologic investigation represents those methods and techniques used to make the differential diagnosis, to determine the etiology, and to evaluate the selected therapy in patients suffering from conduction disturbances and/or tachyarrhythmias. After a brief overview of these investigational techniques, a description of the hardware will be given, followed by a discussion of the influence the application of additional computer techniques could have.

INVASIVE CARDIAC ELECTROPHYSIOLOGY: METHODS

During invasive electrophysiological investigations, a number of electrode catheters are introduced percutaneously into a vein and/or artery and fluoroscopically positioned at predefined positions in the heart. These electrodes can be used to record the local electrical activity at that site of the heart or to stimulate the heart electrically from there. A number of programmed stimulation sequences are commonly used, like the extra stimulus technique or overdrive pacing, to initiate and/or terminate the arrhythmia so that its mechanism and site of origin can be studied.

Electrophysiological investigations can be divided into two subgroups:

1. Programmed electrical stimulation to study the electrophysiological parameters of specific parts of the conduction system or to evaluate the initiation and termination of tachycardias and the protective effect of antiarrhythmic medication on these arrhythmias
2. Mapping techniques, to determine the earliest activation in just a small part of the heart, the focus of a tachycardia, or the ventricular end of

an accessory pathway in WPW patients. These techniques include pace mapping.

Programmed stimulation

Using the extra stimulus technique, after synchronizing with the patient's own rhythm or after a paced basic rate, one or more extra stimuli are delivered and the activation sequence of these stimuli determined. In this way, electrophysiological properties like the conduction times through the AV node and the bundle of His or the refractory period of accessory connections in Wolff-Parkinson-White syndrome (WPW) patients can be determined compared to different basic cycle lengths. Also, the initiation and termination of tachycardias can be studied, together with the protective effect of medication given to change the electrophysiological properties [1,2].

The output is composed of a registration of the electrical activity of the intracardiac recordings together with the surface electrocardiogram (ECG) as a function of time. A 12-lead ECG is needed to detect small changes in QRS morphology, which are important but would not have been picked up if only a few leads were used. Although the number of channels that can be reproduced by the paper recorder has a maximum value, the limiting factor of this technique is formed by the number of catheters that can be introduced and manipulated in the heart and whose exact position can be determined.

An example of such a registration is shown in Figure 1.

Mapping

During programmed stimulation of the heart, the user is interested in conduction on the macro level and in the inducibility of tachycardias. During mapping procedures, interest is concentrated on a small part of the heart where the focus of the tachycardia, or the exit point of a reentrant circuit, is located.

One of the treatment modalities is surgical dissection of the site of the tachycardia. Since this necessitates thoracotomy, mapping of the electrical activation from a large number of sites on the epicardial surface is possible. The introduction of transcatheter ablation of tachycardias (using at first DC current and now radiofrequency energy) has made the surgical approach to arrhythmias almost obsolete [4–9]. This new technique has limited the need for multichannel mapping equipment but has generated a new procedure: pace mapping. During pace mapping, the cardiologist positions the catheter as close as possible to the focus of the tachycardia. By stimulating this site at the rate of the tachycardia from which the patient is suffering, an ECG can be recorded and compared to the one recorded during tachycardia, to uncover similarities. As the focus is approached, the differences between these two ECGs diminish.

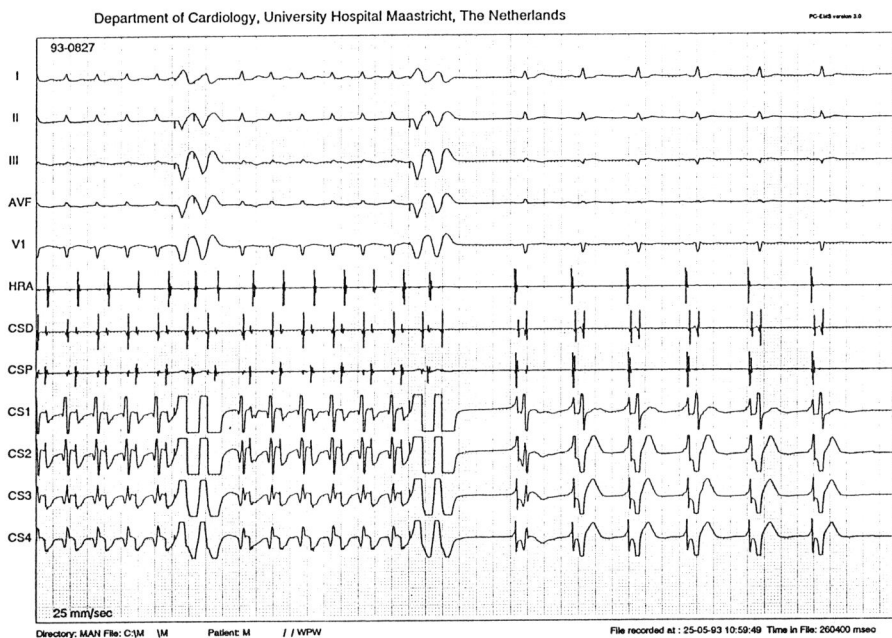

Figure 1. Termination of a tachycardia by two electrical stimuli. HRA = high right atrium, CSD = coronary sinus distal, CSP = coronary sinus proximal, all measured bipolar. CS1 to CS4 = coronary sinus, unipolar recording. Recordings are made using the PC-EMS version 3.0 system [3].

The number of intracardiac signals during pace mapping is relatively small, since all electrodes have to be manipulated from outside the heart.

A disadvantage of classical systems is that the original and the stimulated tachycardia cannot be visualized simultaneously and therefore are difficult to compare. In more recent systems, a template of the original tachycardia is reproduced on the same screen that displays the tachycardia while pace mapping the endocardium (Figure 2). It is possible to superimpose these complexes in all 12 leads to detect even very small differences. Changes in amplification or paper speed of the paced tachycardia should be compensated by adjusting the templates accordingly. To find the exact location, it is essential to display and compare all 12 leads of the ECGs [10].

INVASIVE CARDIAC ELECTROPHYSIOLOGY: HARDWARE

Electrophysiological investigations have been performed in man for more than 25 years [11]. At the beginning, equipment was not commercially avail-

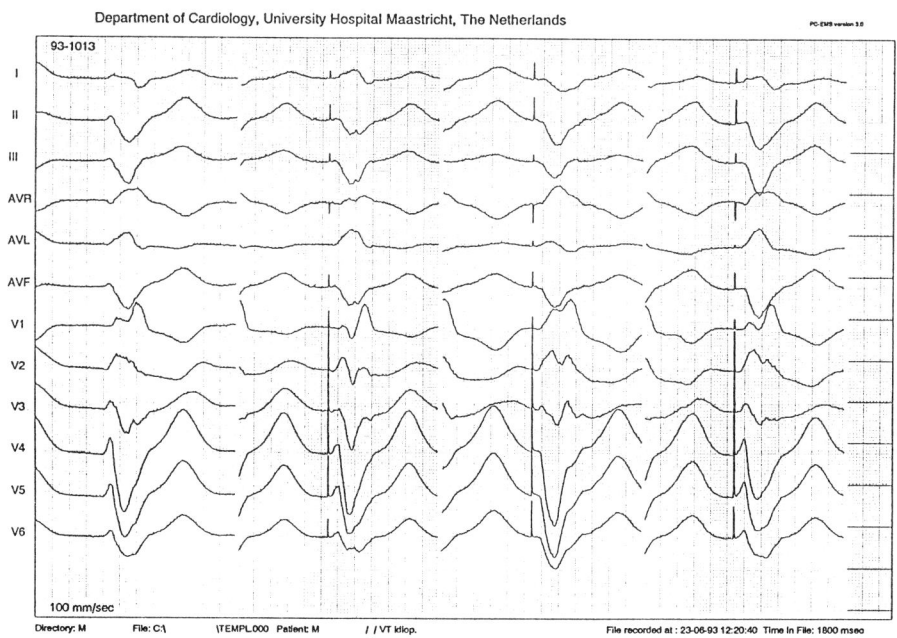

Figure 2. The output of the system during catheter pace mapping, depicted after the recording of the third template. Simultaneously, up to three template ECGs (tachycardia or paced beats) can be reproduced. From left to right: the template representing the original tachycardia, a frozen ECG during pace mapping near the focus of the tachycardia; note the difference in leads V1 and V2, the next frozen ECG during pacing closer to the site of the focus, the actual ECG obtained during pacing. Only this window is refreshed every beat, to enable comparison with one of the three frozen ECGs to the left.

able, and all centers entering this field had to build their own tools [12,13]. The equipment for programmed electrical stimulation of the heart could be subdivided into two parts: the electrical stimulator and the registration equipment.

The programmable stimulator is used to stimulate the heart in a predefined way, to initiate and terminate arrhythmias from which the patient is suffering, under controlled conditions. The registration part visualizes the activation of the different parts of the heart to enable study of the mechanism of the arrhythmia and to select the most optimal treatment. Originally these two functions, registration and stimulation, were separated. Using a locally developed programmable stimulator based on analog electronic technology, the heart was stimulated, while a separate set of amplifiers and recorders made the registrations. Even in the early days of clinical electrophysiology, special attention was paid to the electrical hazards and safety aspects of these procedures [14,15]. The standard configuration for electrophysiologic investi-

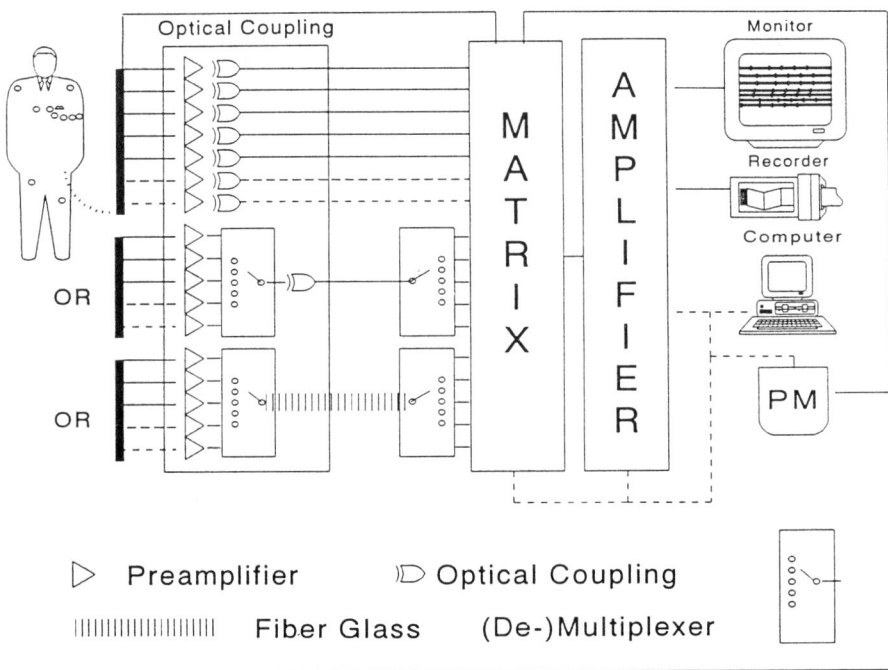

Figure 3. The layout of a modern electrophysiological pacing and measurement unit.

gations using programmed stimulation of the heart has not changed significantly since the first experiments and is schematically depicted in Figure 3.

Registration

Under local anesthesia, fluoroscopic control is used to manipulate the catheters in a predefined location in the heart or to follow the position of the electrode during mapping of the endocardium. The catheters, unipolar or bipolar, are connected to a switch box and from there attached to either the output of the stimulator or the input of the intracardiac amplifiers. The preamplifiers should be mounted as close as possible to the patient to improve the signal/noise ratio. Subsequently, for safety reasons, the patient must be separated from the potentially dangerous recording equipment. These signals should be electrically isolated. This is usually done by using optical coupling. This coupling can take place in each preamplifier, or all preamplified signals can be multiplexed and isolated using one opto coupler. If the recording site and the interpretation site are not adjacent, a fiberglass connection can be used. This fiber serves as an insulator and is insensitive to electromagnetic fields. After preamplification, the signals are filtered, amplified, and reproduced. Normally, a selection has to be made as to which signals should appear on a monitor and which should be written on paper. The number of channels the paper recorder can handle is normally the limiting factor. Furthermore, the 12-lead surface electrocardiogram is recorded using nonradioopaque electrodes for the precordial leads. Finally, all analog signals can be stored on magnetic tape for future processing and retrieval. In this chapter, only recordings made by catheters will be discussed. If the thorax has been opened during surgery and the epicardial surface is accessible, two-dimensional mapping could be performed. Representation of these two-dimensional recordings requires the construction of activation maps, with the help of a computer [16–19].

Stimulation

To be useful in clinical electrophysiology, the pacing equipment should fulfill the following requirements. The system should be able to generate a variety of pulse trains, synchronized to the patient's own rhythm or using a paced basic rate. This basic rate should be followed by at least three extra stimuli. All intervals in the pacing train should be selectable with a 1-ms resolution and allow automatic increments and decrements of the coupling interval to be scanned. Furthermore, burst pacing should be possible. The actual stimuli should be delivered by one of the two available selectable output channels and should be adjustable in duration and amplitude.

FUTURE IMPROVEMENTS

Using the equipment described above, most electrophysiological investigations can be performed. However, the increasing interest in cardiac electrophysiology has led to a growing number of investigations and more complex stimulation protocols [20] to be followed during these investigations. In addition, these techniques have proved to be very manpower, equipment, and time consuming [21]. These growing demands have led to the introduction of the computer in the electrophysiology lab to facilitate a number of tasks: (a) to improve the signal logistics, (b) to control the stimulator, (c) to visualize the results, (d) to archive data and results, and (e) to help interpret complex tracings. In particular, the diagnosis and surgical treatment of the WPW syndrome and ventricular tachycardia have stimulated the application of computers in clinical electrophysiology [22–27]. In which way can the different aspects be facilitated by the introduction of computer techniques?

Improvement of the signal logistics. As shown in Figure 3, a number of catheters are positioned in the heart and connected to either the input of the intracardiac preamplifier or the output of the electrical stimulator. Since in many standard pacing protocols the layout of the catheters is predefined, this selection (how to interconnect the catheters) could be performed by computer. This layout then forms a part of the stimulation protocol. The second step that can be automated is the selection of amplification and filtering of all signals. Finally, these signals should be reproduced, normally on both a multichannel monitor and a paper recorder. At this site, the arrangement of all signals can be taken care of by the computer.

Controlling the stimulator. The new programmed stimulation techniques resulted in a large number of stimulation protocols, all requiring the manual selection of a number of intervals and settings. The large diversity of protocols prompted the demand for a flexible system to define, store, reproduce, and modify pacing protocols [28]. At first, the computer assisted the user while programming the original pacemaker, but shortly thereafter the entire pacemaker was modelled in software, and now most computerized programmable stimulators consist of a flexible software package controlling a small impulse generator. In this way, a large number of protocols can be stored in the memory and loaded at will. Multiple stimulation protocols, for instance for the initiation and termination of tachycardia, can be placed in the memory and executed immediately. Although these software-based stimulators are more user friendly and flexible compared with the first analogue devices, the resulting stimulus trains do not differ significantly.

Visualizing the results. By digitizing the signals, it becomes possible to reproduce on the screen a fixed registration, to stretch the time scale to make more accurate measurements, and to use on-screen calipers to measure any interval the user is interested in. Furthermore, signals like the QRS complex can be compared, subtracted, or manipulated. In this way, small changes in morphology or in activation sequences can be detected accurately and easily.

Archiving data and results. If not digitized, these signals could only be stored by using analog magnetic tape. In digital form, all or parts of the results of a stimulation study can be stored on hard disc. After the study, all the information or selected parts of it can be archived in a more permanent memory, like an optical disc or a DAT recorder. In this way, the information from a large number of studies becomes available for reanalysis or reproduction on paper. Research has been performed to evaluate whether the results of these clinical electrophysiologic investigations could be stored automatically and be used for automatic report generation [29–34].

Supporting the interpretation of complex tracings. Although computers successfully support data acquisition, the computerized interpretation of these signals remains cumbersome. Using a digitizing tablet, the first systems allowed a computerized measurement of intervals whose onset and offset were determined by the user manually. In some systems, the conduction intervals during regular rhythms can be measured or the activation front analyzed automatically, but human overreading remains essential [35–44]. This relative standstill in the computerized interpretation of these studies has a number of causes. Many clinical electrophysiological stimulation and measurement systems are developed locally, and no standardization has been achieved, in contrast to, for example, the interpretation of the resting ECG [45]. Furthermore, the sequence of events which have to be measured cannot always be predicted, so the actual interpretation of these signals remains handwork.

One of the few areas in which progress has been made concerning the automated interpretation of electrophysiological signals is in the automated differentiation of tachycardias. This field of research, stimulated by the development of antitachycardia pacemakers and implantable defibrillators, has recently produced interesting advancements. Algorithms have been developed to differentiate supraventricular from ventricular tachycardia automatically using the electrical activity measured by one atrial and one ventricular lead, or if necessary even by giving one atrial stimulus and monitoring the subsequent ventricular response [46–50].

DISCUSSION

In clinical electrophysiology, the same basic principles and techniques for stimulation and registration of 20 years ago are still being used. However, the introduction of computerized technology has facilitated these investigations, improved the storage and retrieval of a large number of signals and results generated, enabled reanalysis of the signals, and made these procedures more cost effective by decreasing the average time required to perform these studies. Future developments are difficult to predict and will depend largely on new therapeutic possibilities, as demonstrated, for instance, by the introduction of radiofrequency catheter ablation making two-dimensional mapping obsolete in a short period. A breakthrough in automated interpretation would require further standardization before universal criteria could be defined.

ACKNOWLEDGEMENT

We gratefully acknowledge the expert assistance of the AudioVisual Department of the Maastricht University Hospital.

REFERENCES

1. Wellens HJJ. Electrical stimulation of the heart in the study and treatment of tachycardias. Baltimore: University Park Press, 1971.
2. Wellens HJJ. Cardiac pacing in the study and treatment of arrhythmias (tachycardias), in: Thalen, editor, Cardiac Pacing. Assen: Van Gorcum, 1973; 372–5.
3. Van Der Steld B, Dassen W, Den Dull K, Gorgels A, Smeets J, Wellens H. An electrophysi-

ological measurement system especially designed to support ablation procedures. PACE 1993;16:1109.
4. Feld GK, Fleck RP, Chen PS et al. Radiofrequency catheter ablation for the treatment of human type 1 atrial flutter: Identification of a critical zone in the reentrant circuit by endocardial mapping techniques. ClRC 1992;86/4:1233–40.
5. Levy S, Bru P, Cointe R et al. Cardioversion par choc electrique interne de la fibrillation auriculaire permanente. Arch Mal Coeur Vaiss 1989;82/9:1529–32.
6. Ward DE, Rowland E, Wainwright RJ, Camm AJ. Electrical ablation of junctional tachycardias showing a long RP interval. Eur Heart J 1989;10/8:718–24.
7. Lemery R, Talajic M, Roy D et al. Success, safety, and late electrophysiological outcome of low-energy direct-current ablation in patients with the Wolff-Parkinson-White syndrome. CIRC 1992;85/3:957–62.
8. Niwano S, Aizawa Y, Satoh M, Chinushi M, Shibata A. Low-energy catheter electrical ablation for sustained ventricular tachycardia. Am Heart J 1991;122/1:81–8.
9. Aizawa Y, Tamura M, Chinushi M et al. An attempt at electrical catheter ablation of the arrhythmogenic area in idiopathic ventricular fibrillation. Am Heart J 1992;123/1:257–60.
10. Sippens Groenewegen A, Spekhorst H, Van Hemel NM. Localization of the site of origin of postinfarction ventricular tachycardia by endocardial pace mapping. Body surface mapping compared with the 12-lead electrocardiogram. CIRC 1993;88:2290–306.
11. Durrer D, Schoo L, Schuilenburg RM, Wellens HJJ. The role of premature beats in the initiation and the termination of supraventricular tachycardia in the Wolff-Parkinson-White syndrome. CIRC 1967;36:644–62.
12. Scherlag BJ, Lau SH, Helfant RH, Berkowitz WD, Stein E, Damato AN. Catheter technique for recording His bundle activity in man. CIRC 1969;34:13–8.
13. Damato AN, Lau SH, Helfant RH, Stein E, Berkowitz WD. Study of atrioventricular conduction in man using electrode catheter recordings of His bundle activity. CIRC 1969;24:287–96.
14. Stammer CF, Whalen RE, McIntosh HD. Hazards of electric shock in cardiology. Am J Cardiol 1964;14:537–46.
15. Burchell HB, Sturm RE. Electroshock hazards. CIRC 1967;35:227–8.
16. Canavan TE, Schuessler RB, Cain ME et al. Computerized global electrophysiological mapping of the atrium in a patient with multiple supraventricular tachyarrhythmias. Ann Thorac Surg 1988;46:232–5.
17. Witkowski FX, Corr PB. An automated simultaneous transmural cardiac mapping system. Am J Physiol 1984;16:H661–H8.
18. Masse S, Sevaptsidis E, Parson ID, Downar E. A three-dimensional display for cardiac activation mapping. PACE 1991;14:538–45.
19. Laxer C, Alferness CA, Smith WM, Ideker R. The use of computer animation of mapped cardiac potentials in studying electrical conduction properties of arrhythmias. In: Ripley K, editor. Comp in Cardiol. Los Alamitos: IEEE Computer Society Press, 1990:23–6.
20. Elharrar V. A computer-controlled stimulator with applications to cardiac electrophysiology. Am J Physiol 1980;8:H278–H82.
21. Ross DL, Farré J, Bär FW et al. Comprehensive clinical electrophysiological studies in the investigation of documented or suspected tachycardias: Time, staff, problems and costs. CIRC 1980;61:1010–6.
22. Chen PS, Dembitsky WP, Fleck RP, Calisi CM, Feld GK. Demonstration of accessory pathway interaction by computerized mapping in preexcitation syndrome. PACE 1990;13:839–44.
23. Pieper CF, Parsons D, Lawrie GM, Lacy J, Roberts R, Pacifico A. Design and implementation of a new computerized system for intraoperative cardiac mapping. J Appl Physiol 1991;71:1529–39.
24. Buckles DS, Harold ME, Gillette PC, Case CL, Crawford FA. Computer-enhanced mapping of activation sequences in the surgical treatment of supraventricular arrhythmias. PACE 1990;13:1401–7.

25. Canavan TE, Schuessler RB, Boineau JP, Corr PB, Cain ME, Cox JL. Computerized global electrophysiological mapping of the atrium in patients with Wolff-Parkinson-White syndrome. Ann Thorac Surg 1988;46:223–31.
26. Fisher W, Swartz J. Three-Dimensional electrogram mapping improves ablation of left-sided accessory pathways. PACE 1992;15:2344–56.
27. Tweddell JS, Branham BH, Harada A et al. Potential mapping in septal tachycardia: Evaluation of a new intraoperative mapping technique. CIRC 1989;80:I97–I108.
28. Dassen WRM, Van der Steld A, Van Braam W et al. Pactot, a reprogrammable software pacing system. PACE 1985;8:574–8.
29. Kirchner M, Avancini GP, Antolini R. Real-time interval measurement during invasive cardiac electrophysiologic testing. In: Ripley K, editor. Comp in Cardiol New York: IEEE, 1987:93–6.
30. Dijk WA, Kingma JH, Van der Velde W, Lie KI, Van Hemel NM. Computer assisted management of malignant ventricular arrhythmias. In: Ripley K, editor. Comp in Cardiol. Los Alamitos: IEEE Computer Society Press, 1990:93–6.
31. Dijk WA, Kingma JH, Brugada P. Real time data collection during programmed stimulation of the heart. In: Ripley K, editor. Comp in Cardiol. Washington: IEEE Computer Society Press, 1985;177–80.
32. Dijk WA, Kingma JH, Crijns H. Stiekema HR, Van der Velde W. Real time generation of ladder diagrams of arrhythmias during programmed stimulation of the heart. In: Ripley K, editor. Comp in Cardiol. Washington: IEEE Computer Society Press, 1987;89–92.
33. Hieb B, Southworth W, Ruffy R. An electrophysiology report generating system with data base capabilities. PACE 1983;6:708–15.
34. Biallas R, Zinner A, Gilette P. Automated electrophysiologic stimulation and on-line processing. In: Ripley K, editor. Comp in Cardiol. Washington: IEEE Computer Society Press, 1985;181–4.
35. McGillivray R, Wald RW, Budziakowski ME. Technical note: An interval timer with computer interface. J Clin Eng 1987;12:441–5.
36. Pieper CF, Blue R, Pacifico A. Activation time detection algorithms used in computerized intraoperative cardiac mapping. A comparison with manually determined activation times. J Cardiovasc Electrophysiol 1991;2:388–97.
37. Imperiale C. A computerized system for clinical investigations in cardiac electrophysiology. J Clin Eng 1989;14:493–503.
38. Coumel P, Leclercq JF, Maisonblanche P et al. Computerized analysis of dynamic electrocardiograms: A tool for comprehensive electrophysiology. A description of the ATREC II system. Clin Prog Electrophysiol Pacing 1985;3:181–201.
39. D'Alche P, Khayat A, Charon M et al. Cartographie de l'activite electrique cardiaque. Applications à la chirurgie experimentale. Arch Mal Coeur Vaiss 1984;77:969–77.
40. Gillette PC, Garson A Jr, Zinner A, Kugler JD, Kuehneman G, McNemara DG. Automated on-line measurement of electrophysiologic intervals during cardiac catheterization. PACE 1980;3:456–60.
41. Cochrane T, Dunlop AW, Nathan AW, Camm AJ. Cardiac electrophysiological studies: Computer analysis using a digitiser and interactive visual display unit. Clin Phys Physiol Meas 1983;4:321–31.
42. Buckles DS, Harold ME, Gillette PC et al. Real time, automated, interactive cardiac electrophysiology testing. PACE 1990;13:45–51.
43. Gillette P, Zmijewski M, Shelton MB. The evolution of computer application during clinical electrophysiologic testing. J Electrocardiol 1989;22:218–22.
44. Kingma JH, Dijk WA, Wierstra T, Van der Velde W. An interpretation system for cardiac arrhythmias during programmed electrical stimulation of the heart. In: Ripley K, editor Comp in Cardiol. Washington: IEEE Computer Society Press, 1986;667–70.
45. Bailey JJ, Berson AS, Garson A Jr et al. Recommendations for standardization and specifications in automated electrocardiography: Bandwidth and digital signal processing. A report for health professionals by an ad hoc Writing Group of the Committee on Electrocardio-

graphy and Cardiac Electropysiology of the Council on Clinical Cardiology. American Heart Association. CIRC 1990;81:730–9.
46. Lin D, Dicarlo LA, Jenkins JM. Identification of ventricular tachycardia using intracavitary ventricular electrograms: Analysis of time and frequency domain patterns. PACE 1988;11:1592–605.
47. Greenhut SE, Steinhaus BM. Template matching techniques for electrophysiologic signals: A practical, real-time system for detection of ventricular tachycardia. Biomed Sci Instrum 1992;28:37–42.
48. DiCarlo LA, Jenkins JM, Kriegler C. Intraventricular electrogram analysis for discrimination of ventricular tachycardia from ventricular fibrillation. J Electrocardiol 1991;24:135.
49. Noh K, Jenkins J, Bump T, Arzbaecher R. An atrial extrastimulus technique for separating sinus tachycardia from pace-terminable 1:1 tachycardias for use in an antitachycardia pacemaker. J Electrocardiol 1987;20:103.
50. DiCarlo LA, Lin D, Jenkins JM. Automated interpretation of cardiac arrhythmias: Design and evaluation of a computerized model. J Electrophysiol 1993;26:53–63.

2. Vasovagal syncope: clinical presentation, classification and management

RICHARD SUTTON

DEFINITION

Vasovagal syncope of the so-called malignant type may be defined as recurrent syncope with minimal warning, and often associated with self-injury, when conventional investigations are negative and fail to reveal a cause but prolonged head-up tilt testing without drug challenge precipitates the patient's symptoms. The use of the term malignant is especially chosen to distinguish this form of vasovagal syncope from that seen commonly in young people, where there is a significant duration of prodrome. Alternatively, the term malignant is used when asystole is prolonged during tilt-testing [1].

With proper instruction and careful attention paid by the patient to the warning symptoms, syncope can, in these young patients, be avoided. In contrast, the much older sufferers of malignant vasovagal syndrome cannot abort attacks. In youthful vasovagal syncope, the treatment almost always involves just explanation and reassurance, but in malignant vasovagal syndrome (MVVS), other modalities are required. Despite their clinical severity, these attacks are not now thought to be fatal.

INCIDENCE OF MALIGNANT VASOVAGAL SYNDROME

The incidence of MVVS is not yet known. One estimate has been made suggesting that for 70% of those who are not diagnosed by all conventional means of investigation of recurrent syncope or approximately 20% of all patients presenting with recurrent syncope [2], a diagnosis can be made by 60° prolonged head-up tilt testing.

HEAD-UP TILT TESTING METHODOLOGY

Head-up tilt testing at 60° for 45 min following an overnight fast and using a footplate support with a 3-lead ECG and non-invasive blood pressure monitoring is the standard Westminster protocol. A positive test result is the production of syncope [3]. Other methods have been suggested [4,5]. The Cleveland Clinic protocol [4] may lead to some false-negative results as the duration of tilt is only 20 min whereas the mean time to syncope in the Westminster series is 24 min [6]. The Benditt protocol [5] may lead to false-positive results because of the use of isoproterenol as a provocative agent. Raviele et al. [7] have suggested the use of intravenous nitroglycerin (NG) as an alternative to isoproterenol. In a comparative study, fewer false-positive results were found with NG. Employing lower degrees of tilt is likely to lead to false-negative results [3], and use of a saddle support instead of a footplate is likely to lead to false-positive ones [3]. The incidence of positive tilt testing in youthful vasovagal syncope without provocative drugs appears not to be high and may not be different from youthful controls [3]. Isoprenaline challenge probably has value in this context, but the increased sensitivity is tempered by a reduced specificity [8]. The methodology of tilt testing was recently reviewed in detail by Benditt et al. [9].

The value of tilt testing lies not only in the diagnosis of MVVS but also in its classification according to the haemodynamic behaviour prior to and during syncope. Hitherto, an arbitrary classification has been made between cardioinhibitory (CI) and vasodepressor (VD) types. In the former, the heart rate falls below 60 bpm and usually precedes a dramatic fall in arterial pressure, reaching rates of sinus bradycardia < 30 bpm (67%) with sinus arrest (10%), atrioventricular block (13%) and complete asystole (10%) [6]. In the latter, the heart rate does not fall below 60 bpm, but there is a dramatic fall in arterial pressure. Further subclassification will undoubtedly become necessary as understanding of the syndrome increases [10]. In this context, continuous arterial pressure monitoring is essential so that the heart rate change can be matched with the blood pressure fall (Figures 1–4).

In order to achieve adequate arterial pressure monitoring, noninvasive digital plethysmography was selected and has been validated during tilt testing [11]. A print-out of heart rate and arterial pressure monitoring at very slow paper speed is used (Figures 1–4). A large series of tilt tests has now been reported [12], in which all 472 patients suffered no morbidity or mortality. Positive test results occurred in 27.3%, of which 69.8% were cardioinhibitory and 30.2% vasodepressor according to the initial classification (vide supra). Mean time to syncope was 26.1 ± 15 min. The clinical indications for tilt were syncope in 77.5% and presyncope in the remainder. Of the 98 patients who underwent a repeat tilt test, the outcome was concordant in 86%. Furthermore, the various haemodynamic patterns of syncope were also concordant.

Vasovagal syncope 17

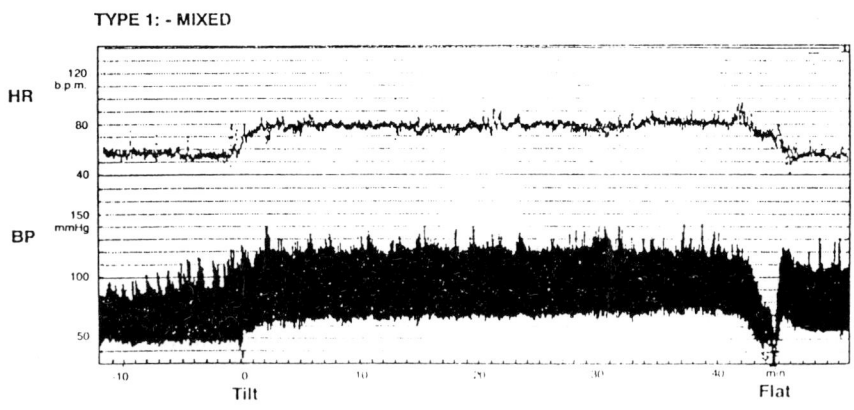

Figure 1. Type 1, mixed: Heart rate rises on tilting to 60° head-up and later falls at the time of syncope, but the ventricular rate does not fall to less than 40 bpm or falls to less than 40 bpm for less than 10 s with or without asystole of less than 3 s. Blood pressure may rise initially during the tilt but then falls before the heart rate falls.

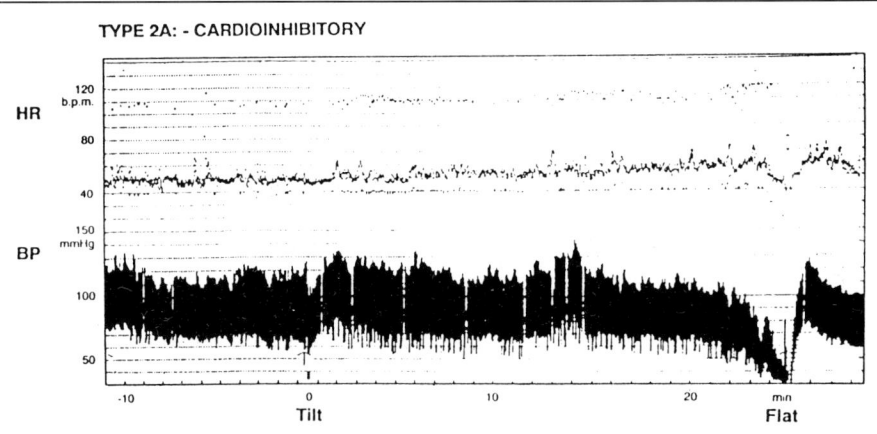

Figure 2. Type 2A, cardioinhibitory: Heart rate rises on tilting to 60° head-up and then falls to a ventricular rate of less than 40 bpm for more than 10 s, or asystole occurs for more than 3 s. Blood pressure may rise initially on tilt but falls before the heart rate falls.

INCIDENCE OF CARDIOINHIBITORY AND VASODEPRESSOR MALIGNANT VASOVAGAL SYNDROMES

The relative frequencies of the subdivisions of MVVS are not yet clearly known. One estimate suggests that approximately two-thirds of patients show CI and one-third, VD [2]. However, patients with type 2 B [10], the group

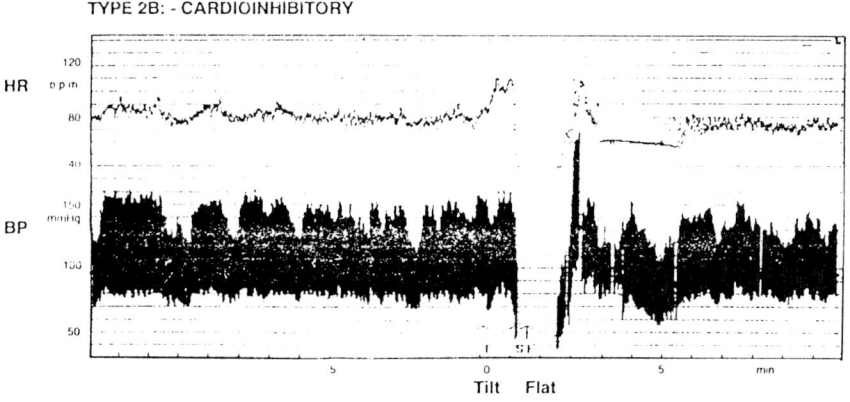

Figure 3. Type 2B, cardioinhibitory: Heart rate rises on tilting to 60° head-up and then falls to a ventricular rate less than 40 bpm for more than 10 s, or asystole occurs for more than 3 s. Blood pressure may rise initially on tilt and only falls to hypotensive levels (less than 80 mmHg systolic) at or after the onset of rapid and severe heart rate fall as defined above.

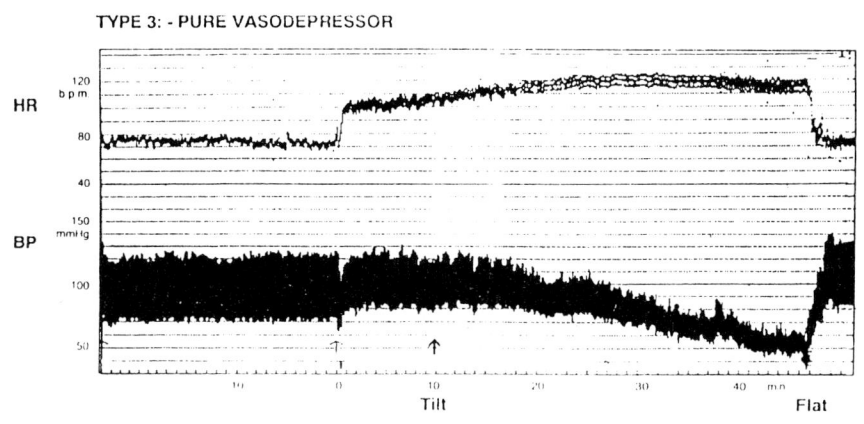

Figure 4. Type 3, pure vasodepressor: Heart rate rises progressively after adoption of the 60° head-up position and does not fall more than 10% from its peak at the time of syncope. Blood pressure falls during tilt to cause syncope.

thought to be most suitable for cardiac pacing, are considered to be much more uncommon amongst those who show cardioinhibition. More studies are necessary to obtain a clear distribution and should take into account the varied nature of positive reactions to tilt testing.

THERAPEUTIC OPTIONS IN CARDIOINHIBITORY MALIGNANT VASOVAGAL SYNDROME

The most effective therapy in bradycardia of any origin is cardiac pacing. In MVVS a similar situation to carotid sinus syndrome pertains. Some patients with CI can be treated by cardiac pacing, whereas VD is presently considered not amenable to it. Patients with MVVS usually have normal hearts with normal heart rate behaviour during exercise and emotion. When a vasovagal attack occurs, there is not only intense bradycardia or asystole but also a fall in arterial pressure which is due to dilatation of the splanchnic venous bed [13] and of the skeletal muscle arterioles [14]. This severely limits venous return. It is, therefore, necessary to use a mode of pacing which maximises the effect of the available returning venous blood, i.e. dual chamber pacing with a physiological atrioventricular delay. Retrograde atrioventricular conduction has been demonstrated despite high vagal tone during ventricular pacing in vasovagal syncope [15]. Thus, it is important to choose a mode of pacing in which retrograde atrioventricular conduction does not lead to pacemaker-mediated tachycardia. The DDI mode with rate hysteresis is advocated in this context, but there is no clinical proof of the efficacy of this mode compared with any other. An external dual chamber pacing study [16] suggested that an observed favourable reduction in the rate of fall of arterial pressure plays an important part in prolonging the prodrome. This, in everyday life, may be sufficient to allow the patient to abort an attack or avoid falls which result in injury. In a recent review of pacing experience using DDI with rate hysteresis in 37 patients with cardioinhibitory MVVS [17] who were followed for 39 ± 19 months, symptomatic improvement was achieved in 84% with a complete resolution of symptoms in 35%. The collective syncopal burden was reduced from 125.8 to 12.6 episodes per year. Clinical features which appeared to favour a successful outcome were relative youth (58 vs 70 years), lower supine systolic blood pressure (135 vs 163 mmHg) and complete absence of prodrome before pacing. Modifications to the presently available pacing behaviour will undoubtedly be made in the future to provide a discrepancy greater than 40 bpm between the trigger and pacing rates and also provide a version of search hysteresis to restore sinus rhythm as soon as it spontaneously occurs at physiological rates. More pacemaker sophistication could involve sensors to allow early pacing intervention prior to the full development of the vasovagal reflex. For example, these could detect activity and respond to an absence of activity combined with an erect posture detector by a mercury switch. These two conditions (stillness and an erect thorax) clinically appear to be invariable in the onset of vasovagal syncope except during medical procedures and in trauma. Thus, their detection by the pacemaker could allow early intervention with the possibility of aborting some or all attacks. There may, however, be limits to this approach, as rapid VVI pacing has been shown not to be helpful [18]. Pacing for this condition has not in the past found favour in the USA where vasovagal syncope was a class III indication, i.e. contraindicated, and therefore not reimbursed by third-party insurance. However, with the latest guidelines of the Joint Task Force of the AHA/ACC, vasovagal syncope is included as a class II indication [19].

THERAPEUTIC OPTIONS IN THE TREATMENT OF VASODEPRESSOR MALIGNANT VASOVAGAL SYNDROME

In vasodepressor MVVS, pacing appears to have nothing to offer the patient and the only available option is pharmacological. Many drugs have been proposed, in particular scopolamine administered by skin patch [4] and beta-blockade in the form of metoprolol [20]. Neither of the groups who performed the studies submitted these drugs to any type of controlled trial. Fitzpatrick et al. [21] performed a randomised controlled trial of scopolamine, atenolol and clonidine and found that none of them offers reliable therapy in MVVS. Thirteen patients completed 6 weeks on each of these three drugs with a repeat tilt challenge in each drug phase. Atenolol fared the worst, with no reduction in syncope and a rapid tilt to syncope time, whilst both scopolamine and clonidine delayed the time to syncope on tilt, but no drug significantly reduced the syncope rate. Disopyramide has been reported to be of benefit, and this has been explained by its negative inotropic effect [22] in addition to its vagolytic properties. This opposes the hypercontractile state of left ventricular function which appears to lead to the paradoxical triggering of both reflex bradycardia and vasodilatation that has been shown to occur in vasovagal syncope [23]. Etilefrine, an alpha- and beta-agonist, has also been reported to be of use [24]. Hypovolaemia was considered important in some of these patients [4,25], but a later study has not supported this [26]. It is possible that fludrocortisone may be helpful when hypovolaemia is present [4]. Partial beta-agonists such as xamoterol and pindolol have clinical advocates, but neither drug has been submitted to a rigorous clinical trial. When so many drugs with different actions are proposed as treatment for a condition, the strong implication is that either there is no effective therapy or that the problem is very complex, or both. The achievement of 100% symptom control may involve the use of an implantable drug dispenser where an infusion is triggered by sensors detecting the early phase of vasovagal syncope.

CONCLUSION

Malignant vasovagal syndrome must be distinguished from youthful vasovagal syncope. Treatment of this condition can be chosen by tilt-testing. Cardioinhibitory vasovagal syndrome, especially when bradycardia has been shown to precede blood pressure fall, can be treated by DDI pacing with rate hysteresis whereas no perfect drug exists for vasodepressor vasovagal syndrome. At present, selection can be made from amongst scopolamine, beta-blockers, clonidine, disopyramide and etilefrine. In the future, early detection of impending syncope even before the patient is aware by means of sensors and application of sophisticated pacing modes appear promising. Although it may ultimately be necessary to combine sophisticated sensors, dual chamber pacing and an implantable drug dispenser releasing small doses of an agent such as dihydroergotamine in order to achieve anything approaching 100% symptom control.

REFERENCES

1. Maloney JD, Jaeger FJ, Fouad-Tarazi FM, Morris HH. Malignant vaso-vagal syncope: Prolonged asystole provoked by head-up tilt. Cleveland Clinic J Med 1988;55:542–8.
2. Fitzpatrick A, Theodorakis G, Vardas P et al. The incidence of malignant vasovagal syndrome in patients with recurrent syncope. Eur Heart J 1991;12:389–94.
3. Fitzpatrick A, Theodorakis G, Vardas P, Sutton R. Methodology of head-up tilt testing in patients with unexplained syncope. J Am Coll Cardiol 1991;17:125–30.
4. Abi-Samra F, Maloney JD, Fouad-Tarazi FM, Castle LW. The usefulness of head-up tilt testing and hemodynamics investigations in the workup of syncope of unknown origin. PACE 1988;11:1202–14.
5. Almquist A, Goldenberg IF, Milstein S et al. Provocation of bradycardia and hypotension by isoproterenol and upright posture in patients with unexplained syncope. N Eng J Med 1989;329:346–51.
6. Fitzpatrick A, Sutton R. Tilting towards a diagnosis in unexplained recurrent syncope. Lancet 1989;1:658–60.
7. Raviele A, Gasparini G, Di Pede F et al. Unexplained syncope. Value of nitroglycerin infusion associated with head-up tilt to disclose a vasovagal reaction. New trends in arrhythmias. 1991;7:561–73.
8. Kapoor WN. Methodology of upright tilt table testing. Eur J Cardiac Pacing Electrophysiol 1992;2:242–6.
9. Benditt DG, Remole S, Bailin S, Dunnigan A, Asso A, Milstein S. Tilt-table testing for evaluation of neurally mediated (cardioneurogenic) syncope: rationale and proposed protocols. PACE 1991;14:1528–37.
10. Sutton R, Petersen MEV, Brignole M, Raviele A, Menozzi C, Giani P. Proposed classification for tilt induced vasovagal syncope. Eur J Cardiac Pacing Electrophysiol. 1992;2:180–3.
11. Imholz BP, Settels JJ, Van Der Meiracker AH, Weseling KH, Wieling W. Non-invasive continuous finger blood pressure measurement during orthostatic stress compared to intra-arterial pressure. Cardiovasc Res 1990;24:214–21.
12. Petersen MEV, Chamberlain-Webber R, Fitzpatrick A, Sutton R. Reproducibility of the Westminster tilt protocol (abstract). J Am Coll Cardiol 1992;19:340A.
13. Fitzpatrick AP, Williams T, Lightman S, Bloom S, Sutton R. Echocardiographic and endocrine changes during vasovagal syncope (abstract). PACE 1989;12:1279.
14. Lewis T. Vasovagal syncope and the carotid sinus mechanism. Br Med J 1932;1:873–4.
15. Fitzpatrick A, Travill CM, Vardas P, Ingram A, Sutton R. Recurrent vasovagal syncope after ventricular pacing. PACE 1990;13:619–24.
16. Fitzpatrick A, Theodorakis G, Ahmed R, Williams T, Sutton R. Dual chamber pacing aborts vasovagal syncope induced by head-up 60° tilt. PACE 1991;14:13–9.

17. Petersen MEV, Chamberlain-Webber R, Morgan JM et al. Permanent pacing for cardioinhibitory malignant vasovagal syndrome. Eur J Cardiac Pacing Electrophysiol 1992;2:100A.
18. Vardas P, Vitakis S, Vemmos C et al. The haemodynamic effects of incremental ventricular pacing during positive tilting test. PACE 1989;12:1169.
19. ACC/AHA Task Force. Guidelines for implantation of cardiac pacemakers and antiarrhythmic devices. J Am Coll Cardiol 1991;18:1-13.
20. Goldenburg IF, Almquist A, Dunbar KN, Milstein S, Pritzker MR, Benditt DG. Prevention of neurally-mediated syncope by selective beta-1 adrenoceptor blockade (abstract). Circulation 1987;76:(Suppl IV):133.
21. Fitzpatrick A, Ahmed R, Williams S, Sutton R. A randomised trial of medical therapy in malignant vasovagal syndrome or neurally-mediated bradycardia/hypotensive syndrome. Eur J Cardiac Pacing Electrophysiol 1991;1:99-102.
22. Milstein S, Buetikofer J, Dunnigan A, Benditt D, Gornick C, Reys W. Usefulness of disopyramide for prevention of upright tilt-induced hypotension-bradycardia. Am J Cardiol 1990;65:1339-44.
23. Thoren P. Role of cardiac c-fibres in cardiovascular control. Physiol Biochem Pharmacol 1979;86:1-94.
24. Raviele A, Gasparini G, Di Pede F, Delise P, Bonso A, Piccolo E. Usefulness of head-up tilt test in evaluating patients with syncope of unknown origin and negative electrophysiologic study. Am J Cardiol 1990;65:1322-7
25. Bergenwald L, Freyshuss U, Sjostrand T. The mechanisms of orthostatic and haemorrhagic fainting. Scand J Clin Lab Invest 1977;37:209-16.
26. Fouad-Tarazi FM, Maloney JD. Vasovagal syncope: lack of relationship between baseline blood volume and presyncopal chronotropic response (abstract). Clin Res 1989;37:880A.

3. Classification of antiarrhythmic drugs in relation to mechanisms of arrhythmias

MICHIEL J. JANSE

INTRODUCTION

For more than 20 years, the classification of antiarrhythmic drugs proposed by Vaughan Williams [1] has held the field. In essence, it is based on the effects of antiarrhythmic agents on the transmembrane potentials of normal, isolated cardiac tissue. In 1972, Singh and Vaughan Williams modified the classification by introducing the calcium entry blocking effect as a fourth class of antiarrhythmic action [2], and in 1992, Vaughan Williams proposed that specific bradycardic agents constitute a fifth class [3]. A modification of the classification of Na^+ channel blocking agents was provided by Harrison et al. [4], who subdivided class I actions into the classes a, b and c, mainly on the basis of the effects on action potential duration. Thus, class Ia agents prolonged the action potential duration, class Ib drugs shortened it, and class Ic components had little effect. Later, more sophisticated subclassifications of drugs that blocked inward currents, either carried by Na^+ or Ca^{2+} ions, were made on the basis of the kinetics of ion channel blockade and by defining the state of the channel (i.e. resting, activated or inactivated) to which drugs bind and unbind [5–7]. An important consequence of these later modifications was the recognition of use or frequency-dependent channel blockade. Drugs with use-dependent action bind to the activated and/or inactivated channel and slowly dissociate from the channel during diastole. They therefore exert their greatest effect at rapid heart rates. The time constants for unbinding are short for class Ib drugs and long for class Ia and Ic drugs. Class Ic drugs, which have the slowest kinetics, can further be subdivided into three groups according to their saturation behaviour at rapid rates [7].

Despite these modifications, the original division of antiarrhythmic drugs into those that block sodium channels (class I), those that block beta-adrenergic receptors (class II), those that prolong the action potential (class III) and those that block calcium channels (class IV) is still widely used. The advantage of this classification is that it is easily learned, as it is based on physiological actions, and that it provides a shorthand for communication among researchers and physicians. One of the attractive aspects of the classification is its simplicity. However, this simplicity also has its disadvantages.

First of all, the classification is one of drug *actions*, not of drugs [3]. In practice, however, the classification is used as a classification of *drugs*. (Incidentally, the title of the original publication [1] is "Classification of antiarrhythmic drugs".) One of the implications of this is that all drugs in the same class have the same beneficial and/or harmful effects. In reality, most antiarrhythmic drugs have more than one action, and the tendency to label drugs as one particular class can be very misleading. In some countries, for example, sotalol is classified as a class II drug, because of its beta-adrenergic blocking effect, while in other countries it is listed as a class III agent because of its ability to prolong the action potential. Amiodarone is usually considered to be a class III agent, whereas it has class I, class II and class IV actions as well. Especially in the post-Cardiac Arrhythmia Suppression Trial (CAST) era, it is important to realize that not all agents listed as class Ic have the same properties [8]. In other words, the apparent simplicity of the classification is not that useful in clinical practice since almost every drug has its own profile and there are very few drugs with a single, "pure" action.

Another limitation of the classification is that it is incomplete. For example, alpha-adrenergic blockers, cholinergic agonists, adenosine, digitalis, potassium channel openers and blockers of stretch-activated channels are not included, and there is no room for the potential antiarrhythmic action of agents that modify gap junctional resistance, biochemical pumps or exchangers.

These and other considerations led a group of basic and clinical investigators to attempt a new approach for classifying antiarrhythmic drug action, known as the Sicilian Gambit [9].

THE APPROACH OF THE SICILIAN GAMBIT

The name refers both to the island where the meeting to consider a new approach was held and to an opening, offering various possibilities. It is not a strict classification, but is open to criticism and revision as more is learned about arrhythmia mechanisms and about ionic channels, pumps, exchangers, receptors, second messengers, etc. The approach of the Sicilian Gambit consists in principle of four steps. First, the mechanism of a particular arrhythmia is defined. Second, a vulnerable parameter is identified as the electrophysiological property most susceptible to modification, which modification will suppress or prevent the arrhythmia. Third, the ionic channel, pump or receptor most likely to modify the vulnerable parameter is selected, and finally, a drug is chosen.

Table 1. Summary of the different mechanisms of arrhythmias and their respective vulnerable parameters.

Mechanism of arrhythmia	Vulnerable parameter
Automaticity	
Enhanced normal	Phase 4 depolarization (decrease)
Abnormal	Phase 4 depolarization (decrease) or maximum diastolic potential (hyperpolarize)
Triggered activity	
Based on early afterdepolarizations (EAD)	Action potential duration (shorten) or EAD (suppress)
Based on delayed afterdepolarizations (DAD)	Calcium overload (unload) or DAD (suppress)
Reentry dependent on Na$^+$ channels	
Long excitable gap	Excitability and conduction (depress)
Short excitable gap	Effective refractory period (prolong)
Reentry dependent on Ca^{2+} channels	Excitability and conduction (depress)

ARRHYTHMIA MECHANISMS AND THEIR VULNERABLE PARAMETER

Table 1 shows the various arrhythmia mechanisms and their vulnerable parameters. The concept of the vulnerable parameter is illustrated in Figure 1. Here, diagrams of action potentials of fibres of the sinus node exhibiting spontaneous diastolic depolarization are shown. Four different ways of slowing the rate of spontaneous impulse formation are indicated:

1. shifting the maximal diastolic potential to a more negative level (hyperpolarization; B)
2. shifting the threshold potential to a more positive level (C)
3. slowing the rate of diastolic depolarization (D)
4. prolonging the duration of the action potential (E)

In theory, therefore, there are four different approaches to slowing a tachycardia caused by enhanced automaticity, and there are many different ways in which this can be achieved. A change in one variable may, however, also change other ones. For example, an increase in potassium currents will hyperpolarize the membrane and thus slow the rate of impulse formation. However, it will also shorten the action potential, which will increase the rate. Moreover, an increase in outward current carried by potassium ions will counteract the depolarizing inward currents and thus slow the rate. For enhanced normal automaticity, the vulnerable parameter is the rate of diastolic (or phase 4) depolarization. The ionic currents most likely to modulate phase 4 depolarization are the pacemaker current I_f and the T-type calcium current I_{Ca-T}. Block of these currents will slow the rate. Agents that do so are beta-adrenergic blocking agents, sodium blocking agents and calcium

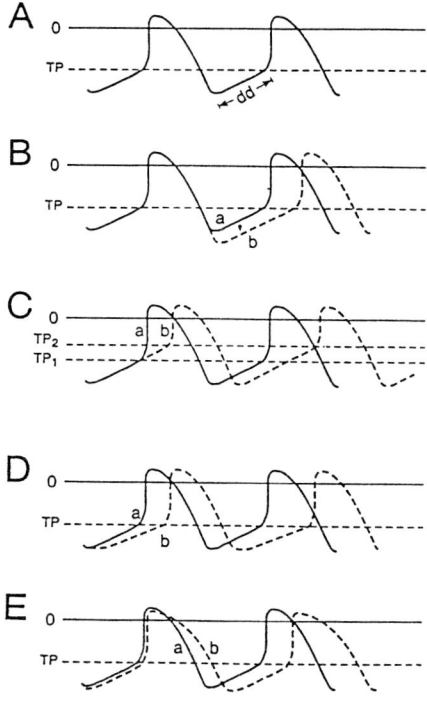

Figure 1. Diagrams of sinus node action potentials illustrating normal automaticity caused by spontaneous diastolic depolarization and the factors that change the rate of impulse initiation. (A) A typical sinus node action potential with spontaneous diastolic depolarization (dd). (B) Change in rate that occurs when the maximum diastolic potential is shifted to a more negative level (from a to b). (C) Change in rate caused by change in threshold potential to a less negative level (from TO_1 to TP_2). (D) Change in rate that occurs when the slope of phase 4 depolarization is decreased (from a to b). (E) Change in rate that occurs when the action potential duration is increased (from a to b). (Reproduced with permission from [12].)

blocking agents. Theoretically, activation of the acetylcholine-sensitive potassium current (I_{K-Ach}) will also slow diastolic hyperpolarization. As already described, activation of the potassium current will also have other effects.

As shown in Table 1, the number of arrhythmia mechanisms and vulnerable parameters is limited. When these are identified, it theoretically becomes easy to establish a hierarchy among the ionic currents and receptors that are responsible for the arrhythmia. By extension, one can then choose among the available antiarrhythmic agents, which, more often than not, influence more than one current and/or receptor. Figure 2 summarizes the actions of a number of antiarrhythmic drugs on channels, receptors and pumps, and in addition briefly indicates their clinical effects.

Classification of antiarrhythmic drugs 27

Drug	Channels						Receptors					Pumps	Clinical effects			ECG effects		
	Na Fast	Na Med	Na Slow	Ca	K	I$_f$	α	β	M$_2$		P	Na/K ATPase	LV FX	Sinus rate	Extra cardiac	PR	QRS	JT
Lidocaine	○												—	—	◉			↓
Mexiletine	○												—	—	◉			↓
Tocainide	○												—	—	●			↓
Moricizine	●												↓	—	—	↑		↑
Procainamide		◐			◎								↓	—	●	↑	↑	↑
Disopyramide		◐			◎				○				↓	—	◉	↑↑	↑	↑
Quinidine		◐			◎		○		○				—	↑	◉	↑↑	↑	↑
Propafenone		◐						◯					↓	↓	○	↑	↑	
Flecainide			◐		○								↓	—	○	↑	↑	
Encainide			◐										↓	—	○	↑	↑	
Bepridil	○			●	○								?	↓	○			↑
Verapamil	○			●				○					↓	↓	○	↑		
Diltiazem				◐									↓	↓	○	↑		
Bretylium					●		▲	▲					—	↓	○			↑
Sotalol					●			●					↓	↓	○	↑		↑
Amiodarone	○			○	●		◎	○					—	↓	●	↑		↑
Alinidine					◎	●							?	↓	●			
Nadolol								●					↓	↓	○	↑		
Propranolol	○							●					↓	↓	○	↑		
Atropine									●				—	↑	◉	↓		
Adenosine										△			?	↓	○	↑		
Digoxin										△		●	↑	↓	●	↑		↓

Figure 2. Summary of the important actions of drugs on membrane channels, receptors and ion pumps in the heart as well as on the ECG, sinus rate and left ventricular function. Most of these drugs are already marketed as antiarrhythmic agents, but some are not yet approved for this purpose, and others are no longer being used. There is no listing for pro-arrhythmia because, under appropriate circumstances, all antiarrhythmic drugs may be pro-arrhythmic. With this in mind, be aware that this figure, like all drugs, should be used with caution; it is certain to raise some controversy. For areas such as the clinical and ECG effects, the information available is so voluminous and diverse that the data here unavoidably includes some degree of subjectivity. Accordingly, the shading of the symbols and the direction of the arrows should not be taken as absolute. Moreover, the clinical information presented refers to the patient who does not have importantly compromised left ventricular function prior to drug administration.

For the section on channels, receptors and pumps, the actions of drugs on the sodium (Na), calcium (Ca), potassium (I_K) and I_f channels are indicated. Sodium channel blockade is subdivided into three groups of actions characterized by fast ($\tau < 300$ ms), medium ($\tau = 200$–1500 ms) and slow ($\tau > 1500$ ms) time constants for recovery from block. This parameter is a measure of use dependence and predicts the likelihood that a drug will decrease conduction velocity of normal sodium-dependent tissues in the heart and perhaps the propensity of a drug for causing bundle branch block or pro-arrhythmia. The rate constant for onset of block might be even more clinically relevant. Blockade in the inactivated (I) or activated (A) state is indicated.

Drug interaction with receptors (alpha, beta, muscarinic 2 [M_2], A_1, purinergic [P]) and drug effects on the sodium/potassium pump [Na/K ATPase] are indicated. Solid triangles indicate antagonist or inhibitory actions; open triangles indicate direct- or indirect-acting agonists or stimulators. The intensity of the action is indicated by the various shadings.

(*Legend continues on p. 28*)

LIMITATIONS OF THE SICILIAN GAMBIT

Despite the relative simplicity of the approach of the Sicilian Gambit, there are difficulties in applying the Gambit's philosophy in clinical practice.

Table 2 assigns a variety of clinical arrhythmias to the different arrhythmia mechanisms. The first difficulty in applying the principles of the Sicilian Gambit is the identification of the mechanism of a particular arrhythmia. Possibly the greatest difficulty is encountered when a distinction must be made between a re-entrant tachycardia with a long excitable gap and one with a short excitable gap. The tools to define an arrhythmia mechanism are the electrocardiographic characteristics, the history, and the response of an arrhythmia to electrical stimulation and to drugs. None of these approaches is foolproof, and even when all are used, one may still be left with uncertainties about the mechanism.

The distinction between re-entrant tachycardias with a short and with a long excitable gap was made because in the former, drugs that prolong the refractory period would be chosen, while in the latter, it would be drugs that depress excitability and conduction.

When invasive studies are performed, a tachycardia that can be entrained or terminated by electrical stimuli [10] is most likely caused by a long excitable gap re-entry. Thus, type I flutter [11], which has an atrial rate of 240–338 per min and which can be entrained, is considered to be due to a long excitable gap re-entry; type II flutter, which has an atrial rate of 340–433 per min and which cannot be influenced by atrial pacing, is characterized as short excitable gap re-entry. Of course, invasive electrophysiological testing is not always performed, and then identification of a short or long excitable gap re-entry becomes very difficult indeed. Certain clues may be derived from the response to drugs: tachycardias that are easily abolished or prevented by drugs that prolong the refractory period are likely to be due to short excitable gap re-entry, whereas those that respond well to sodium channel blocking

---

Figure 2 (continued).

The absence of a symbol indicates a lack of effect. The use of a question mark indicates uncertainty concerning the effect. The arrows in the clinical effect and ECG section indicate direction; no quantitative differentiation has been made between weak and strong effects. The effects listed for ECG, left ventricular function (LVFX), sinus rate and 'extracardiac' are those that may be seen at therapeutic plasma levels. Deleterious effects that may appear with concentrations above the therapeutic range are not listed. Antiarrhythmic drug actions, relative potency: ○ = low; ◐ = moderate; ● = high; △ = agonist; ▲ = agonist/antagonist; A = activated state blocker; I = inactivated state blocker; LVFX = left ventricular function. (Reproduced with permission from [13].)

Table 2. Association of arrhythmia and mechanism.

Arrhythmia	Mechanisms
	Automaticity
	Enhanced normal
Inappropriate sinus tachycardia	
Some idiopathic ventricular tachycardias	
	Abnormal
Ectopic atrial tachycardia	
Accelerated idioventricular rhythms	
	Triggered activity EAD
Torsade de pointes	
	DAD
Digitalis-induced arrhythmias	
Certain autonomically mediated ventricular tachycardias	
	Reentry
	(sodium channel dependent)
	Long excitable gap
Atrial flutter type I	
Circus movement tachycardia in WPW	
Sustained monomorphic ventricular tachycardia	
	Short excitable gap
Atrial flutter type II	
Atrial fibrillation	
Circus movement tachycardia in WPW	
Polymorphic and sustained monomorphic ventricular tachycardia	
Bundle branch reentry	
Ventricular fibrillation	
	Reentry
	(calcium channel dependent)
AV nodal reentrant tachycardia	
Circus movement tachycardia in WPW	
Verapamil-sensitive ventricular tachycardia	

drugs are likely to be caused by long excitable gap re-entry. Rapid and/or polymorphic tachycardias are more likely due to short excitable gap re-entry, whereas stable, relatively slow tachycardias are most probably caused by long excitable gap re-entry.

Whilst it is important to recognize the limitations of the Sicilian Gambit, it should also be recognized that the future development of antiarrhythmic drug treatment largely depends on acquiring more complete knowledge about arrhythmia mechanisms and the specific actions of antiarrhythmic drugs. The Sicilian Gambit provides an opportunity for a more rationalistic approach, based on arrhythmia mechanisms and the identification of vulnerable parameters. It is to be hoped that future research will close the gap between theory and practice.

REFERENCES

1. Vaughan Williams EM. Classification of antiarrhythmic drugs. In: Sandoe E, Flensted-Jensen E, Olsen KH, editors. Cardiac Arrhythmias. Sodertalje, Sweden: Astra, 1970:449–72.
2. Singh BN, Vaughan Williams EM. A fourth class of antidysrhythmic action? Effect of verapamil on ouabain toxicity, on atrial and ventricular intracellular potentials, and on other features of cardiac function. Cardiovasc Res 1972;6:109–19.
3. Vaughan Williams EM. Classifying antiarrhythmic actions: by facts or speculation. J Clin Pharmacol 1992;32:964–77.
4. Harrison DC, Winkle RA, Sami M, Mason JW. Encainide: A new and potent antiarrhythmic agent. In: Harrison DC, Hall GK, editors. Cardiac Arrhythmias, a Decade of Progress. Boston: Medical Publishers 1981:315–30.
5. Hondeghem LM, Katzung BG, Antiarrhythmic agents: the modulated receptor mechanism of action of sodium and calcium blocking drugs. Annu Rev Pharmacol Toxicol 1984;24:387–423.
6. Starmer CF, Grant AO, Strauss HC. Mechanisms of use dependent block of sodium channels in excitable membranes by local anesthetics. Biophys J 1984;46:15–27.
7. Weirich J, Antoni H. Differential analysis of the frequency-dependent effects of class I antiarrhythmic drugs according to periodical ligand binding: implication for antiarrhythmic and proarrhythmic activity. J Cardiovasc Pharmacol 1990;15:998–1009.
8. Vaughan Williams EM, Significance of classifying antiarrhythmic actions since the Cardiac Arrhythmia Suppression Trial. J Clin Pharmacol 1991;31:123–35.
9. Task Force of the Working Group on Arrhythmias of the European Society of Cardiology. The Sicilian Gambit. A new approach to the classification of antiarrhythmic drugs based on their action on arrhythmogenic mechanisms. Circulation 1991;84:1831–51; Eur Heart J 1991;12:1112–31.
10. Waldo AL, Olshansky B, Okumura K, Henthorn RW. Current perspectives on entrainment of tachyarrhythmias. In: Brugada P, Wellens HJJ, editors. Cardiac Arrhythmias: Where to go from Here? Mount Kisco, NY: Futura, 1987:171–89.
11. Wells JL, MacLean WAH, James TN, Waldo AL. Characterization of atrial flutter. Studies in man after open heart surgery using fixed atrial electrodes. Circulation 1979;60:665–73.
12. Wit AL, Janse MJ. The ventricular arrhythmias of ischemia and infarction. Electrophysiological mechanisms. Mount Kisco, NY: Futura, 1993.
13. Schwartz PJ, Zaza A. The Sicilian Gambit revisited – theory and practice. Eur Heart J 1992;(Suppl F):23–9.

4. Electrophysiological characteristics in arrhythmogenic right ventricular dysplasia and dilated cardiomyopathies

GUY FONTAINE, R. FRANK, R. TSEZANA, J. TONET, E. VELASQUEZ & G. LASCAULT

INTRODUCTION

Arrhythmogenic right ventricular dysplasia (ARVD) is now classified under "cardiomyopathies" as it is a disease of the myocardial muscle of unknown etiology [1]. However, the term cardiomyopathy by itself has been criticized since it covers a wide group of clinical entities, and progress in that field seems to involve identifying subgroups [2]. In this view, ARVD appears to be a subgroup of arrhythmogenic right ventricular cardiomyopathies (ARVC), although the distinction between these two subgroups deserves further definition. Right ventricular dysplasia, as well as right ventricular cardiomyopathy are associated with different forms of arrhythmogenicity which are not completely understood, especially in the latter [3,4].

HISTOLOGICAL BACKGROUND OF ARRHYTHMOGENIC RIGHT VENTRICULAR DYSPLASIA

In arrhythmogenic right ventricular dysplasia the typical histological structure consists of strands of surviving cardiomyocytes located in a large amount of surrounding fatty tissue [5]. These strands of fibers are edged by a thin rim of fibrosis (Figure 1). The presence of fibrosis is indispensable for the positive histological diagnosis of the disease [6]. It is thought that these surviving fibers which are still interconnected with normal tissue are the site of a delayed activation and unidirectional block which could lead to the development of a reentrant mechanism [7].

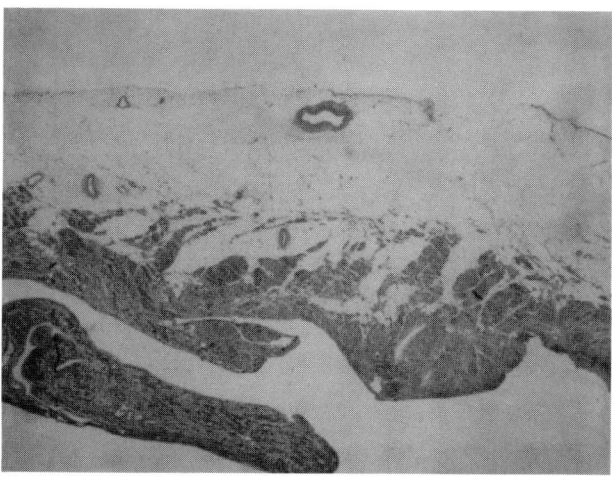

Figure 1. Typical aspect of the free wall of the right ventricle in a case of arrhythmogenic right ventricular dysplasia. The endocardial layers and trabeculations are spared. Many of the subepicardial layers are replaced by fatty tissue. Inside this fat strands of surviving fibers connected with normal endocardium are clearly seen (G ×10).

HISTOLOGICAL BASIS OF ARRHYTHMOGENIC RIGHT VENTRICULAR CARDIOMYOPATHY

The situation is less clear in the arrhythmogenic forms of idiopathic dilated cardiomyopathy. However, in some cases histological study demonstrates surviving myocardial fibers embedded in a large amount of fibrous interstitial tissue (Figure 2) [8,9]. Eventually, this produces the same histopathological background for the development of cardiac arrhythmias as the situation observed in arrhythomogenic right ventricular dysplasia. As fat cell or fibrosis is not arrhythmogenic, we are forced to conclude that the arrhythmogenicity is the result of the peculiar electrophysiological properties of the surviving myocardial fibers provided that they demonstrate ectopic impulse formation or slow conduction [10,11].

GENERAL BACKGROUND FOR THE DEVELOPMENT OF CARDIAC ARRHYTHMIAS

The general mechanism for the development of cardiac arrhythmias is frequently explained by three factors:

1. The existence of an arrhythmogenic substrate based on the anatomical structure which has been just described in dysplasia or cardiomyopathies.

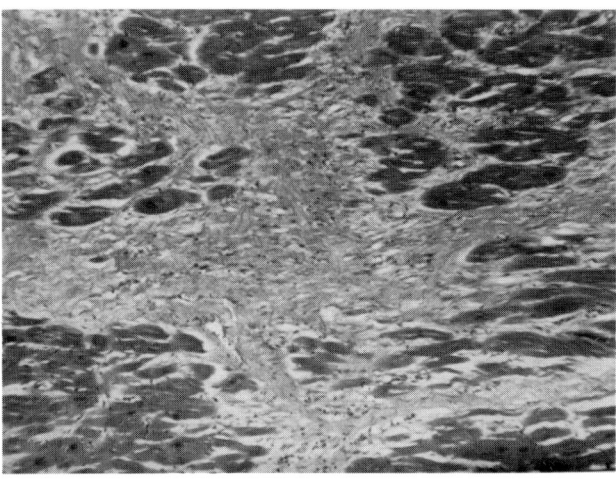

Figure 2. Typical pattern of the fibrous form of idiopathic dilated cardiomyopathy. Strands of surviving fibers are clearly seen within a major area of substitution by fibrous tissue (G ×120).

2. A triggering factor like a spontaneous extrasystole.
3. The modulator role of the autonomous nervous system. Minor but consistent variations of the cycle length are frequently observed before the inception of major ventricular arrhythmias [12].

CLINICAL ELECTROPHYSIOLOGY OF CARDIAC ARRHYTHMIAS IN ARVC AND ARVD

Some characteristics have been observed in abnormal myocardium in patients with arrhythmogenic right ventricular dysplasia as well as idiopathic dilated cardiomyopathy:

1. The observation of delayed potentials, which means the demonstration of a local potential recorded by epicardial map or endocardial electrograms, observed after the end of the QRS complex, strongly suggests a slowdown of conduction in some areas of the myocardial fibers (Figure 3) [13,14].
2. The effect of pacing in this zone, showing an isoelectric line between the pacing stimulus and the ventricular activation, is the reverse proof of delayed conduction in this structure, but also demonstrates that from the area of slow conduction, the activation could be transmitted to the rest of myocardium [15].
3. The time-dependent properties of this structure are also striking. Increasing the rate of pacing or the use of premature stimulation on a stable

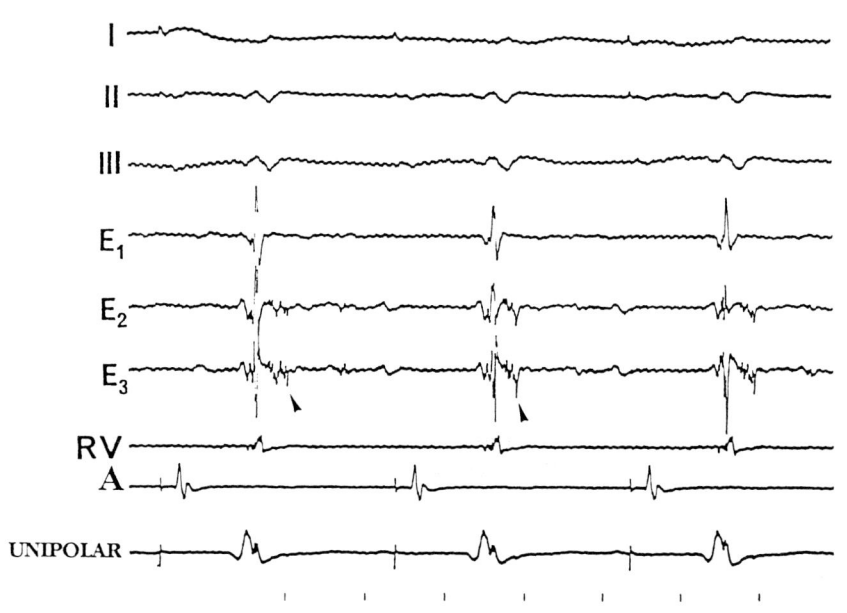

Figure 3. Recording of late potentials on the epicardium, in a patient with arrhythmogenic right ventricular dysplasia, during surgery for ventricular tachycardia. Surface ECG leads from I to III. Three epicardial leads recorded from a roving probe with electrodes 1.5 mm apart located at the angles of an equilateral triangle. RV = right ventricle, A = atrium; UNIPOLAR = unipolar recording from one of the epicardial electrodes. Delayed potentials (arrowheads) occur after the end of the QRS complex recorded on the surface tracing.

basic cycle length demonstrates an increase in the coupling interval of these delayed potentials (Figure 4). The time-dependent properties of this anatomic structure are closer to those observed in the AV node [15].

As a result, the delayed potential occurring long after the end of the QRS complex could lead to the development of arrhythmias when the coupling interval exceeds the refractory period of the adjacent healthy myocardium. This is a spectacular explanation for the development of a re-entrant mechanism [11].

Beside these features, the reentrant nature of the arrhythmia has been clearly demonstrated by data obtained at the time of surgery in patients with intractable forms of this arrhythmia [16]. After a precise epicardial map, our group demonstrated for the first time the delineation of the reentrant pathway on the epicardium in a case of Uhl's anomaly which provides a two-dimensional structure of the myocardium [13]. In this patient as well in other forms of ventricular tachycardia (VT), the "site of origin" was identified. Pressure at this point with the finger or a blunt instrument, repeatedly interrupted the

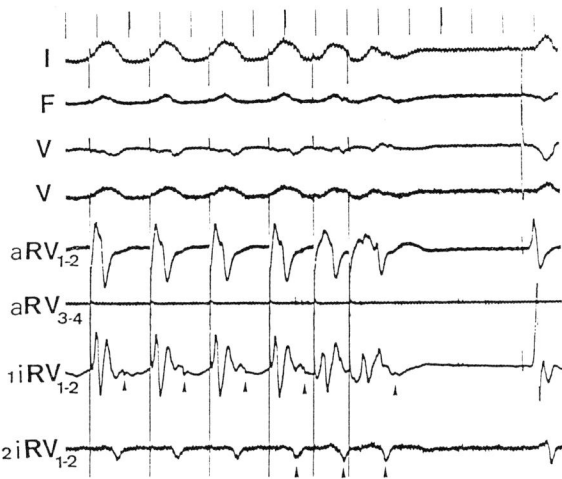

Figure 4. Effect of pacing on the endocardial fibers in a patient with arrhythmogenic right ventricular dysplasia, showing the time-dependent properties of the abnormal zone. Note that the coupling interval between the pacing stimulus and the delayed potentials (arrowheads) increases when two premature stimuli are delivered. aRV_{1-2} = apex right ventricle, electrodes 1 and 2; 1iRV = infundibular area, catheter no. 1.

arrhythmia. Also, simple transmural incision at this particular point proved to be effective for the long-term prevention of the arrhythmia.

Our first case had VT in the clinical setting of idiopathic dilated form of cardiomyopathy (this patient had two morphologies of VT, and thus two simple ventriculotomies of 2 and 5 cm long were performed at the site of origin on the free wall of the left ventricle). This patient died of acute heart failure 9 months later without any new episode of VT. Complete disappearance of the ventricular extrasystoles was also observed. The second case was our first case of ARVD. The site of origin was located in the middle of the acute margin of the right ventricle where a simple ventriculotomy proved to be effective. This patient is still alive (20 years later) and does not require any antiarrhythmic therapy [17].

INDUCTION OF CARDIAC ARRHYTHMIAS

For quite a long time, the alternation of long and short cycles leading to ventricular arrhythmias has been reported [18]. In addition, we have observed data suggesting that inside the abnormal myocardium, independently of other factors, the blocking of conduction could occur spontaneously.

The first observations were made during an EP study of patients with

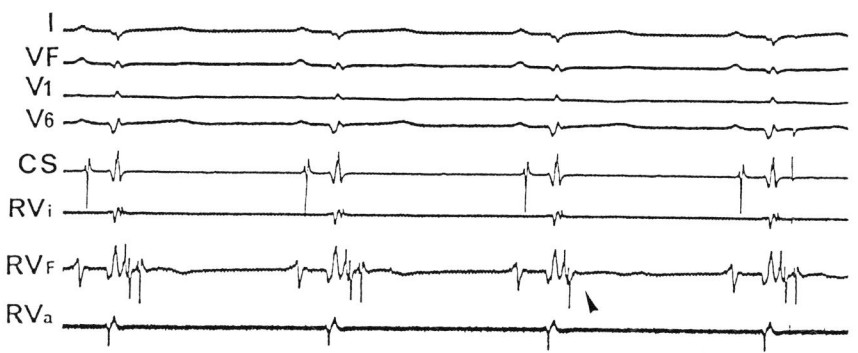

Figure 5. Spontaneous block observed in the right ventricle in a zone of abnormal conduction in a case of idiopathic dilated cardiomyopathy, showing the spontaneous disappearance of endocardial potential (arrowhead), suggesting a local block in the area of delayed activity.

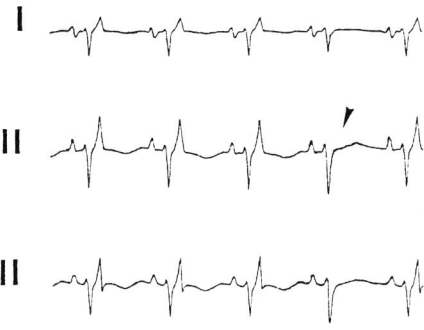

Figure 6. Spontaneous block affecting a large enough amount of myocardium to be clearly visible on the surface recording in a severe form of arrhythmogenic right ventricular dysplasia. Note the spontaneous disappearance of the last part of the rapid phase of the QRS complex which occurs spontaneously (arrowhead).

arrhythmogenic right ventricular dysplasia or idiopathic dilated cardiomyopathy, showing that episode of conduction block could occur without a clear-cut modification of the basic cycle length. An example of this phenomenon is provided in Figure 5.

The second observation was taken from the surface ECG in a patient with a severe form of ARVD in whom a part of the ventricular activation seemed to disappear spontaneously (Figure 6). In this case, a quite significant amount of myocardium which was no longer activated is blocked without triggering any form of arrhythmia. However, demonstration of a spontaneous block by itself is one of the prerequisites for the inception of the reentrant phenomenon [11].

Therefore, the unidirectional block of conduction which was generally the result of a change in the cardiac cycle or a spontaneous extrasystole or the introduction of a premature activation by programmed pacing could also be the result of a spontaneous defect of conduction inside the myocardial fibers. Recent data suggest that an abnormal longitudinal conduction in myocardial fibers is replaced by transversal conduction at a much slower speed, with a decrease of the safety factor for the propagation of conduction [19].

EFFECT OF CONDUCTION TROUBLE IN THE MYOCARDIUM

The recording of late potentials in patients with chronic reentrant VT is an important concept for the understanding of cardiac arrhythmias. However, it is a particularly striking example of a more general aspect of abnormal myocardial activation in patients who exhibit a more global phenomenon of slow conduction.

It is predictable that delayed conduction in some part of the right ventricular musculature in patients with ARVD will affect the electrocardiogram in a different way as compared with patients with dilated cardiomyopathy, which involves both right and left ventricles. In a preliminary study of 43 ECGs of patients with ARVD compared with a control group, it was demonstrated that:

1. The duration of the QRS complex in all leads in patients with ARVD is prolonged compared with the control group.
2. The prolongation of the QRS complex duration was longer in the right precordial leads from V1 to V3, and V1 demonstrated the longest prolongation. This simple sign could be used to identify the disease in the population since it appears that the sensitivity of this sign is 55% for a specificity of 100%. If the three precordial leads are included, the sensitivity goes up to 60% [20].

Abnormal activation of the ventricular myocardium could also affect the repolarisation, and in a second group of patients with ARVD, it was observed that inversion or flatness of the T wave in lead V2 gives a sensitivity of 66% for a specificity of 100%. Finally, the combination of these two criteria and other minor signs which could be observed on the ECGs led to a sensitivity of close to 80% for a specificity of 100% [21].

This result is consistent with a previous analysis performed to explain the delayed activation of the right ventricle in 7 patients with ARVD. Epicardial mapping in sinus rhythm demonstrated that in most of them the time of arrival of the activation of the right ventricular free wall was normal in time and location. From this point, a slow speed of progression of the ventricular

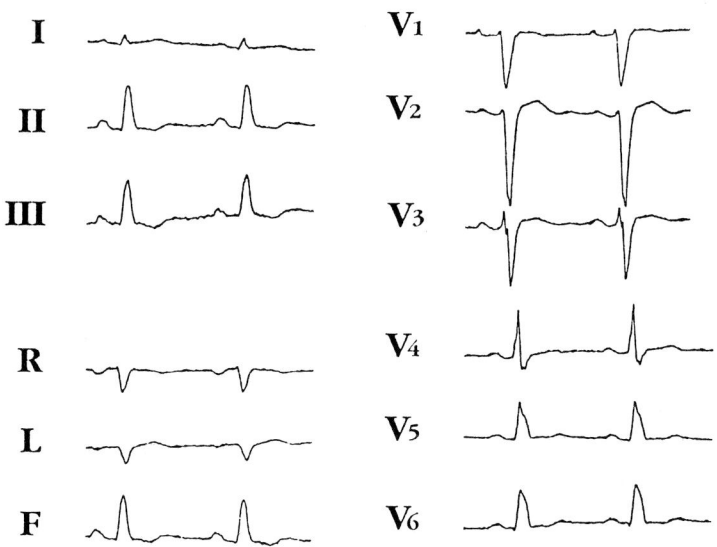

Figure 7. Electrocardiogram in sinus rhythm in a patient referred for ventricular tachycardia of right origin and who had a poor function of the left ventricle. The tracing suggests a left bundle branch block pattern. This case was finally considered not as a form of ARVD but of IDCM, with ventricular tachycardia originating from the right ventricle.

activation was suggested by tightly bunched isochrones. It was therefore concluded that in ARVD, a pattern of right bundle branch block was not in most cases the result of a block of conduction in the right branches of the AV conduction system but a slow-down of conduction in the ventricular musculature [22].

DILATED CARDIOMYOPATHY

In patients with idiopathic dilated cardiomypathy, there is a prolongation of the QRS complex which affects all the leads. This is probably the result of a more diffuse phenomenon involving both ventricular musculatures. This observation, which has to be confirmed in a further study, could help in the differential diagnosis between ARVD and IDCM. When the ECG exhibits an intraventricular block, its classification should be closer to a left as opposed to a right bundle branch block pattern.

We recently observed a patient referred with the diagnosis of ARVD because the VT of right ventricular origin demonstrated all the criteria of a reentrant mechanism. However, the ECG in sinus rhythm was close to a left bundle branch block pattern (Figure 7). In fact, the angiogram of this patient demonstrated a poor contraction of the left ventricle in addition to a typical pattern of ARVD of the right ventricle. We therefore concluded that this patient was not a case of ARVD showing involvement of the left ventricle [23] but rather of idiopathic dilated cardiomyopathy with ventricular tachycardia of right ventricular origin. The evolution of this case over a period of several years demonstrated the development of generalised heart failure.

CONCLUSION

In conclusion, the abnormal behaviour of local ventricular activation studied by recordings of the epicardial and endocardial signals as well as epicardial mapping has demonstrated that most VT in arrhythmogenic right ventricular dysplasia and idiopathic dilated cardiomyopathy are related to a reentrant mechanism, leading to a better understanding of the genesis of ventricular arrhythmias in these situations which will enable their prevention by surgical treatment and later ablative techniques.

The global phenomenon of intraventricular conduction delay provides differential diagnostic signs between arrhythmogenic right ventricular dysplasia and normal subjects and probably arrhythmogenic right ventricular dysplasia and arrhythmogenic right ventricular cardiomyopathy, which could be deduced from a regular 12-lead ECG recording. This could provide an interesting tool to perform a prospective study of these diseases in the population at risk (public transport drivers, sportsmen) at a reasonable cost. Correctly controlled preventive treatment is supposed to be able to prevent sudden cardiac death, which is the major complication in this group of young patients with an otherwise normal heart.

REFERENCES

1. Thiene G, Nava A, Corrado D, Rossi L, Pennelli N. Right Ventricular Cardiomyopathy and sudden death in young people. N Engl J Med 1988;318:129–33.
2. Olsen EGJ. Fundamentals of clinical cardiology. The pathology of cardiomyopathies. A critical analysis. Am Heart J 1979;98:385–92.
3. McKenna WJ, Krikler DM, Goodwin JF. Arrhythmias in dilated and hypertrophic cardiomyopathy. Med Clin North Am 1984;68:983–1000.
4. Poll DS, Marchlinski FE, Buxton AE, Doherty JU, Waxman HL, Josephson ME. Sustained ventricular tachycardia in patients with idiopathic dilated cardiomyopathy: Electrophysiologic testing and lack of response to antiarrhythmic drug therapy. Circulation 1984;70:451–6.
5. Marcus FI, Fontaine G, Guiraudon G et al. Right ventricular dysplasia: A report of 24 cases. Circulation 1982;65:384–99.
6. Fontaliran F, Fontaine G, Fillette F, Aouate P, Chomette G, Grosgogeat Y. Frontieres nosologiques de la dysplasie arythmogene. Variations quantitatives du tissu adipeux ventriculaire droit normal. Arch Mal Coeur 1991;84:33–8.
7. Fontaine G, Frank R, Tonet JL, Guiraudon G, Cabrol C, Grosgogeat Y. Arrhythmogenic

right ventricular dysplasia: A clinical model for the study of chronic ventricular tachycardia. Jpn Circ J 1984;48:515-38.
8. Hasumi M, Sekiguchi M, Yu ZX, Hirosawa K, Hiroe M. Analysis of histopathologic findings in cases with dilated cardiomyopathy with special reference to formulating diagnostic criteria on the possibility of postmyocarditic change. Jpn Circ J 1986;50:1280-7.
9. Baandrup U, Olsen EGJ. Critical analysis of endomyocardial biopsies from patients suspected of having cardiomyopathy. I. Morphological and morphometric aspects. Br Heart J 1981;45:475-86.
10. Cranefield PF, Wit AL, Hoffman BF. Genesis of cardiac arrhythmias. Circulation 1973;47:190.
11. Wellens HJJ. Pathophysiology of ventricular tachycardia in man. Arch Intern Med 1975;135:473.
12. Coumel P, Rosengarten MD, Leclercq JF, Attuel P. Role of sympathetic nervous system in non-ischaemic ventricular arrhythmias. Br Heart J 1982;47:137-47.
13. Fontaine G, Guiraudon G, Frank R et al. Stimulation studies and epicardial mapping in ventricular tachycardia: Study of mechanisms and selection for surgery. In: Kulbertus HE, editor. Reentrant Arrhythmias. Lancaster: MTP, 1977:334-50.
14. Fontaine G, Guiraudon G, Frank R. Intramyocardial conduction defects in patients prone to ventricular tachycardia. I. The postexcitation syndrome in sinus rhythm. In: Sandoe E, Julian DG, Bell JW, editors. Amsterdam: Excerpta Medica 1978:39-55.
15. Fontaine G, Guiraudon G, Frank R. Intramyocardial conduction defects in patients prone to ventricular tachycardia. II. A dynamic study of the post-excitation syndrome. In: Sandoe E, Julian DG, Bell JW, editors. Management of ventricular tachycardia. Role of mexiletine. Amsterdam: Excerpta Medica 1978:56-66.
16. Guiraudon G, Fontaine G, Frank R, Leandri R, Barra J, Cabrol C. Surgical treatment of ventricular tachycardia guided by ventricular mapping in 23 patients without coronary artery disease. Ann Thorac Surg 1981;32:439.
17. Fontaine G, Guiraudon G, Frank R et al. La cartographie epicardique et le traitement chirurgical par simple ventriculotomie de certaines tachycardies ventriculaires rebelles par reentree. Arch Mal Coeur 1975;68:113-24.
18. Zoll PM, Linenthal AJ, Zarsky RN. Ventricular fibrillation treatment and prevention by external electric currents. N Engl J Med 1960;262:105.
19. De Bakker JMT, van Capelle FJL, Janse MJ et al. Reentry as a cause of ventricular tachycardia in patients with chronic ischemic heart disease: Electrophysiologic and anatomic correlation. Circulation 1988;77:589-606.
20. Fontaine G, Umemura J, Di Donna P, Tsezana R, Cannat JJ, Frank R. La duree des complexes QRS dans la dysplasie ventriculaire droite arythmogene. Un nouveau marqueur diagnostique non invasif. Ann Cardiol Angeiol (Paris) 1993;42:399-405.
21. Fontaine G, Tsezana R, Lazarus A, Lascault G, Tonet J, Frank R. Troubles de la repolarisation et de la conduction intraventriculaire dans la dysplasie ventriculaire droite arythmogene. Ann Cardiol Angeiol (Paris) 1994, (in press).
22. Fontaine G, Frank R, Guiraudon G. Pavie A, Tereau Y, Grosgogeat Y. The significance of intraventricular conduction defects in arrhythmogenic right ventricular dysplasia. In: Levy S, Scheinman M, editors. Cardiac arrhythmias, from diagnosis to therapy. Mount Kisco: Futura, 1984:233-9.
23. Pinamonti B, Sinagra G, Salvi A et al. Left ventricular involvement in right ventricular dysplasia. Am Heart J 1992;123:711-24.

5. Classification of death in patients under antiarrhythmic treatment

RALPH ROGERS, HUGO ECTOR, ANN RUBENS,
CARL TIMMERMANS, HEIN HEIDBÜCHEL
& HILAIRE DE GEEST

INTRODUCTION

A new effective therapy for an important disease completely changes the clinical spectrum. This is also true for sudden arrhythmic death. The introduction of the implantable cardioverter-defibrillator (ICD) poses the question for every case of sudden death, whether or not it could have been prevented by the device. For patients treated with the ICD or with antiarrhythmic drugs, survival analysis requires an adequate reporting of the cause of death.

The World Health Organization, in an attempt to standardize research, has defined sudden death as occurring within 24 h of the onset of symptoms [1]. It is clear that this definition cannot be used when research is focusing on the aspect of arrhythmic death. Death from arrhythmia was the primary end point in the CAST study [2]. This definition includes witnessed instantaneous death in the absence of severe congestive heart failure or shock, unwitnessed death with no preceding change in symptoms and for which no other cause can be ascribed, and cardiac arrest. These criteria had been developed in CAPS [3]. Arrhythmic death or cardiac arrest was defined in CAPS as the abrupt spontaneous cessation of respiration and blood circulation (pulse) and loss of consciousness in the absence of other severe medical conditions likely to cause death. Arrhythmic death was subclassified as "proven" if ventricular tachycardia (VT) or fibrillation was recorded within 10 min of clinical death. Otherwise, the event was classified as "presumed arrhythmic" if death was observed visually without immediate electrocardiographic documentation. Death was classified as "instantaneous" if witnessed and if occurring <5 min from the onset of symptoms or witnessed and having no premonitory symptoms. In the presence of other severe disease such as class III or IV congestive heart failure, arrhythmia was chosen as the major immediate cause of death only if the Events Committee judged that the patient would probably have survived at least 4 months had the arrhythmia not occurred [3].

An event that led to clinical death within 60 min of the onset of symptoms was classified as "sudden" and an event that led to clinical, biologic, or clinical/biologic death in > 60 min from the onset of symptoms was defined as "nonsudden" cardiac death.

The CAPS and CAST investigators [2,3] have discussed the method used to classify deaths/cardiac arrests as cumbersome and time-consuming. They conclude with the statement that the combination of a time-based and etiology-based assessment of the cause of death will be necessary, since "sudden" death is not equivalent to "arrhythmic" death. Considering all of the possible effects of antiarrhythmic drugs as well as the difficulty in classifying events, they suggest that it may be more practical simply to evaluate total cardiac mortality in the conduct of any future, randomized, intervention trial. Also, the CASCADE [4] investigators have taken total cardiac mortality as the end point, because of the difficulty and potential bias in assigning the cause of death (arrhythmic vs. nonarrhythmic). Total cardiac mortality is an end point difficult to misclassify. This total cardiac mortality will be the most important and final measurement in a survival analysis.

In a cohort of patients under antiarrhythmic treatment, total mortality was analyzed in detail. According to currently accepted definitions, we have reviewed the problems of cardiac death classification. For a concise summary of cause and circumstances of death, a new coding system is presented.

METHODS AND DEFINITIONS

This observational study concerns a group of 129 patients treated for VT and/or ventricular fibrillation. All patients took amiodarone as a substantial part of their therapy. In 84 patients the administration of amiodarone was started without electrophysiological testing. In 45 high-risk patients, antiarrhythmic therapy was tested by programmed electrical stimulation (PES): 1 and 2 extrastimuli at 100 and 150 bpm, RV apex, and RV outflow tract. All these 45 patients received amiodarone as therapy of first choice. At the time of the first PES, 34 patients were on amiodarone for 4–6 weeks. In the other patients amiodarone was started after the initial PES, and the PES was repeated after 4–6 weeks. For chronic therapy, a dose of 400 mg per day was preferred. When inducible, some patients underwent repeated testing with the addition of a class I antiarrhythmic agent. When inducibility with haemodynamic collapse persisted, the implantation of an ICD was considered. When appropriate, drug therapy was combined with surgical treatment. The baseline characteristics are listed in Table 1. Patients were not entered in this study, unless their initial condition was stabilized. Five patients received an ICD.

Sudden arrhythmic death: This definition includes witnessed instantaneous death in the absence of severe congestive heart failure or shock, unwitnessed death with no preceding change in symptoms and for which no other cause can be ascribed, and cardiac arrest (CAST [2] definition).

Table 1. Baseline characteristics of study patients

	Male	Female	All
Number of patients	104	25	129
Age Mean	62.4	64.9	62.9
SD	11.9	14.9	12.6
Amiodarone treatment			
Duration (in months) Mean	36.1	26.2	34.2
SD	31.2	28.5	30.9
Follow-up[a] (in months) Mean	43.9	35.2	42.2
SD	33.8	33.2	33.8
Number of deaths	19	4	23
Initial arrhythmia diagnosis			
VT	95	24	119
VF	37	7	44
Out of hospital resuscitation	19	4	23
In-hospital resuscitation	43	13	56
DC-shock	56	17	73
Associated structural heart disease			
Myocardial infarction	66	12	78
Ischaemic heart disease	71	14	85
Myoc inf norm cor arteries	1		1
Dilated cardiomyopathy	18	2	20
Valvular heart disease	5	5	10
RV dysplasia	1		1
Hypertrophic obstructive CM		1	1
No structural disease	7	3	10
Functional class			
1 NYHA	31	7	38
2 NYHA	53	11	64
3 NYHA	18	7	25
4 NYHA	2		2
Surgical treatment			
ICD + cryoablation	1		1
ICD	3	1	4
Aortic valve replacement	1		1
Aortic + mitral valve replacement		1	1
Aortic valve replacement + PM	1		1
Mitral valve replacement	1		1
Aneurysmectomy	1		1
Aneurysmectomy + CABG	2		2
Aneurysmectomy + endoc resection	4		4
Aneurysmectomy + endoc resect + CABG	1		1
CABG	6	1	7
CABG + PM	1		1
CABG + PTCA	1		1
PTCA	2		2
PM	6	6	12
Heart transplant	1		1
All	32	9	41

[a] Follow-up duration = time in months between first administration of amiodarone and last control or death.

Table 2. Classification of death in cardiac patients

Sudden death (SD)

Subscripts
For D: 1–4   referring to functional class 1–4
For S: 1–4   1 instantaneous
             2 < 60 min
             3 unwitnessed
             4 other

When suddenness is not relevant
 HF: heart failure for in-hospital deaths
 MI: myocardial infarction
 CA: malignant disease
 CVA: cerebrovascular accident
 . . . . .

Extension
 letter code for drug treatment at the time of death

Functional status: The cardiac status of each patient was classified according to the criteria of the New York Heart Association [5]: class 1 = uncompromised; class 2 = slightly compromised; class 3 = moderately compromised; class 4 = severely compromised.

Cardiac death code: In view of the need to identify arrhythmic deaths possibly preventable by an ICD, a new letter code is presented in Table 2. This letter code describes sudden cardiac deaths with an indication for suddenness of death and for functional class. When the suddenness of death is not at all relevant, a letter code can indicate conditions such as heart failure (HF), myocardial infarction (MI), and carcinoma (Ca). We propose to use HF for in-hospital deaths of patients with end-stage cardiac failure, who are considered as "not to be resuscitated". For other patients SD can be used. After "D" subscripts 1–4 indicate functional class 1–4. After "S", subscript "1" indicates instantaneous death, "2" refers to death within 60 min, "3" stands for unwitnessed death, and "4" points to other conditions.

Statistics

Survival analysis was performed with the program of SPSS/PC+ Advanced Statistics 4.0 (SPSS Inc., Chicago). This program calculates a life table with the cumulative proportion of surviving at the end, and the standard error (S.E.) of the cumulative proportion surviving. Survival analysis between groups is calculated according to the algorithm of Lee and Desu. Survival time is calculated in months between the first administration of amiodarone and last-check-up or death.

Table 3. Study results and details of patients: age at time of death, cause of death, time of follow-up between first administration of amiodarone and death, surgical treatment, proposed code

Case	Age, death	Time	Surgical treatment	Code
1	66, CA	81		CA, DIS
2	55, CA	17	AN, ER	CA, AM
3	62, Card shock IH	99	AN	HF, AM
4	68, Card shock IH	9		HF, AM
5	64, Card shock IH	17		HF, AM
6	81, Card shock IH	117		HF, NO
7	70, Card shock IH	29		HF, AM
8	56, Card shock IH	9	AN, ER	HF, NO
9	60, Card shock IH	94	ICD	HF, AM
10	65, HF IH	3		HF, AM DIS
11	58, HF IH	15	ICD, CABG, CRYO	HF, NO
12	69, HF IH	8		HF, AM, PRF
13	82, HF IH	10		HF, AM, APR
14	76, HF IH	21	PM	HF, AM
15	71, HF IH	5	PM	HF, NO
16	62, HF VT IH	22		HF, LIDOC
17	79, HF Pneumonia IH	36	PM	HF, AM
Classification problematic				
18	68, HF OH inst death	30		S_1D_4, AM DIS
19	72, HF OH unwitnessed	34		S_3D_3, AM
20	47, HF OH inst death	4	AO V REPL	S_1D_3, NO
21	46, HF OH inst death	17	PM	S_1D_4, AM
22	62, HF OH inst death	10		S_1D_4, AM
23	61, OH unwitnessed	115		S_3D_1, NO

IH = in-hospital, OH = out of hospital, HF = heart failure, Inst = instantaneous, AN = aneurysmectomy, ER = endocardial resection, CRYO = cryoablation, AO V REPL = aortic valve replacement, AM = amiodarone, APR = aprindine, DIS = disopyramide, PRF = propafenone. Code: see Table 2.

RESULTS

Twenty-three deaths occurred: 2 cases of malignant disease and 21 of cardiac death (Table 3). For the whole group the cumulative cardiac survival at 60 months was 83% (SE 3.9). Eight of the cardiac deaths occurred in the group of 102 class 1–2 patients; 13 cardiac deaths were observed in the group of 27 class 3–4 patients. For class 1–2 patients, the cumulative cardiac survival at 60 months was 91% (SE 3.6); for class 3–4 patients, 52% (SE 10, $p < 0.001$). In the group of 45 patients with previous PES, 9 died of cardiac causes and 2 of non-cardiac causes (60 months' cardiac survival 73%, SE 7.8). In the other group of 84 patients, 12 cardiac deaths occurred (60 months' cardiac survival 86%, SE 4.4). The difference between these two groups was not statistically significant. In the group with PES, 20 patients were or became non-inducible (no sudden death, 4 VT recurrences), and 25 remained inducible (3 instances of sudden death, one device-rescued sudden death, 2 VT recurrences). The difference in survival for inducible and non-inducible patients was not statistically significant. No death occurred in the group of ten patients without structural heart disease. Heart failure was the cause of death in 2/5 patients with the ICD. Presumedly appropriate shocks were delivered by the ICD in 2 patients. Amiodarone-related side effects occurred in 22 patients: hyperthyroidism 11; hypothyroidism 5; severe skin discoloration 3; lung 2; eye 1. Amiodarone was withdrawn in 15 patients because of the side effects. After withdrawal, specific therapy was required in 5 patients (hyperthyroidism 4, lung 1). In 4 cases amiodarone was continued but combined with specific treatment (hyperthyroidism 3, hypothyroidism 1).

In the 21 cases of cardiac death, with respect to the notion "sudden arrhythmic death" classification was problematic in 6 patients. According to a different interpretation, the number of deaths listed as such could vary between 1 and 6. If the absence of severe progressive heart failure were required for the diagnosis of sudden arrhythmic death, only case 23 could be classified as such. Another approach would classify all 6 patients as suffering sudden arrhythmic deaths. Four deaths were instantaneous: all 4 occurred in class 3–4 patients. Two deaths were unwitnessed: one in class 1 patient with triple vessel disease and diminished left ventricular function found dead in bed in the morning (case 23), the other in a class 3 patient found dead 24 h after he had been seen for the last time (case 19).

The proposed code summarizes these deaths as: CA 2, HF 15, SD 6. SD can be subdivided in: S_3D_1 1, S_1D_3 1, S_3D_3 1, S_1D_4 3.

DISCUSSION

There is a need for a careful description of the patient's condition before the start of a treatment and at the time of death. The success or failure of specialized treatments is another incentive for such a description, especially when large randomized trials are designed. Identifying patients for prophylactic ICD therapy will remain a provocative issue for the next decade [6]. For socioeconomic and financial reasons worldwide, only a minority of patients will have access to the ICD.

This observational study reflects recent clinical practice in our institution. We have used amiodarone as the first-choice drug for malignant arrhythmias in high-risk patients. The low incidence of proarrhythmia and the lack of haemodynamic complications [7] outweigh its side-effects. In patients with congestive heart failure, even a beneficial effect was observed [8]. The efficacy of amiodarone in the prevention of sudden arrhythmic death was and will remain a matter of discussion for years. In clinical practice today, amiodarone is used for short-term [9,10] as well as for long-term treatment [11–14]. Electrophysiological testing during amiodarone treatment appears useful in identifying patients who are prone to suffer catastrophic arrhythmia recurrences and could allow for the institution of additional or alternative modes of therapy [15]. Among the clinical variables, an ejection fraction of less than or equal to 30% is a significant predictor of arrhythmia recurrence [16]. Table 1 illustrates the complex clinical picture of our patients. Besides the implantation of the ICD, other therapeutic options complicate the choice of treatment.

We had difficulties with cardiac death classification in 6/21 patients. These difficulties are likely to arise in patients with heart failure dying outside the hospital. Most of the patients at risk for sudden death have structural heart disease. If heart failure is progressive with disabling symptoms, in our health care system with free treatment the patient will be admitted recurrently to the hospital. This explains in this study group the high number of witnessed in-hospital deaths (15 patients). In a study group with most of the deaths occurring outside the hospital, the incidence of difficulties in classification will be even higher than in our patient population. This problem has been commented on extensively by the CAST and CAPS investigators [2,3]. A clear definition of sudden death is always difficult. In CAPS the on-site principal investigator was required to gather an extensive amount of data in addition to completing many forms and composing a letter explaining the circumstances surrounding the death or cardiac arrest event. The review of this information led to frequent disagreement. They stated that a less complex process would be advantageous. Also, the subjectivity in the assessment of the contribution of "end-stage" left ventricular failure to the fatal event was discussed. Both the CAPS and CASCADE investigators came to the conclusion that total mortality was the only reliable end point [4]. This conclusion would compromise reporting on sudden arrhythmic death.

We propose a new coding system giving a concise description of cardiac death. This code is applicable for both device-treated and drug-treated patients. The subscripts of SD show suddenness of death and NYHA functional class at the time of death. In the case of end-stage heart failure, two codings are possible: SD_4 or HF. We would use HF for in-hospital deaths, considered as not to be resuscitated, and SD_4 in other cases. The proposed cardiac death code allows a very short notation.

An appropriate code, together with total mortality and with total cardiac mortality, may contribute to adequate reports on the natural history of life-threatening arrhythmias and on the results of modern treatment.

ACKNOWLEDGEMENT

This study was supported by a grant from Lotto Nationale Loterij, België.

REFERENCES

1. WHO Scientific Group. The pathological diagnosis of acute ischaemic heart disease. WHO Rep Ser 1970;441:5.
2. The CAST Investigators. Effect of encainide and flecainide on mortality in a randomized trial of arrhythmia suppression after myocardial infarction. N Engl J Med 1989;321:406–12.
3. Greene HL, Richardson DW, Barker AH et al. Classification of deaths after myocardial infarction as arrhythmic or nonarrhythmic (The Cardiac Arrhythmia Pilot Study). Am J Cardiol 1989;63:1–6.
4. The CASCADE Investigators. Cardiac arrest in Seattle: Conventional versus amiodarone drug evaluation (The CASCADE Study). Am J Cardiol 1991;67:578–84.
5. The Criteria Committee of the New York Heart Association. Nomenclature and Criteria for Diagnosis of Diseases of the Heart and Great Vessels. Boston: Little, Brown, 1973:286.
6. Nisam S, Thomas A, Mower M, Hauser R. Identifying patients for prophylactic automatic implantable cardioverter defibrillator therapy: status of prospective studies. Am Heart J 1991;122:607–12.
7. Cleland JG, Dargie HJ, Findlay IN, Wilson JT. Clinical, haemodynamic, and antiarrhythmic effects of long term treatment with amiodarone of patients in heart failure. Br Heart J 1987;57:436–45.
8. Hamer AWF, Arkles LB, Johns JA. Beneficial effects of low dose amiodarone in patients with congestive cardiac failure: a placebo-controlled trial. J Am Coll Cardiol 1989;14:1768–74.
9. Nalos PC, Ismail Y, Pappas JM, Nyitray W, DonMichael TA. Intravenous amiodarone for short-term treatment of refractory ventricular tachycardia or fibrillation. Am Heart J 1991;122:1629–32.
10. Ochi RP, Goldenberg IF, Almquist A et al. Intravenous amiodarone for the rapid treatment of life-threatening ventricular arrhythmias in critically ill patients with coronary artery disease. Am J Cardiol 1989;64:599–603.
11. Herre JM, Sauve MJ, Malone P et al. Long-term results of amiodarone therapy in patients with recurrent sustained ventricular tachycardia or ventricular fibrillation. J Am Coll Cardiol 1989;13:442–9.
12. Myers M, Peter T, Weiss D et al. Benefit and risks of long-term amiodarone therapy for sustained ventricular tachycardia/fibrillation: minimum of three-year follow-up in 145 patients. Am Heart J 1990;119:8–14.
13. Burkart F, Pfisterer M, Kiowski W, Follath F, Burckhardt D. Effect of antiarrhythmic therapy on mortality in survivors of myocardial infarction with asymptomatic complex ventricular arrhythmias: Basel antiarrhythmic study of infarct survival (BASIS). J Am Coll Cardiol 1990;16:1711–8.
14. Neri R, Mestroni L, Salvi A, Pandullo C, Camerini F. Ventricular arrhythmias in dilated cardiomyopathy: efficacy of amiodarone. Am Heart J 1987;113:707–15.
15. Kadish AH, Buxton AE, Waxman HL, Flores B, Josephson ME, Marchlinsky FE. Usefulness of electrophysiologic study to determine the clinical tolerance of arrhythmia recurrences during amiodarone therapy. J Am Coll Cardiol 1987;10:90–6.
16. Manolis AS, Uricchio F, Estes NA III. Prognostic value of early electrophysiologic studies for ventricular tachycardia recurrence in patients with coronary artery disease treated with amiodarone. Am J Cardiol 1989;63:1052–7.

6. Heart rate variability

Methodology and physiological basis

LÜ FEI & MAREK MALIK

INTRODUCTION

It is well-known that the autonomic nervous system plays an important role in the regulation of activities of the heart. The assessment of autonomic function has been a challenging problem confronting cardiologists for many years. Sinus respiratory arrhythmia has also been known for a long time, but the importance of heart rate variability (HRV) was not recognised until recently. The study in 1981 by Akselrod et al. [1] showed that different components of spectral HRV could be suppressed by muscarinic parasympathetic and/or β-adrenergic blockade and provided a cornerstone for the physiological basis of HRV. HRV has since been studied by several investigators in both animals and humans [2–6]. In 1987 Kleiger and colleagues [7] demonstrated that HRV is a useful risk predictor following myocardial infarction. At present, it is generally accepted that HRV reflects the autonomic modulation of firing of the sinus node and that the analysis of HRV is an established non-invasive method for the assessment of autonomic influence on the heart. In this chapter, we will review the methodology of HRV measurement, the physiological basis of HRV and the factors influencing HRV.

METHODOLOGY OF HRV MEASUREMENT

Simple methods

Using simple methods, HRV can be computed and expressed as a ratio (minimum RR interval/maximum RR interval), as an absolute difference (maximum RR − minimum RR), or as this difference in relative terms, i.e. ([maximum RR] − [minimum RR])/[mean RR]), etc. In fact, many similar formulae have been proposed and used, ranging from the very simple to the

Table 1. The most commonly used time domain methods of HRV measurement.

Statistical methods

sdRR:	standard deviation of all normal RR intervals
SD:	mean of all 5-min standard deviations of R–R intervals
pNN50:	proportion of adjacent intervals more than 50 ms different

Robust geometrical methods

HRV index:	total number of RR intervals divided by the height of the RR interval histogram
TINN:	baseline width of the triangular interpolation of the RR interval histogram

somewhat more complicated. Although specialised technical studies have been conducted to examine the accuracy of these methods with computer-generated signals of known variability, these simplest methods are now of limited practical value.

Comprehensive time domain methods

Basic time domain methods use simple statistical measures to express the variability of the RR interval sequence. The most commonly used statistical measure is the standard deviation of all normal RR intervals (sdRR). Other statistical measures of HRV are shown in Table 1.

The statistical time-domain methods are dependent on the accuracy of the analysed RR interval sequences. Unfortunately, misrecognitions occur frequently in the processing of long-term electrocardiograms (ECGs). Therefore, it has been proposed that the statistical methods should be combined with various "filters", e.g. by excluding all the RR intervals which differ by > 20% from the preceding normal RR interval. However, technical evaluations of such filters have shown that they frequently fail [8]. In order to overcome the difficulty of obtaining precise RR interval data from long-term ECGs, geometrical time-domain methods (based on the evaluation of the histograms of the RR interval durations) have been proposed. These have been shown to be less affected by artefacts in the RR interval sequence. The simplest geometrical method (called the HRV index) expresses HRV as the relative number of RR intervals with the most frequent duration (i.e. the fraction of *total/maximum*; where *maximum* is the maximum number of computer-recognised RR intervals with the same duration; and *total* is the total number of all RR intervals recognised in a Holter recording). A more complicated artefact-robust method interpolates the histogram of the RR interval durations with a triangle and expresses HRV as the baseline width of this triangle (TINN, Figure 1) [9].

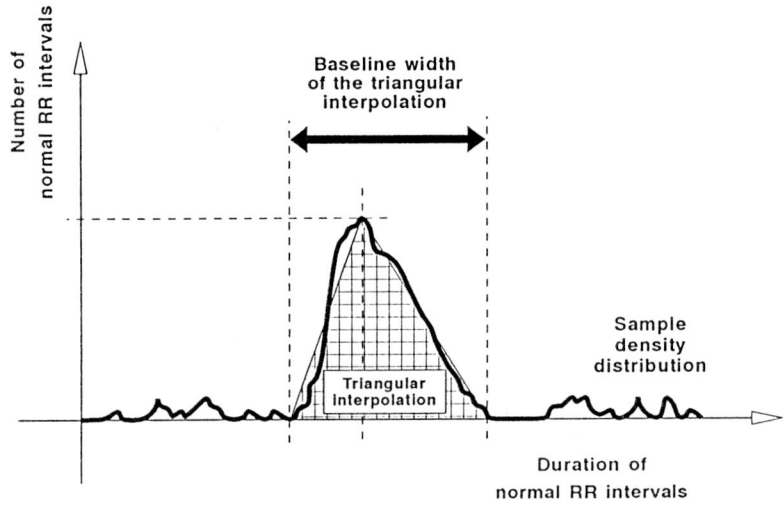

Figure 1. The triangular HRV index. The frequency distribution histogram is constructed from the number of RR intervals. The triangular index is the baseline width of the triangle that has the same maximal point and is the nearest to the frequency histogram as measured by the integral of the square difference.

Spectral methods

The spectral analysis of HRV aims at distinguishing all frequency components of sinus rhythm variations and quantifying each of them separately. There are two main technical approaches for calculating the spectra of HRV. *Fourier transformation* expresses the analysed data as a sum of sine functions with different periods and uses the degree of contribution of each of the sine functions to the total signal as an estimate of the spectral component corresponding to the given period [10]. *Autocorrelation methods* provide estimates of spectral components as correlations of the sequence of RR interval data with itself, shifting one of the sequences along the time axis [11]. There are several technical differences between these two methods, but there are no known important practical advantages of one over the other for the assessment of HRV spectra.

Like the time domain analysis, the spectral analysis of HRV is highly dependent on the accuracy and quality of the analysed data and requires special techniques to exclude the influence of cardiac arrhythmias. Usually, the RR interval preceding and following ectopic beats is excluded and replaced by interpolation of the durations of genuine RR intervals before and after the episode. However, it is impractical to exclude more than two RR intervals surrounding the ectopic beat because of the loss of continuity of the analysed signal. Thus, an accurate spectral assessment of HRV from rhythms containing many ectopic beats (e.g. bigeminy) is difficult. Adjustment of the low and high frequency bands in the spectral analysis of HRV may occasionally be necessary under certain conditions [12].

Chaos and Poincaré plots

Kobayashi and Musha [13] first noted that the heart rate power spectrum decays as the reciprocal of frequency rises to a power close to 1. This 1/f decay could reflect the fractal nature of HRV [14]. In theory, a system which exhibits a deterministic chaos includes a large or eventually infinite number of unstable periodic cycles. The system never remains long in any of these cycles but continuously switches from one motion to another such that it appears as completely random behaviour. The investigation of such systems is based on mathematical models which identify the key parameters, that is, localise the most important periodic components.

There are several ways of investigating a chaotic system; the most commonly used one employs the so-called attractors. A two-dimensional attractor is composed of lines which connect points defined by the i-th and (i + 1)-th, (i + 1)-th and (i + 2)-th, (i + 2)-th and (i + 3)-th, etc. stages of the system. True attractors, which are composed of lines, are difficult to perceive if the system has a high number of periodic components and if the recorded sequence of its stages is very long. This is frequently the case with sequences of RR intervals. Thus, it has been proposed that the Poincaré plots (also called the Lorentz plots), which are only composed of points defined by the i-th and (i + 1)-th, (i + 1)-th and (i + 2)-th, etc. RR intervals without the interconnecting lines, should be used (Figure 2).

Although several technical studies have been devoted to HRV measurement using the chaos theory, a practical method has not yet been established. It has been reported that using a method derived from nonlinear dynamics to analyse complex HRV may provide a more sensitive marker of physiological changes than conventional statistical methods [15,16]. However, these methods should be used cautiously since the mathematical procedures behind fractal and chaos analysis of HRV are still under investigation.

The major differences in methodology of published HRV studies are the length of the observation window (minutes to days), the rules for dealing with non-sinus data (ectopics and artefacts) and the method of data processing (statistical summary and spectral analysis). Different methods could provide complementary information [17], but they may also bias the results achieved when comparing HRV calculated using different methods and different lengths of observation. When artefact-free data are analysed, there is a strong correlation between the standard statistical methods, artefact-robust methods and spectral frequency components. HRV parameters in the time-domain and frequency-domain correlate well with each other (most correlation coef-

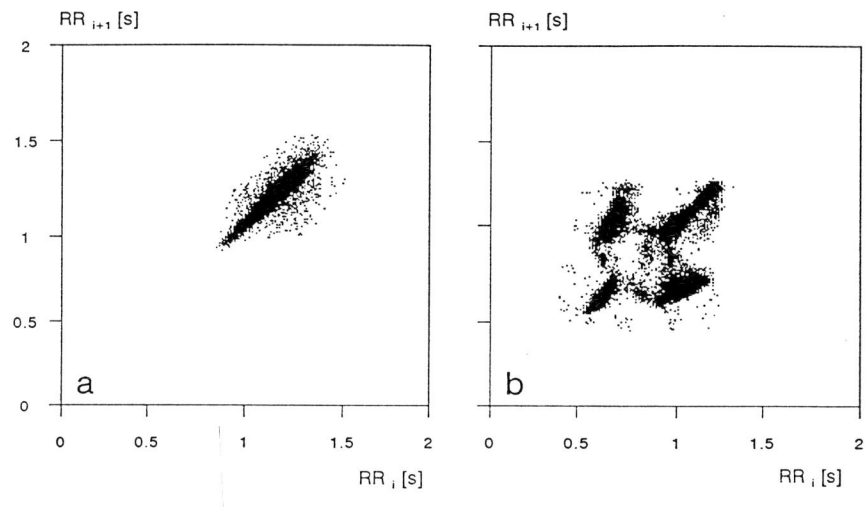

Figure 2. Poincaré plots of supraventricular RR intervals recorded in two survivors of acute myocardial infarction. Plot **a** shows one component of heart period variation, whilst several components are distinguishable in plot **b**. The rhythm in plot **b** was distorted by supraventricular ectopic activity (Post-Infarction Survey Programme of St. George's Hospital Medical School).

ficients range from 0.70 to 0.98). It has been shown that there is little influence of investigator bias [18].

Although there are intra-individual and temporal variations in HRV, both long- and short-term HRV is generally reproducible under comparable conditions [19]. For example, the correlation coefficients of HRV between two different days of 0.88 for SDANN and 0.89 for SD in normal subjects, and 0.85 for SDANN and 0.97 for SD in patients with congestive heart failure were observed [20]. Akselrod and colleagues [1] demonstrated that the spectral peak areas varied by no more than 5–10%.

PHYSIOLOGICAL BASIS OF HRV

The physiological significance of HRV has been studied mainly by autonomic interventions (including blocking or stimulating drugs, physiological provocative manoeuvres and stress tests). It has been shown that direct electrical stimulation of the vagus nerve causes a decreased low-frequency component of HRV, an increased high-frequency component and a decreased low to high ratio. Akselrod et al. [1] observed that in the power spectrum of HRV obtained from a 5 min recording of adult conscious dogs, three distinct components could be distinguished: a high-frequency peak at approximately

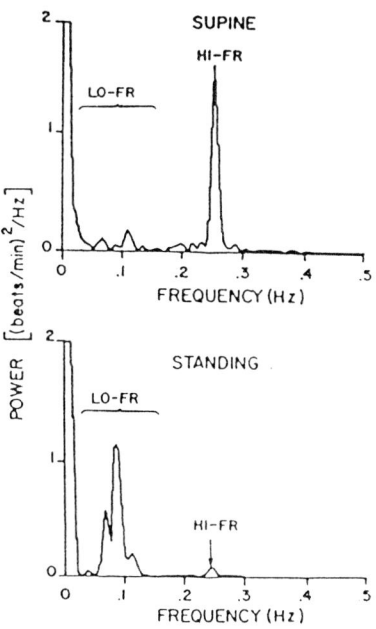

Figure 3. Power spectrum of HRV recorded in man in supine (top) and standing (bottom) positions. Note that there is a prominent high-frequency peak and a small low-frequency peak in the supine position, whereas there is a small high-frequency peak and a prominent low-frequency peak in the standing position. HI-FR = the high-frequency component, LO-FR = the low-frequency component. Reproduced with permission from Pomeranz et al. [5].

0.4 Hz, a mid-frequency peak at approximately 0.15 Hz and a low-frequency peak at approximately 0.05 Hz. The high- and mid-frequency peaks were abolished and the power of the low-frequency peak was reduced by selective parasympathetic blockade, while combined beta-sympathetic and parasympathetic blockade abolished all variations of heart rate. Modulations of the low-frequency peak due to blockade of the renin-angiotensin system were also noted in this study. These findings by Akselrod et al. were later confirmed by others in both animals and humans [2–6].

The low-frequency component (0.04–0.15 Hz) of HRV in the frequency domain is thought to provide a measure of sympathetic activity with some influence from vagal activity, while the high-frequency component (0.15–0.40 Hz) is almost exclusively mediated by vagal activity and the low to high ratio has been hypothesized to represent the sympathovagal balance of the heart. The overall HRV is believed to be mainly influenced by cardiac vagal activity because of the vagal predominance under normal conditions. The contribution of sympathetic activity to HRV is relatively small, particularly in the resting supine position (Figure 3). The physiological significance of the very or ultra low-frequency component (< 0.04 Hz) is less well understood and should be addressed with caution. Nonetheless, the analysis of HRV has provided a non-invasive method for the assessment of sympathovagal interaction at the level of the sinus node of the heart.

HRV and arterial baroreflex sensitivity (BRS) represent the "tonic" and "phasic" activity of the autonomic nervous system, respectively. Although the relationship between them is still disputed, HRV and BRS are complementary to each other in the assessment of cardiac autonomic activity [21,22].

Physiological diurnal variation in humans has been noted for a long time [23]. There may be an association between circadian variation and a trigger for the onset of acute cardiovascular disease [24]. Reports concerning the diurnal variation of HRV in relation to cardiovascular events are scarce. However, currently available data suggest that an alteration of the circadian rhythm of HRV may be of clinical significance [25–27].

It is well-known that the innervation of the heart is asymmetrical. Therefore, one challenge confronting the clinical application of HRV as a non-invasive tool for quantifying autonomic nervous system activity is that autonomic activity at the sinus node may not necessarily be a faithful "autonomic barometer" of sympathetic/vagal drive to the ventricle. However, the bulk of evidence has revealed the important clinical significance of HRV. The mechanism inside this "black box" remains to be fully elucidated, although there is increasing evidence that vagal innervation does exist in the ventricle.

FACTORS INFLUENCING HRV

HRV has been shown to be influenced by many physiological and pathological factors including age, gender, mean heart rate, posture, exercise, drugs, emotion and other behavioural factors (such as alcohol and smoking), cardiac function and underlying heart disease. Ventricular arrhythmias themselves may also have a notable impact on HRV values [28].

Effects of age and gender

In normal subjects, HRV decreases with age. The relationship between HRV and age is non-linear [29] and is not affected by deep breathing, standing up or the Valsalva manoeuvre. In the study by Korkushko and colleagues [30], the spectral analysis of HRV was performed in 354 apparently healthy individuals, ranging in age from 3 months to 89 years. It was demonstrated that in the early years of life, there is a prevalence of parasympathetic activity. In infancy and after the age of 50 years, sympathetic activity predominates against a background of weak parasympathetic activity. The reduction in HRV in elderly subjects is consistent with the known age-related decline in cardiac responsiveness to sympathetic activation [31]. The mid-frequency component of HRV has been shown to be related to the frequency response of the baroreceptor reflex [1]. There is evidence that nervous reflexes, such as the baroreceptor reflex [32] and the bradycardia response to the Valsalva manoeuvre [33] are significantly depressed in the elderly. These observations suggest that aging is characterised by a new equilibrium between the two sections of the autonomic nervous system rather than by alterations of sympathetic activity alone [34,35]. However, the relationship between age and HRV may be altered under abnormal conditions [36].

It has been shown that there is a significant difference in HRV between male and female subjects. Both time- and frequency-domain HRV parameters are significantly higher in males than in females, although no significant difference is observed in the high-frequency component of HRV [29,37].

Effect of heart rate

HRV is significantly related to mean heart rate [19,38]. When multivariate analyses were performed after adjusting for features reflecting left ventricular function, heart rate, exercise testing and early post-infarction angina, the strongest association was found between HRV and the average heart rate over 24 h from the same Holter recording in patients with myocardial infarction [7]. This association may be largely accounted for by a purely mathematical effect. However, it is also likely to be caused by decreased vagal and/or increased sympathetic activity at higher heart rate. It has been shown that an increased heart rate itself may be associated with an increased propensity to ventricular tachyarrhythmias and sudden cardiac death [39]. Despite the dependence on heart rate, HRV provides more information about the autonomic function of the heart than the mean heart rate alone.

Effect of posture

Pomeranz et al. [5] demonstrated that sympathetic influences are normally present only in the low-frequency component of HRV in the standing posture (and not in the high-frequency component), whereas vagal activity influences the low- and high-frequency components in both supine and standing postures. It has been shown that during head-up tilting, the high-frequency component is decreased and the low-frequency component increased, while the standard deviation of the RR intervals remains unchanged [40]. The effects of orthostasis on HRV is independent of the depth and frequency of respiration [41].

Effect of exercise

It has been shown that the response time to electrical stimulation of the parasympathetic nervous system is much shorter than that of the sympathetic nervous system [42]. Exercise elicits reductions in both the low- and high-frequency components of HRV (especially the high-frequency component) [11]. This reduction is accentuated by β-adrenergic receptor blockade. Orthostatic stress produces a significant increase in the ratio of low- to high-frequency peak power, while steady-state exercise causes a significant suppression of both the low and high components, followed by a significant rise in the low-frequency peak power in the first 15 min of the post-exercise recovery period. The low-frequency component peak shifted to the left during exercise and to the right during the supine recovery period. It has been postulated that neuroregulatory control of heart rate may play a major role in adaptive responses to orthostatic stress and post-exercise recovery, while humoral factors are probably more important in maintaining heart rate during steady-state exercise [43].

Comparative studies of HRV in normal subjects and heart transplant recipients have revealed that at peak exercise a non-autonomic mechanism, possibly intrinsic to the heart muscle, may determine heart rate fluctuations in synchrony with ventilation in the intact as well as in the denervated human heart [44]. This suggests that HRV may not be modulated by the autonomic nervous system alone.

Effect of long-term physical training

The influence of long-term exercise on HRV has been studied in athletes [45]. The average RR interval was significantly longer, and the low- and high-frequency components of HRV were significantly higher in athletes than in controls, but there were no significant differences in the low to high ratio or the normalised low- and high-frequency components between athletes and controls. These observations suggest that the higher HRV observed in athletes reflects a higher parasympathetic tone without reduction of the sympathetic tone. It has been shown that physical training may increase vagal tone without altering the arterial baroreflex control of heart rate in normal subjects [46].

The fact that physical training has a distinct impact on HRV in healthy subjects infers that physical training may be of value in the modification of cardiac autonomic activity in patients with depressed HRV [47]. This has been demonstrated in patients with depressed HRV following acute myocardial infarction [48].

Effects of emotion and mental stress

Many studies have been conducted to investigate the effects of stress on HRV [49]. Recently, Pagani et al. [50] observed that psychological stress induced marked changes in the sympathovagal balance, mainly characterised by sympathetic predominance. A significant difference in HRV changes induced by stress has been observed between groups of highly anxious and less anxious women. The influence of emotion should also be taken into account when interpreting the results of animal experiments or comparing HRV between different groups of patients.

Effects of alcohol and smoking

HRV has been shown to be significantly lower in alcohol-dependent patients than in normal subjects [51]. HRV was also depressed in chronic alcoholic neuropathy. However, the effects of acute alcohol ingestion on the different spectral components of HRV are diverse [52]: the medium-frequency component is significantly reduced, whilst the high-frequency parasympathetic component is only minimally decreased.

It has been reported that smoking causes an acute and transient decrease in the vagal component and an increase in the sympathetic component of HRV. Heavy smokers also exhibit depressed behavioural variations of HRV, such as those induced by postural changes [53].

Effects of drugs

It has been shown that many drugs have a significant influence on HRV directly or indirectly (e.g. through drug-induced haemodynamic changes) [54,55]. The majority of these findings can be explained by the known parasympathetic and/or sympathetic blocking or stimulating effects of these drugs. However, the results of different studies do not always agree. This may be due to a different basal state of vagal tone of the heart. In addition, other factors influencing drug effects (such as underlying heart disease and left ventricular dysfunction) may also significantly influence pharmacological effects on HRV.

The effect of antiarrhythmic drugs on HRV may be of special clinical interest. Most antiarrhythmic agents decrease HRV. This may be attributed to their vagolytic or β-blocking properties. For instance, Zuanetti et al. [56] found no significant change in HRV in patients with ventricular arrhythmias treated with amiodarone, whereas a significant decrease in HRV was noted in patients treated with flecainide or propafenone. The decreased HRV was reversible when treatment was discontinued and was not related to the suppression of arrhythmias since HRV over the 24-h period was similar during treatment irrespective of the presence or absence of frequent arrhythmias. To date, there are no reports concerning the relationship between the alterations of HRV induced by antiarrhythmic agents and their antiarrhythmic and proarrhythmic actions. It would be of clinical interest to classify antiarrhythmic drugs according to their effects on autonomic activity. There is evidence that chronic β-adrenergic blockade leads to a reduction in sympathetic efferent activity, whereas acute blockade may not have the same effect [57]. It has been shown that both acute and chronic administration of propranolol significantly alter HRV [1,6,58–60].

In conclusion, the analysis of HRV provides a useful non-invasive measure of autonomic influence of the heart. Although HRV shows inter- and intra-individual (or temporal) variations, it does not change significantly during periods of clinical steady state in either normal subjects or patients with structural heart disease. HRV has been shown to be decreased in conjunction with major cardiovascular events [15,61,62]. However, the physiological mechanisms underlying HRV need to be fully elucidated, and the methodology of HRV analysis needs to be standardised.

REFERENCES

1. Akselrod S, Gordon D, Ubel FA, Shannon DC, Barger AC, Cohen RJ. Power spectrum analysis of heart rate fluctuations: a quantitative probe of beat-to-beat cardiovascular control. Science 1981;213:220–2.
2. Eckberg DL. Human sinus arrhythmia as an index of vagal cardiac outflow. J Appl Physiol 1983;54:961–6.
3. Mancia G, Ferrari A, Gregorini L et al. Blood pressure and heart rate variabilities in normotensive and hypertensive human beings. Circ Res 1983;53:96–104.
4. Ewing DJ, Neilson JMM, Travis P. New method for assessing cardiac parasympathetic activity using 24 hour electrocardiograms. Br Heart J 1984;52:396–402.
5. Pomeranz B, Macaulay RJB, Caudill MA et al. Assessment of autonomic function in humans by heart rate spectral analysis. Am J Physiol 1985;248:H151–3.
6. Pagani M, Lombardi F, Guzzetti S et al. Power spectral analysis of heart rate and arterial pressure variabilities as a marker of sympatho-vagal interaction in man and conscious dog. Circ Res 1986;59:178–93.
7. Kleiger RE, Miller JP, Bigger JT Jr, Moss AJ, and The Multicenter Post-Infarction Research Group. Decreased heart rate variability and its association with increased mortality after acute myocardial infarction. Am J Cardiol 1987;59:256–62.
8. Malik M, Farrell T, Cripps T, Camm AJ. Heart rate variability in relation to prognosis after myocardial infarction: selection of optimal processing techniques. Eur Heart J 1989;10:1060–74.
9. Farrell TG, Bashir Y, Cripps T et al. Risk stratification for arrhythmic events in post-infarction patients based on heart rate variability, ambulatory electrocardiographic variables and the signal-averaged electrocardiogram. J Am Coll Cardiol 1991;18:687–97.
10. Lipsitz LA, Mietus J, Moody GB, Goldberger AL. Spectral characteristics of heart rate variability before and during postural tilt. Relations to aging and risk of syncope. Circulation 1990;81:1803–10.
11. Arai Y, Saul JP, Albrecht P et al. Modulation of cardiac autonomic activity during and immediately after exercise. Am J Physiol 1989;256:H132–41.

12. Osaka M, Saitoh H, Sasabe N et al. Personal adjustment of low and high frequency bands (PAB) in spectral analysis of heart rate variability (HRV). J Ambulatory Monitoring 1992;5(Suppl):30.
13. Kobayashi M, Musha T. 1/f Fluctuation of heartbeat period. IEEE Trans Biomed Eng 1982;29:456–7.
14. Goldberger AL, West BJ. Application of nonlinear dynamics to clinical cardiology. Ann N Y Acad Sci 1987;504:195–213.
15. Skinner JE, Pratt CM, Vybiral T. A reduction in the correlation dimension of heartbeat intervals precedes imminent ventricular fibrillation in human subjects. Am Heart J 1993;125:731–43.
16. Goldberger AL, Mietus JE, Rigney DR, Wood ML, Fortney SM. Short-term bedrest deconditioning causes a loss of complex heart rate variability. J Am Coll Cardiol 1992;19:371A.
17. Singer DH, Martin GJ, Magid N et al. Low heart rate variability and sudden cardiac death. J Electrocardiol 1988;21:S46-S55.
18. Ohler JP, Abel T, Höpp HW, Hilger HH. Day-to-day-reproducibility of heart-rate-variability with Holter-ECG in patients with coronary heart disease. J Ambulatory Monitoring 1992;5(Suppl):6.
19. Huikuri HV, Kessler KM, Terracall E, Castellanos A, Linnaluoto MK, Myerburg RJ. Reproducibility and circadian rhythm of heart rate variability in healthy subjects. Am J Cardiol 1990;65:391–3.
20. van Hoogenhuyze D, Martin GJ, Weiss JS, Schaad J, Fintel D, Singer DH. Heart rate variability 1989. An update. J Electrocardiol 1989;22(Suppl):204–8.
21. Bigger JT Jr, La-Rovere MT, Steinman RC et al. Comparison of baroreflex sensitivity and heart period variability after myocardial infarction. J Am Coll Cardiol 1989;14:1511–8.
22. Farrell TG, Paul V, Cripps TR et al. Baroreflex sensitivity and electrophysiological correlates in patients after acute myocardial infarction. Circulation 1991;83:945–52.
23. Aschott J. Day-night variations in the cardiovascular system. Historical and other notes by an outsider. In: Schmidt TFH, Engel BT, Blümchen G, Editors. Temporal variations of the cardiovascular system. Berlin: Springer-Verlag, 1992:3–14.
24. Muller JE, Tofler GH, Stone PH. Circadian variation and triggers of onset of acute cardiovascular disease. Circulation 1989;79:733–43.
25. Malik M, Farrell T, Camm AJ. Circadian rhythm of heart rate variability after acute myocardial infarction and its influence on the prognostic value of heart rate variability. Am J Cardiol 1990;66:1049–54.
26. Huikuri HV, Linnaluoto MK, Seppänen T et al. Circadian rhythm of heart rate variability in survivors of cardiac arrest. Am J Cardiol 1992;70:610–5.
27. Bernardi L, Ricordi L, Lazzari P et al. Impaired circadian modulation of sympathovagal activity in diabetes. A possible explanation for altered temporal onset of cardiovascular disease. Circulcation 1992;86:1443–52.
28. Vybiral T, Bryg RJ, Maddens MA. Impact of arrhythmias on heart rate variability. Strategies to deal with imperfect clinical data. Comput Cardiol 1990;251–4.
29. O'Brien IAD, O'Hare P, Corrall RJM. Heart rate variability in healthy subjects: effect of age and the derivation of normal ranges for test of autonomic function. Br Heart J 1986;55:348–54.
30. Korkushko OV, Shatilo VB, Plachinda YuI, Shatilo TV. Autonomic control of cardiac chronotropic function in man as a function of age: assessment by power spectral analysis of heart rate variability. J Auton Nerv Syst 1991;32:191–8.
31. Lakatta EG. Age-related alterations in the cardiovascular response to adrenergic mediated stress. Fed Proc 1980;39:3173–7.
32. Kawamoto A, Shimada K, Matsubayashi K et al. Cardiovascular regulatory functions in elderly patients with hypertension. Hypertension 1989;13:401–7.
33. Shimada K, Kitazumi T, Ogura H, Sadakane N, Ozawa T. Effects of age and blood pressure

on the cardiovascular responses to the Valsalva manoeuvre. J Am Geriatr Soc 1986;34:431–4.
34. Rodeheffer RJ, Gerstenblith G, Becker LC, Fleg JL, Weisfeldt ML, Lakatta EG. Exercise cardiac output is maintained with advancing age in healthy human subjects: Cardiac dilatation and increased stroke volume compensate for a diminished heart rate. Circulation 1985;69:203–13.
35. Sever PS, Osikowska B, Birch M, Tunbridge RDG. Plasma noradrenaline in essential hypertension. Lancet 1977;1:1078–81.
36. Saul JP, Arai Y, Berger RD, Lilly LS, Colucci WS, Cohen RJ. Assessment of autonomic regulation in chronic congestive heart failure by heart rate spectral analysis. Am J Cardiol 1988;61:1292–9.
37. Brüggemann T, Andersen D, Völler H, Schröder R. Heart rate variability from Holter monitoring in a normal population. Circulation 1990;84:II-595.
38. Fleiss JL, Bigger JT Jr, Rolnitzky LM. The correlation between heart period variability and mean period length. Stat Med 1992;11:125–9.
39. Gillman MW, Kannel WB, Belanger A, D'Agostino RB. Influence of heart rate on mortality among persons with hypertension: The Framingham Study. Am Heart J 1993;125:1148–54.
40. Vybiral T, Bryg RJ, Maddens ME, Boden WE. Effect of passive tilt on sympathetic and parasympathetic components of heart rate variability in normal subjects. Am J Cardiol 1990;63:1117–20.
41. Weise F, Heydenreich F. Effects of modified respiratory rhythm on heart rate variability during active orthostatic load. Biomed Biochim Acta 1989;48:549–56.
42. Warner HR, Cox A. A mathematical model of heart rate control by sympathetic and vagus efferent information. J Appl Physiol 1962;17a:349–55.
43. Kamath MV, Fallen EL, McKelvie R. Effects of steady state exercise on the power spectrum of heart rate variability. Med Sci Sports Exerc 1991;23:428–34.
44. Bernardi L, Salvucci F, Suardi R et al. Evidence for an intrinsic mechanism regulating heart rate variability in the transplanted and the intact heart during submaximal dynamic exercise? Cardiovasc Res 1990;24:969–81.
45. Costa O, Freitas J, Puig J et al. Spectrum analysis of the variability of heart rate in athletes. Rev Port Cardiol 1991;10:23–8.
46. Seals DR, Chase PB. Influence of physical training on heart rate variability and baroreflex circulatory control. J Appl Physiol 1989;66:1886–95.
47. Molgaard H, Sorensen KE, Bjerregaard P. Circadian variation and influence of risk factors on heart rate variability in healthy subjects. Am J Cardiol 1991;68:777–84.
48. La-Rovere MT, Mortara A, Sandrone G, Lombardi F. Autonomic nervous system adaptations to short-term exercise training. Chest 1992;101:299S–303S.
49. Langewitz W, Ruddel H. Spectral analysis of heart rate variability under mental stress. J Hypertens 1989;7:S32–3.
50. Pagani M, Mazzuero G, Ferrari A et al. Sympathovagal interaction during mental stress. A study using spectral analysis of heart rate variability in healthy control subjects and patients with a prior myocardial infarction. Circulation 1991;83:II-43–II-51.
51. Malpas SC, Whiteside EA, Maling TJ. Heart rate variability and cardiac autonomic function in men with chronic alcohol dependence. Br Heart J 1991;65:84–8.
52. Gonzalez-Gonzalez J, Mendez-Llorens A, Mendez-Novoa A, Cordero-Valeriano JJ. Effect of alcohol ingestion on short term heart rate fluctuations. J Stud Alcohol 1992;53:86–90.
53. Hayano J, Yamada M, Sakakibara Y et al. Short- and long-term effects of cigarette smoking on heart rate variability. Am J Cardiol 1990;65:84–8.
54. Lombardi F, Torzillo D, Sandrone G, Dalla Vecchia L, Cappiello E. Autonomic effects of antiarrhythmic drugs and their importance. Eur Heart J 1992;13(Suppl F):38–43.
55. McCabe PM, Yongue BG, Ackles PK, Porges SW. Changes in heart period, heart-period variability, and a spectral analysis estimate of respiratory sinus arrhythmia in response to pharmacological manipulations of the baroreceptor reflex in cats. Psychophysiology 1985;22:195–203.

56. Zuanetti G, Latini R, Neilson JMM, Schwartz PJ, Ewing DJ. Heart rate variability in patients with ventricular arrhythmias: effect of antiarrhythmic drugs. J Am Coll Cardiol 1991;17:604–12.
57. Wallin BG, Sundlöf G, Strömgren E, Åberg H. Sympathetic outflow to muscles during treatment of hypertension with metoprolol. Hypertension 1984;6:557–62.
58. Syutkina EV. Effect of autonomic nervous system blockade and acute asphyxia on heart rate variability in the fetal rat. Gynecol Obstet Invest 1988;25:249–57.
59. Hayano J, Sakakihara Y, Yamada A et al. Accuracy of assessment of cardiac vagal tone by heart rate variability in normal subjects. Am J Cardiol 1991;67:199–204.
60. Filipecki A, Trusz-Gluza M, Szydlo K, Giec L. Effect of propranolol and propafenone on heart rate variability in patients with ventricular arrhythmias. PACE 1993;16:1157.
61. Huikuri HV, Valkama JO, Airaksinen KEJ et al. Frequency domain measures of heart rate variability before the onset of non-sustained and sustained ventricular tachycardia in patients with coronary artery disease. Circulation 1993;87:1220–8.
62. Monir G, Fintel D, Weiss J et al. Long term reproducibility of heart rate variability. J Am Coll Cardiol 1992;19:369A.

7. Heart rate variability and QT interval: their relationships with the cardiac frequency

PHILIPPE COUMEL & PIERRE MAISON-BLANCHE

INTRODUCTION

The influence of the autonomic nervous system (ANS) on cardiac functions can be evaluated in ambulatory surface ECG recordings by two different approaches; the heart rate variability (HRV) and the QT interval dynamicity. HRV specifically evaluates the modulation of the sinus node automatism by the ANS, whereas QT dynamicity is related to the ANS influence on the ventricular myocardium. One expects that under physiological conditions in normal hearts the indications yielded by these two approaches will probably be consistent. However, this is probably no longer the case when a structural heart disease is present. As a matter of fact, HRV is only affected by the impact of the heart disease on the ANS, whereas QT dynamicity is involved by the disease itself.

The important issue we intend to deal with in the present chapter is the influence of the rate itself on these two parameters, a problem that is very much overlooked in the literature. Cardiac frequency and the ANS are not synonymous terms, and their respective impact on the HRV on the one hand and the QT dynamicity on the other are not easy to dissociate clearly by non-invasive methods.

HEART RATE VARIABILITY

Methodology

Numerous techniques of evaluation of HRV have been developed in the frequency as well as in the time domain. The heart rate modulation of vagal origin is responsible for the respiration-related short-term variations of cycle length that occur about 15–20 times per minute and cover 2–6 cardiac cycles. This influence is present in the 0.25 Hz band of the power spectrum, and it can be assessed by measuring differences between the cycle length duration of consecutive beats or short sequences of a few beats. The sympathetic modulation has a longer wavelength of the order of 10-15 s that represents the time response of the baroreflex, and is expressed in the 0.10 Hz band of the power spectrum. Humoral influences have much longer wavelengths that may range from a few minutes to 24 h or probably even longer.

Direct evaluation of the heart rate oscillations

The method we have developed for evaluating HRV in the time domain is based on the detection and quantification of the heart rate oscillations of different wavelengths. A heart rate oscillation is defined as the succession of an increase and a decrease of the frequency over a certain number of cycles. Respiration-related oscillations cover 2-6 cycles, whereas sympathetically mediated modulation covers longer sequences. Once detected, the oscillations are numbered per time unit, and their amplitude is defined by the

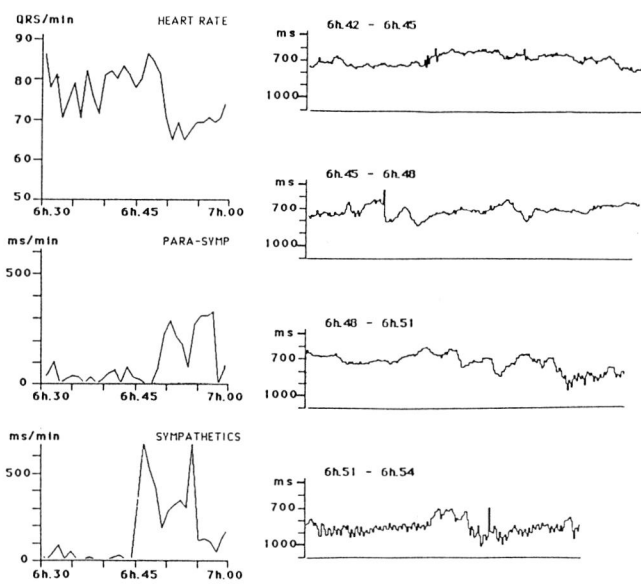

Figure 1. Quantitation of HRV by the evaluation of heart rate oscillations. The right panels display the beat-by-beat tachograms between 06.42 h and 06.54 h. The three upper strips clearly involve sympathetic influences: the oscillations are prolonged, covering 10-20 cycles or more. In contrast, the bottom panel shows a predominance of short-term, respiration-related, vagally mediated oscillations. The left panels give for the 30-min period the value of the heart rate (in QRS/min), the para-sympathetic and the sympathetic activity in ms/min (product amplitude times number). Note that dissociations are visible with time between the different variables, so that information about the autonomic nervous system is not identical to the heart rate.

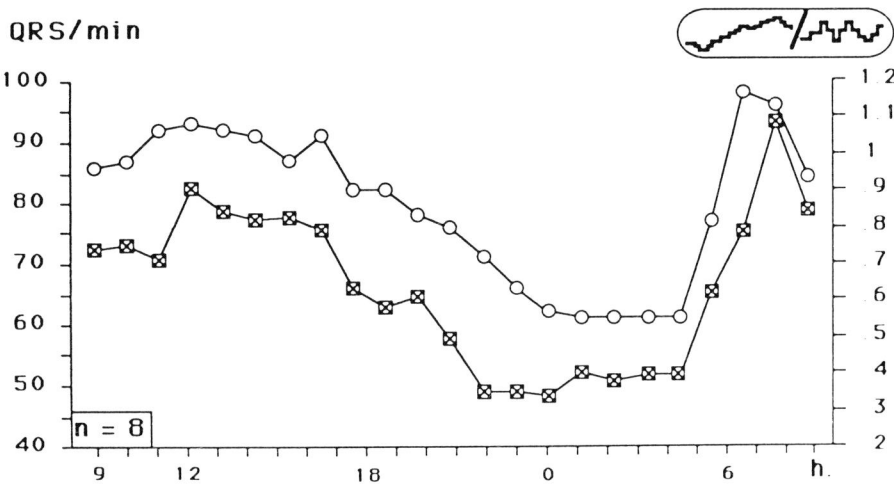

Figure 2. Correlation between heart rate and HRV in a group of 8 normal subjects. The hourly values of heart rate (QRS/min, left scale) and sympathovagal ratio (right scale) are closely parallel over the 24-h period. This pattern gives the impression that the two parameters are directly correlated, whereas in fact the heart rate acts rather as a marker of clockwise variations (see the text for discussion).

difference between the shortest and the longest cardiac cycle within an oscillation: the product amplitude times number is expressed in ms/min.

This method has been described in detail previously [1], and the correlations between 'short' vagally mediated and 'long' sympathetically mediated oscillations and the corresponding peaks of high and low frequency in the power spectrum are excellent [2]. In contrast to the spectral analysis, this method is not sensitive to the lack of constancy of the cardiac frequency, a necessary but rarely fully respected condition for using the fast Fourier transform, and this is well-adapted to studying HRV in Holter recordings. A demonstrative example is given in Figure 1, in which frequent and marked changes in heart rate and HRV occur during a 30-min period. The various types of oscillations are clearly visible in the beat-by-beat tachograms displayed on the right panels, and their quantification is represented on the left.

The ratio between the sympathetic and the parasympathetic activity can be calculated over long periods of time, and Figure 2 represents the pooled data of eight normal subjects. There is a close parallelism between the hourly values of the heart rate and those of the sympathovagal ratio. The strong correlation between these two variables is not surprising at all at first glance, precisely because the ANS balance is supposed to condition the heart rate. However, Figure 3 shows that the relationships between heart rate and HVR

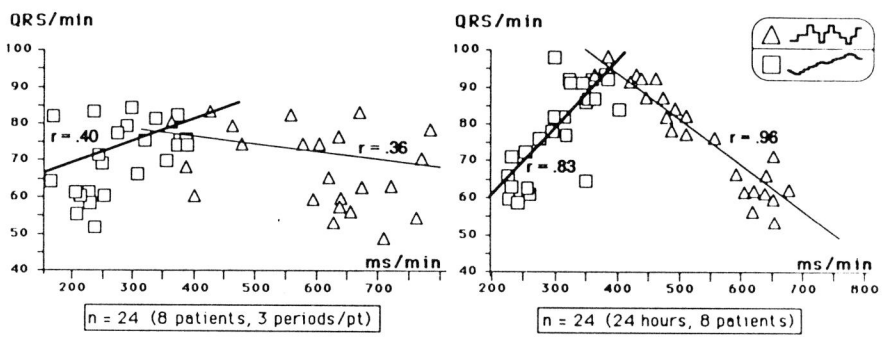

Figure 3. Correlations between heart rate and HRV. On the right part, the data represent the 24 pooled hourly values of the 8 individuals. Close correlations are apparent between heart rate and the 'long' sympathetically mediated and 'short' vagally mediated types of oscillations: the former increase as the rate accelerates, whereas the latter decrease with good correlation coefficients. From this pattern, one could conclude that a direct relationship exists between heart rate and HRV. However, the left part of the figure demonstrates that this is not the case, using 24 values quite differently pooled values from the same data. Three periods (day, night and intermediate) have been defined for each of the 8 subjects according to the heart rate levels, so that the interindividual differences in the mean level of heart rates are not blurred as in the right part of the figure. In other words, an individual may well have at night the same cardiac frequency as another person in the daytime: the clearly poor correlations observed with heart rate for both types of oscillation demonstrate that the latter relate in fact not to the cardiac frequency as such but to the circadian period.

are not obvious and are in fact very complex: the notion of circadian variations of the heart rate is essential to understanding this figure.

In the right panel of Figure 3, the data from the eight subjects have been pooled in terms of hourly values of the short and long oscillations, so that each symbol represents the averaged value of eight individuals for every hour in the 24-h period. Plotting these hourly values with the corresponding heart rate shows a very good correlation between the two variables, either positive (Pearson correlation coefficient $r = 0.83$) or negative ($r = -0.96$) according to the respective significance of the oscillations.

One is tempted to conclude that the meaning of this correlation is the cardiac frequency itself and the ANS balance, but the left panel of Figure 3 demonstrates that this is not the correct interpretation. Here, the same data have been rearranged in the different way. For every subject, the 24 hourly values have been grouped into three categories of upper, middle and lower rates, no matter the time of measurement. Thus, in contrast to the right panels in which each subject is plotted 24 times, on the left each of the eight subjects is represented by three points, with a total of 24 points for the whole group. With this representation, it appears that the correlations between HRV and the heart rate are much weaker ($r = 0.40$ rather than 0.83, and

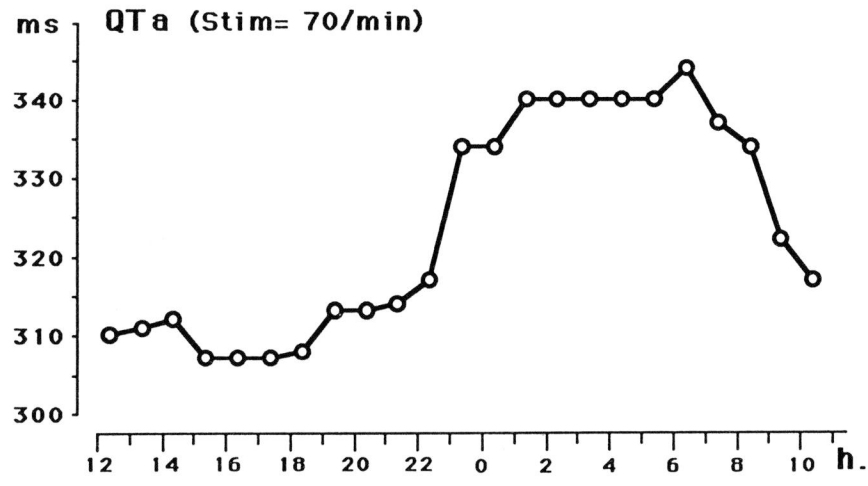

Figure 4. Purely automatic modulation of the QT interval. In a patient with a fixed rate ventricular pacemaker set at 70/min, the QTa (T apex) interval varies from day to night by about 30 ms, and this variation can be ascribed exclusively to the ANS-related modulation of the ventricular repolarization.

− 0.36 rather than − 0.96). The conclusion is that the relationships between heart rate and HRV over the 24-h period are closely linked to the time: the value of cardiac frequency forms in fact a marker of the circadian period, a surrogate of clockwise variations of the ANS balance rather than a true variable. Pooling the values on an hourly basis or on a frequency basis totally changes the apparent relationships: pooling the hourly values just makes in fact the heart rate a biological marker of time. The fundamental reason for this state of affairs is that the level of the cardiac frequency is proper to each individual, but that the circadian variations are common to all subjects.

DYNAMIC VARIATIONS OF THE QT INTERVAL

The Holter technique allows a new approach to the dynamicity of ventricular repolarization, with the present but not definitive technical limitation of using the apex of T rather than the end of T for the evaluation ('QTa' rather than the QT interval). It is well-known that the QT duration diminishes as the heart rate increases, and although everyone agrees that it is imperfect, the Bazett formula ($QTc = QT/\sqrt{RR}$) is still largely employed to normalize the QT value at a rate of 60/min in order to compare various individuals. It happens, however, that it is not appropriate to use this formula, or probably any formula, to evaluate the dynamic changes of QT in a single individual.

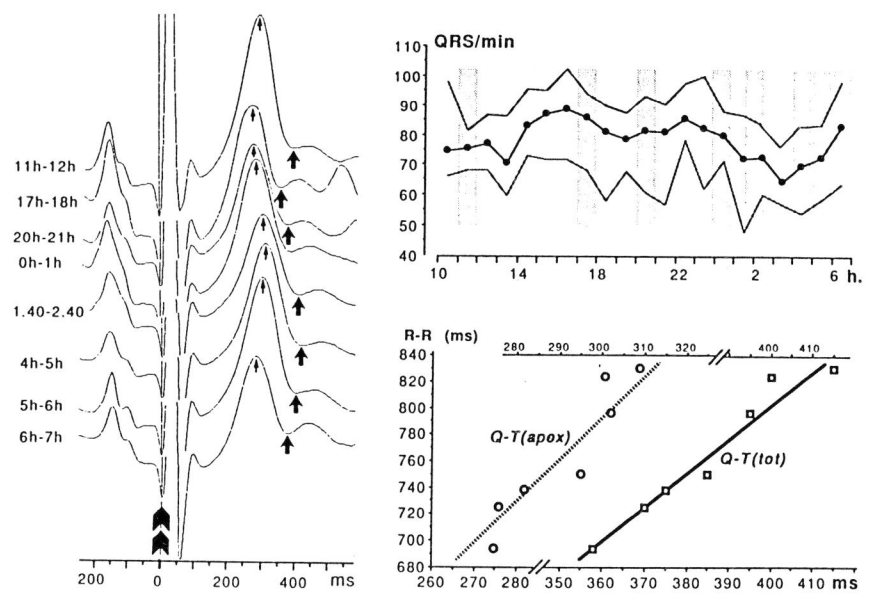

Figure 5. QT variations in Holter recordings. Averaged QRS-T complexes are collected for 1-h periods over the whole tracing, and they are displayed in the left panel. The corresponding hourly heart rate is figured in the right upper panel, where the mean heart rate is bounded by the maximal and minimal cardiac frequencies. In the lower right panel, the QTa (apex of T) and QT (end of T) values are plotted against the heart rate. The regression is linear, and the correlation is good, but its meaning is not so evident. In fact, the rate dependence and the ANS dependence cannot be dissociated in this figure (see the text for discussion).

A striking example is given in Figure 4, where the QTa interval was determined in the hourly averaged QRS-T complexes in a patient paced at a constant rate of 70/min: the presence of circadian variations of the QT interval implies that they are indeed related to the vagosympathetic balance instead of the heart rate. On the other hand, studies in the literature have frequently documented that the QT interval does vary as a function of the heart rate as such when one changes the pacing rate over a short period of time. Thus, the problem is to differentiate in the 24-h recordings what is linked to the heart rate as such, and what is related to the ANS balance.

If one examines the hourly values of QT over 24 h, as in Figure 5, it is obvious that there is a linear and strong correlation between the heart rate and the QT interval. Again, as in the case of HRV, the question is to distinguish which meaning should be attributed to the heart rate: a marker of the timing or the real determinant? This information cannot be obtained from the hourly values, because the high rates represent the daytime period, whereas the slow rates represent the night, so that using any correction

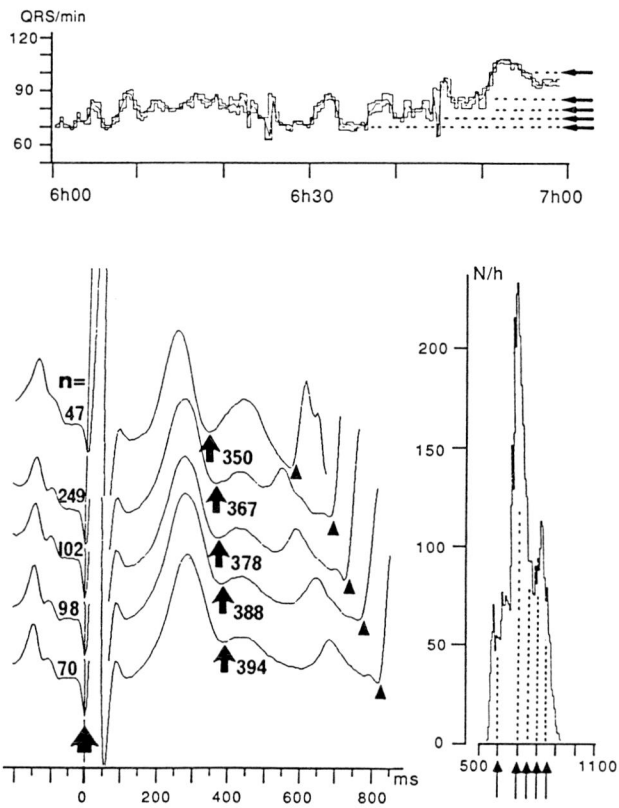

Figure 6. Rate dependence of the QT interval. During a 1-h period, QRS-T complexes were averaged according to the preceding RR interval ranging from 500 to 750 ms, as shown in the upper diagram of heart rate trends, and the lower right panel displays the RR interval histogram. The number 'n' of beats is indicated for each family, as well as the QT interval (in ms).

formula would be nonsensical because it would presuppose that the heart rate is the exclusive determinant.

To obviate this difficulty, we have designed a particular approach using the facilities of the ATREC program of processing of the Holter tapes [3]. The principle is to collect individual QRS-T complexes as a function of their environment in terms of the preceding heart rate over a certain number of cycles (up to 18) or of mean frequency over minutes (up to 10). Figure 6 displays the type of results that can be obtained during a predefined period of time: 'slices' of constant RR cycles are distinguished in the RR interval histogram, and the averaged values of the QT interval can then be ascribed essentially to the heart rate rather than to the supposedly stable ANS variations. Then, if the values of the QT interval at a certain rate are compared

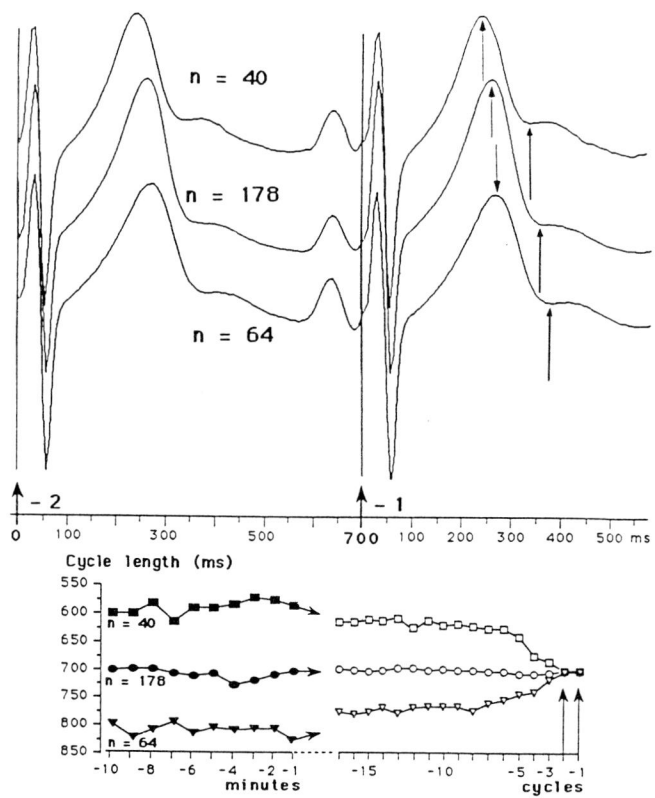

Figure 7. Variations of QT interval according to environmental conditions. The upper part superimposes three populations of QRSs averaged through the ATREC system. The number of beats (n) collected in the 24-h recording is indicated for each population. The QRS-T studied (labelled beat ' − 1') follows a cardiac cycle (' − 2' to ' − 1' cycle) uniformly set at 700 ms. The lower diagram displays the value of the 17 preceding cycles, and the preceding 10 min. The mean RR interval during the last minute (' − 1' minute) was chosen to be shorter (less than 600 ms) or longer (more than 800 ms) than the value of 700 + 7 ms taken for the 'middle' population. The different preceding rates (about 100, 70 and 85 bpm) explain the shorter or longer repolarization durations in the different groups. The QTa and the QT intervals have different increments, and the differences may reach up to 50 ms for the same 700 ms last cycle value.

over different periods of time, their differences can be ascribed to variations of the vagosympathetic balance at fixed rates and without using any correction formula. For instance, comparing the day and night values of QT at a rate of 75/min, we found in normal individuals a physiological difference of the order of 20 ms.

It is a well-established fact that a sudden, stimulation-induced change in heart rate does not modify the QT interval immediately: a 1-min period elapses before the QT values stabilizes at its new level when the pacing rated is kept constant. This phenomenon was verified in the setting of the Holter technique thanks to the ATREC program. Figure 7 shows that some precautions must be taken when determining the QT interval and its relationships with the environment. The upper part of the figure superimposes three populations of averaged QRSs. The number of beats (n) collected in the 24-h recording is indicated for each population. The QRS-T studied (labelled as beat ' − 1') follows a cardiac cycle (' − 2' to ' − 1' cycle) uniformly set at 700 ms. The lower diagram displays the value of the 17 preceding cycles, and the preceding 10 min. The mean RR interval during the last minute (' − 1' min) was chosen to be shorter (less than 600 ms) or longer (more than 800 ms) than the value of 700 ± 7 ms taken for the 'middle' population with a stable environmental rate. The different preceding rates (about 100, 70 and 85 bpm) explain the shorter or longer repolarization durations in the different groups. The QTa and the QT intervals have different increments, and the differences may reach up to 50 ms for the same 700 ms last cycle value.

The dynamicity of the QT interval progressively diminishes with age, a phenomenon already well-established for heart rate variability and which is related to the senescence of the ANS. QT dynamicity also dramatically decreases in any structural heart disease, a phenomenon which is in our experience much more marked than the reduction of HRV, probably because the alteration of the myocardium itself has a much earlier and stronger direct impact on ventricular repolarization than through the sinus node automatism and its autonomic modulation. There is no doubt that in the future, studying the QT interval will become extremely important as a prognostic marker as well as for assessing the impact of drugs. The present technical limitations of signal processing will be progressively overcome [4] now that 3-lead recordings are available and that sophisticated morphological analyses are developing. Time and space dimensions must be controlled in order to draw upon all the relevant information contained in the ECG signal [5].

REFERENCES

1. Coumel P, Hermida JS, Wennerblöm B, Leenhardt A, Maison-Blanche P, Cauchemez B. Heart rate variability in myocardial hypertrophy and heart failure, and the effects of beta-blocking therapy. A non-spectral analysis of heart rate oscillations. Eur Heart J 1991;12:412–22.
2. Kauffmann, Maison-Blanche P, Cauchemez B et al. A study of a non stationary phenomena of heart rate variability during ECG ambulatory monitoring. Med Bio Eng Comput 1988;26:303–6.
3. Coumel P, Leclercq JF, Maison-Blanche P, Attuel, Cauchemez B. Computerized analysis

of dynamic electrocardiograms: a tool for comprehensive electrophysiology. Clin Prog 1985;3:181–201.
4. Fayn J, Hamidi S, Maison-Blanche P, Bozza F, Rubel P, Coumel P. Quantitative assessment of changes in the repolarization phase in Holter recordings using CAVIAR. Computers in Cardiology 1992.
5. Coumel P, Maison-Blanche P. Electrocardiography and computers. J Ambul Monit 1992;5:265–72.

8. Role of dynamic QT interval in Holter tapes to stratify risk in postmyocardial infarction patients

E. RODRIGUEZ FONT, E. HOMS, J. GUINDO, V. MARTÍ, X. VIÑOLAS, A. BAYÉS GENÍS & A. BAYÉS DE LUNA

According to Moss et al. [1], the value of Holter monitoring for identifying those patients with congenital long-QT syndrome at risk for malignant ventricular arrhythmias is unclear. Such patients have few, if any, premature ventricular contractions on a 24-h recording. Heart rate fluctuations, quantification of heart rate variability through power spectrum analysis techniques, and variability in the QT interval and T wave morphology may provide some electrophysiological insight into the dynamic aspects of this disorder, but the clinical value of this information has not been substantiated. Nevertheless, a study has recently been published indicating that non-invasive ECG techniques in combination with autonomic manoeuvres may contribute significant information towards a precise diagnosis in patients with suspected long-QT syndrome [2]. The greatest diagnostic impact lies in the significant prolongation of QTc duration at rest and during a provocation test.

In our opinion Holter monitoring could be quite useful in patients with various types of acquired QT prolongation. Such patients often have underlying myocardial disorders with a relatively high frequency of isolated and repetitive premature ventricular contractions. Holter monitoring can provide a quantitative evaluation of the antiarrhythmic effects of the drugs being administered. In addition, information could be obtained concerning fluctuating changes in the QT interval, the T wave morphology, and the long-short ventricular cycle length sequence which commonly initiates more dangerous forms of repetitive premature ventricular contractions.

The QT interval is a parameter modulated by the autonomic nervous system, and it has been demonstrated that transient factors (such as nervous impulse to the heart) can induce ventricular fibrillation [3]. Therefore, changes in the dynamic QT interval which may be induced by sudden changes of the autonomic nervous system may be markers or triggering mechanisms of sudden death. There are several studies which have demonstrated that QT lengthening can trigger 'torsades de pointes', possibly induced by afterpotentials. Therefore, although the relationship between the autonomic nervous system and QT is complex, there is clinical and experimental evidence that this exists.

An important limitation of the research into the QTc value in a surface ECG is the fact that only one measurement is performed. Nevertheless, several authors [4–6] consider the serial measurement of the QT interval to be more useful, and when this is performed, we can use the QTc to stratify the prognosis. For this reason our group [7–10] and Algra [11] have studied the role of serial QTc measurements in Holter tapes in order to determine the possible implications of dynamic QT.

Algra [11] performed a follow-up study in postinfarction patients in whom the values for the different parameters were studied to detect markers of sudden death, including QTc in the surface ECG and the dynamic QTc in Holter tapes. It was seen that a QTc > 440 ms in the surface ECG in patients without ventricular dysfunction (heart failure or EF < 40%) represented 2.3 times higher risk for sudden death in comparison to a QTc < 440 ms. On the contrary, coronary patients with evidence of cardiac dysfunction had a relative risk of 1.0. Therefore, in patients with ventricular dysfunction, the risk of sudden death is independent of the prolongation of the QTc.

Concerning the dynamic measurement of the QTc over 24 h in the Holter tapes, it was demonstrated [11] that patients with a long QTc (> 440 ms; mean value) and short QTc (< 440 ms) had twice the risk of sudden death compared with mean values (400–440 ms). That QTc values > 440 ms increase the risk of sudden death is to be expected, but it is difficult to understand that a short QT could provoke sudden death. However, 22% of the patients were taking digitalis. It was not observed that peaks of QTc above 440 ms enabled patients with and without risk to be distinguished, as demonstrated elsewhere [7–10]. The Algra study [11] has several limitations: (1) It is is a retrospective study, and in the study cohort there were patients who had undergone 24-h Holter ECG in any of four Holter laboratories of Rotterdam hospitals. (2) Not all cases of sudden death were within 1 h. More than 25% died within 24 h. (3) The group was heterogeneous, only 32% of patients had suffered a myocardial infarction, and a large proportion of patients did not suffer from ischaemic or other heart disease. (4) A large proportion of patients had taken drugs which modified the repolarization (23% digitalis, 25% beta-blockers, 23% diuretics, 22% antiarrhythmic), and the follow-up data were not supplied.

We conducted different studies to demonstrate the value of the dynamic behaviour of QT in evaluating risk in postmyocardial patients. We measured the QT interval manually [7,9] every hour in the Holter tapes of three different patient groups: (A) postinfarction patients with malignant ventricular arrhythmia (sustained ventricular tachycardia or ventricular fibrillation outside the acute phase of myocardial infarction), (B) postmyocardial infarction patients with similar characteristics (age, sex, infarction location and degree of heart failure) to group A, but without malignant ventricular arrhythmias in the subacute phase, and (C) a control group without heart

Role of dynamic QT interval 75

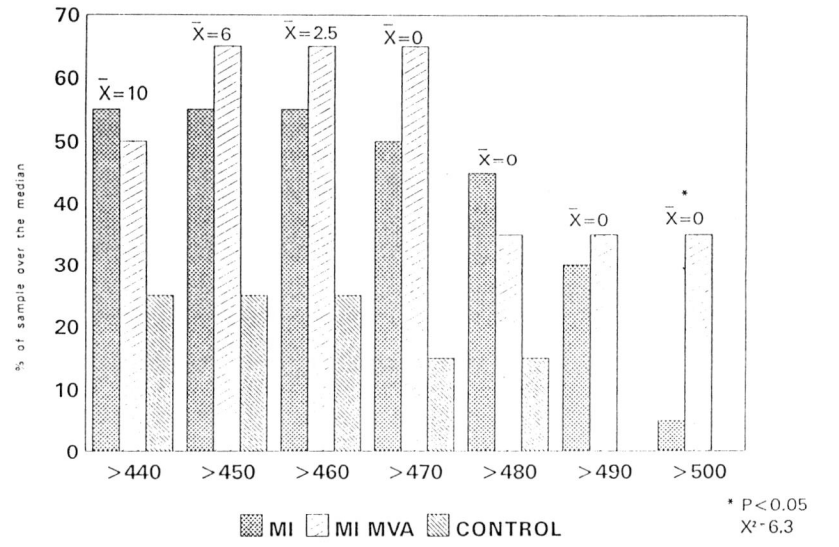

Figure 1. Relative frequencies of QT intervals measurements in three groups of patients using different cutoff values (see text). MI = myocardial infarction, MVA = malignant ventricular arrhythmia, abscissa = length of QT interval (in ms).

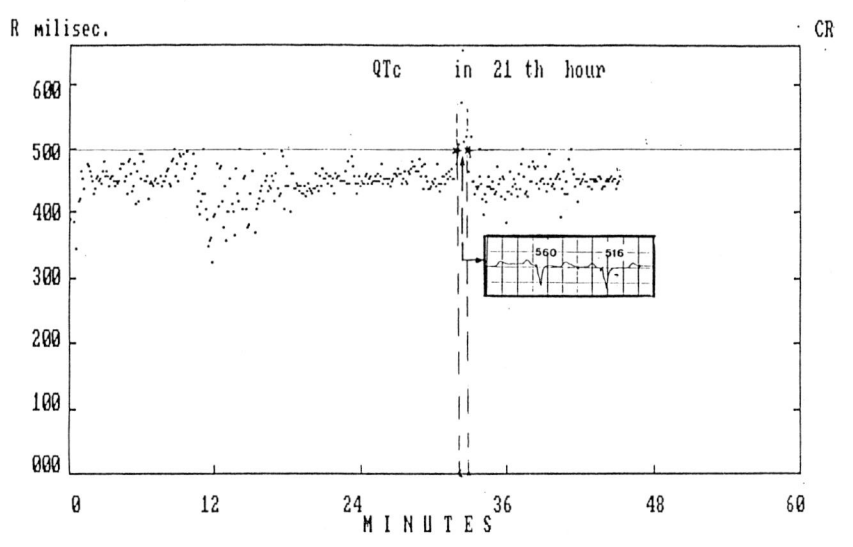

Figure 2. One-hour automatic recording of QT, showing the variations in the QT measurements. Around minute 30, there are peaks of QT higher than 500 ms.

Table 1. Validation results with two manual measurements and between observers on 18 Holter tapes.

Tape	n	Automatic-Expert 1				Automatic-Expert 2				Expert 1-Expert 2	
		d*	d	SD*	SD	d*	d	SD*	SD	d*	SD*
1	34	4.3	2.4	33.9	16.9	7.0	−0.8	36.0	12.6	3.6	12.6
2	42	3.5	3.0	15.1	12.0	1.7	−0.1	11.5	9.8	−0.3	14.7
3	26	−5.9	−8.5	21.0	19.5	−7.7	−7.4	18.8	20.9	2.7	18.5
4	19	−2.3	−2.8	7.7	7.3	−7.2	−7.5	7.3	8.1	4.7	6.8
5	38	4.5	3.2	10.3	8.6	4.5	3.2	10.3	8.6	1.9	10.2
6	49	−21.0	−20.0	10.4	9.0	−22.0	−21.0	14.4	15.4	0.0	10.7
7	39	−7.2	−10.0	20.4	15.0	−26.0	−28.0	23.7	17.4	19.2	14.4
8	41	1.0	2.4	13.1	13.3	−1.1	−1.2	14.6	14.5	2.1	14.1
9	29	16.5	16.8	18.7	19.3	16.7	16.5	16.9	17.7	−1.0	5.5
10	39	−8.8	−8.5	13.1	12.4	−7.1	−7.3	14.1	14.9	−1.3	7.6
11	42	9.5	9.1	14.0	11.6	6.8	6.3	11.0	7.5	2.6	7.9
12	45	−17.0	−16.0	16.7	14.6	−18.0	−15.0	19.1	16.9	0.9	8.4
13	36	8.8	9.4	17.8	15.2	9.4	11.4	19.0	17.5	−0.6	5.7
14	34	7.7	10.9	17.0	14.8	12.3	14.6	17.7	15.7	−4.4	7.3
15	37	8.2	5.1	44.7	22.1	6.1	5.8	39.8	21.9	2.2	15.4
16	35	11.7	11.7	16.0	16.0	9.7	8.5	12.5	11.5	1.7	12.8
17	40	19.6	17.9	13.2	12.9	21.9	21.6	12.3	11.9	−0.2	6.5
18	35	9.5	9.3	15.9	17.5	9.9	8.4	14.8	16.7	−0.3	5.0
Mean	37	2.4	2.0	17.7	14.3	0.9	0.4	17.4	14.4	1.9	10.2

n = Number of beats measured on each tape, d* = mean difference between automatic and manual QT interval measurements, SD* = standard deviation. d and SD are the values remaining after rejection of the maximum and minimum QT values in each five-beat set. Unit for d, SD, d* and SD* is ms.

disease matched for age and sex ratio to the other groups. Corrected QT was measured every hour according to the Bazett formula, each value being the result of an average of five measurements, representing 120 QT measurements for each tape. The global mean value of QT in the Holter tapes, although longer in group A than in group B, did not present statistically significant differences between the groups. When we examined only the number of measurements above a certain corrected QT value, we found that patients with malignant ventricular arrhythmias (group A) had a higher QT (> 500 ms) than other groups, and this was statistically significant. Figure 1 shows the relative frequencies of measurement of particular QT intervals in the three groups of patients. The controls seem to be different in all cases, and the two groups of MI vary only above 500 ms.

Due to the extremely laborious nature of manual measurement, it would be better to automate the measurement. Our objectives are to develop a new signal processing of Holter ECGs [8] and to obtain QT segment trends, RR interval, QT and QTc measurements. We have already achieved automatization of the trends of QTc and performed a clinical validation (Table 1) [8].

Regarding the clinical results, we have demonstrated that postmyocardial infarction patients with malignant ventricular arrhythmias present the following characteristics: a higher mean value of QT and higher incidence in the number of peaks of QT > 500 ms than other postmyocardial patients (Figure 2).

CONCLUSION

The role of the dynamic behaviour of QT as a marker of malignant ventricular arrhythmias in postmyocardial infarction patients seems promising. It is necessary to implement these results with other markers in order to increase the possibility of predicting new arrhythmic events in postmyocardial infarction patients.

REFERENCES

1. Moss A, Schwartz P, Crampton R, Locati E, Carleen E. The long QT syndrome: a prospective international study. Circulation 1985;17:17.
2. Eggeling T, Hoeher M, Osterhues H-H, Weismueller P, Hombach V. Significance of noninvasive diagnostic techniques in patients with long QT syndrome. Am J Cardiol 1992;70:1421–6.
3. Lown B, Verrier RL. Neural activity and ventricular fibrillation. N Engl J Med 1976;294:1165.
4. Cripps T. The QT interval and its relationship to heart rate in patients after acute myocardial infarction. In: Butrous GS, Schwartz PJ, editors. Clinical Aspects of Ventricular Repolarization. London: Farrand Press, 1989:369.
5. Schwartz PJ. Clinical significance of QT prolongation: a personal view. In: Butrous, GS, Schwartz PJ, editors. Clinical Aspects of Ventricular Repolarization, London: Farrand Press, 1989:343.
6. Puddu DE, Bourassa MG. Prediction of sudden death from QTc interval prolongation in patients with chronic ischemic heart disease. J Electrocardiol 1986;19:203.
7. Martí V, Bayés de Luna A, Arriola J et al. Value of dynamic QTc in arrhythmology. New Trends in Arrhythmia 1988;4:683–7.
8. Laguna P, Taker NV, Caminal P, Jané R, Hyung Ro Yoon, Bayés de Luna A. New algorithm for QT interval analysis in 24 hour Holter ECG: performance and applications. Med Biol Eng Comput 1990;28:67–73.
9. Martí V, Guindo J, Homs E, Viñolas X, Bayés de Luna A. Peak of QTc lengthening measured in Holter recordings as a marker of life-threatening arrhythmias in postmyocardial infarction patients. Am Heart J 1992;124:234–5.
10. Homs E, Viñolas X, Guindo J, Laguna P, Maid G, Bayés de Luna A. Automatic QTc lengthening measured in Holter ECG as a marker of life-threatening arrhythmias in post-myocardial infarction patients. Eur Heart J 1993;14(Abstr. suppl.):1201.
11. Algra A. Electrocardiographic Risk Factors for Sudden Death. Alblasserdam: Drukkerij Haveka, 1990.

9. Heart rate variability in patients with angina pectoris

NINA REHNQVIST, INGE BJÖRKANDER, LENNART FORSLUND, CLAES HELD & PAUL HJEMDAHL

INTRODUCTION

Ambulatory ECG recordings are used in patients with ischemic heart disease to study factors of prognostic importance, such as ST depressions in patients with angina pectoris. In patients after myocardial infarction and those with arrhythmia, the ambulatory monitoring gives information on ectopic beats and heart rate variability. Patients with a higher number of ectopic beats and more complex forms have a worse prognosis after myocardial infarction than patients without such findings. A low heart rate variability measured in the time or frequency domain also indicates a worse prognosis after myocardial infarction. Furthermore, it has been hypothesized and demonstrated that quantitative differences in various frequency domain measures of heart rate variability may exist before the onset of episodes of ventricular tachycardia in patients with symptomatic arrhythmia. The aim of the present study was to evaluate heart rate variability in patients with chronic stable angina pectoris and to relate these findings to other prognostic variables and treatment [1–5].

PATIENTS

The 790 patients participating in a single-center long-term follow-up study of stable angina pectoris are included in this APSIS study. The one inclusion criterion is the presence of stable angina pectoris. Exclusion criteria are recent myocardial infarction within 3 years, age over 70 years, and contraindications for either verapamil or metoprolol. Patients are investigated before the start of treatment and then after 1 month of either metoprolol 200 mg od or verapamil 240 mg bid. The patients are investigated yearly thereafter. Long-term ECG recordings are analyzed with an Oxford Medilog Excel system, and the number of episodes of 1 mm ST depression lasting more than 1 min, number and type of premature ventricular complexes (PVCs),

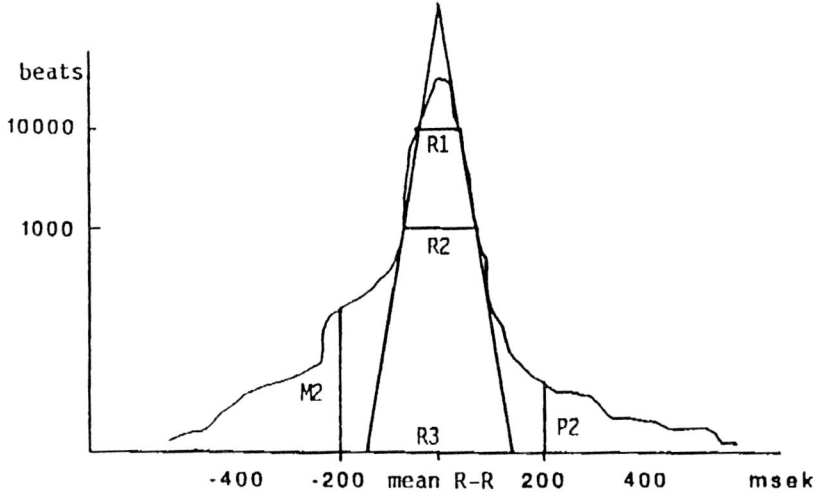

Figure 1.

minimal and maximal heart rate, and heart rate variability are measured. The long term ECG recordings were computer analyzed, and an annual overview was done to consider heart rate, PVCs, and heart rate variability. Heart rate variability was measured graphically from the histogram of relative RR differences according to Figure 1, using the values for at least 10 000 beats per 24 h, for 1000 beats per 24 h, and along the abscissa.

During the same 24 h the urinary excretion of adrenaline and noradrenaline was measured to estimate the sympathetic tone.

RESULTS

The minimal heart rate was 48 and 49 bpm in men and women, respectively, at baseline. After 1 month of treatment, it was 45 in men, while in women it continued to be 49 bpm ($p < 0.05$). The median number of PVCs was significantly higher in men (16 versus 1; $p < 0.001$). The total duration of ST depression during 24 h was the same in men and women (median 5 and 5.5 min, respectively). The urinary excretion of adrenaline and noradrenaline and the heart rate variability were evaluated in 123 patients (82 men). There was a significant correlation between noradrenaline and maximal heart rate. The minimal heart rate correlated inversely to noradrenaline excretion ($p < 0.05$). There was no relationship between adrenaline excretion and the maximal or minimal heart rate. The heart rate variability was slightly higher in women (407 ± 182 ms compared to 349 ± 163 in men). Measured as heart rate variability for 1000 beats, the difference was significant. There was a strong negative correlation between the number of PVCs and heart rate variability ($r = -0.78$). There was no correlation between the heart rate variability and duration of ST depression. The heart rate variability correlated significantly and inversely to noradrenaline excretion. The duration of ST depression was significantly correlated to adrenaline excretion but not to noradrenaline excretion. Heart rate variability and number of PVCs did not vary between the 4 risk groups, but the total duration of ST depression was longer in the high-risk patient group (median 14 versus 4 and 1 min, respectively, in the high-, intermediate- and low-risk groups; $p < 0.05$). After 1 month of treatment there were no changes in the number of PVCs. However, there was a reduction in the duration of ST depression. The heart rate variability increased from 369 ± 171 to 425 ± 198 ms after 1 month of treatment ($p < 0.05$).

DISCUSSION

The heart rate variability may be measured in different ways. The frequency domain takes into consideration the high frequency changes induced by altering vagal tone and the low frequency changes induced by more complex mechanisms through the baroreflex mechanism and sympathetic tone. In the time domain, the heart rate variability may be measured manually using a triangular method as done in our study or as indicated by Malik where the absolute RR intervals are used from the histogram. The 24-h time domain heart rate variability measurements take into consideration the overall autonomic tone and may be used as a marker of overall prognosis. The frequency domain analysis may be better employed to elucidate the direct mechanisms and especially for predisposing elements for arrhythmia and ischemia.

In this study, angina pectoris patients exhibited differences in heart rate variability in the time domain. Women had a higher heart rate variability in spite of a higher mean heart rate. This may reflect their better prognosis and also the lower frequency of previous myocardial infarctions and heart failure than in men. Men had a higher number of PVCs and accordingly a lower heart rate variability. The prognostic information of the PVCs is mainly applicable in men, while the prognostic aspect and PVCs in women are either non-existent or negligible. Further follow-up of the APSIS study will elucidate whether the prognostic information from heart rate variability measured in our study will contribute independently when other measures are used.

The treatment for angina pectoris is symptomatic through prophylaxis with either calcium antagonists or beta-blockers. Comparative studies have been made concerning these two types of drugs, and the beta-blockers seem to be more beneficial in terms of changes in ST depression than the dihydropyridine calcium antagonists or the benzothiazepines. Verapamil may be different. The influence on the prognosis is, however, not known, and the present study will hopefully give information on this. In this study the study codes have so far not been broken, and therefore no conclusions can be made as regards the different influences of verapamil and metroprolol.

CONCLUSION

Heart rate variability in angina pectoris patients is higher in women, correlates negatively to the number of PVCs but does not correlate to duration of ST depression. Heart rate variability in the time domain is related to overall sympathetic activity and increases, with treatment, with either metoprolol or verapamil.

REFERENCES

1. Huikuri HV, Valkama JO, Airaksinen KEJ et al. Frequency domain measures of heart rate variability before the onset of nonsustained and sustained ventricular tachycardia in patients with coronary artery disease. Circulation 1993;87:1220–8.
2. Pagani M, Lombardi F, Guzzetti S et al. Power spectral analysis of heart rate and arterial pressure variabilities as a marker of sympathovagal interaction in man and conscious dog. Circ Res 1986;59:178–93.
3. Kleiger RE, Miller JP, Bigger JT, Moss AJ, and the Multicenter Post-Infarction Research Group. Decreased heart rate variability and its association with increased mortality after acute myocardial infarction. Am J Cardiol 1987;59:256–62.
4. Farrell TG, Bashir Y, Cripps T et al. Risk stratification for arrhythmic events in postinfarction patients based on heart rate variability, ambulatory electro-cardiographic variables and the signal-averaged electrocardiogram. J Am Coll Cardiol 1991;18:687–97.
5. Bigger JT, Fleiss JL, Steinman RC, Rolnitzky LM, Kleiger RE, Rottman JN. Frequency domain measures of heart period variability and mortality after myocardial infarction. Circulation 1992;85:164–72.

10. Time and frequency domain analysis of heart rate variability after myocardial infarction

FEDERICO LOMBARDI, GIULIA SANDRONE & ALBERTO MALLIANI

INTRODUCTION

Despite the significant reduction in mortality which has been obtained over the last few years, the identification of patients at risk after a myocardial infarction remains one of the most important objectives for clinical cardiology. In addition to the more traditional techniques based upon the evaluation of residual left ventricular dysfunction or ischemia and upon the characterization of cardiac electrical instability, as indicated by the presence of ventricular arrhythmias or ventricular late potentials, new approaches have been recently proposed to evaluate the alterations of neural regulatory mechanisms and to identify patients at risk. Among them, the study of heart rate variability has provided the most relevant clinical results.

In patients after acute myocardial infarction, Kleiger et al. [1] observed that a decreased heart rate variability was associated with increased mortality. In particular, these authors reported that patients who at the time of discharge had a standard deviation of the 24-h Holter recording of less than 50 ms exhibited a relative risk of mortality 5.3 times higher than that of patients with a standard deviation greater than 100 ms. A reduced heart rate variability remained a significant predictor of mortality after adjusting for clinical, demographic and Holter features, and ejection fraction. To explain their findings, Kleiger et al. [1] advanced the hypothesis that a decreased heart rate variability correlated with an increased sympathetic or decreased vagal tone, which could predispose to ventricular fibrillation.

In the same year we published an article [2] about a smaller group of patients whose RR interval variability during 10-min controlled resting conditions was analyzed with spectral techniques 2 weeks, 6 and 12 months after an acute myocardial infarction. In comparison to an age-matched control group, patients 2 weeks after myocardial infarction presented with a significant increase in the low-frequency (LF) and a marked decrease of the high-frequency (HF) component of RR variability that were consistent with a shift of sympathovagal balance towards sympathetic predominance. The alteration in neural regulatory mechanisms was even more evident when considering the LF/HF ratio, which was markedly augmented in these patients. Conversely, the RR variance was slightly but not significantly reduced. A progressive reduction of LF and increase in HF were observed within 6 months of the acute event; such changes determined a quite complete normalization of the LF/HF ratio within 1 year. Three additional patients who died in the first 3 months after the acute event exhibited a very reduced heart rate variability [2], thus confirming the negative predictive value of a diminished heart rate variability as suggested by Kleiger et al. [1]. However, it is worth noting that in these three patients, the spectral profile was characterized by a reduced total power which was mainly distributed below 0.03 Hz and in the HF range, whereas an LF component was practically undetectable. Thus, our limited observations based on the short time spectral analysis of R-R variability, while confirming the negative predictive value of a reduced heart rate variability, seemed to contradict the interpretation provided by Kleiger et al. [1] that a reduced heart rate variability could be simply interpreted as evidence of a diminished vagal tone.

We therefore evaluated 75 consecutive patients in whom the RR variability was analyzed with spectral techniques 2 weeks after the first myocardial infarction and attempted to correlate the observed results with long-term survival as well as with the occurrence of cardiac events in the first 3 years after the acute event.

METHODS

We studied 75 patients discharged from the Coronary Care Unit of our hospital with the diagnosis of acute myocardial infarction based on clinical, electrocardiographic, and enzymatic criteria. Criteria for inclusion were the following: (1) under 70 years of age; (2) low frequency of ventricular arrhythmias on Holter monitoring performed 12–14 days after admission; (3) absence of concomitant alterations known to affect heart rate variability directly (e.g. diabetes). The group included 66 men and 9 women; their mean age was 52 ± 1 years. Of these 75 patients, 40 had had an anterior and 35 an inferior myocardial infarction. At the time of the study, all patients were in sinus rhythm and were not taking any beta-blockers.

In all subjects, an electrocardiographic signal with a prominent R wave was recorded in the late morning for 15–20 min during controlled resting conditions in a quiet isolated room. Arterial blood pressure was measured using a conventional sphygmomanometer.

In order to obtain information on the post-infarction period, all patients underwent periodic ambulatory examination for a period of 3 ± 1 years (range 1–5 years). The following cardiovascular events were taken into consideration: post-infarction angina, sustained ventricular tachycardia, post-infarction heart failure, and cardiac death.

Data analysis off-line was performed on a Microvax 3400 computer. Briefly, as previously reported [3–5], the electrocardiographic signals were played back from the FM tape and digitized at 300 samples/s. The software used for data acquisition and analysis has been previously described [4–6]. Stationary sections of data of appropriate length were selected for the analysis. The computer program first calculates the interval tachogram. From sections of tachogram of 256 or 512 interval values, the simple statistics (mean and variance) of the data are computed. Then the program automatically calculates the autoregressive coefficients necessary to define the power spectral density estimate and prints out the power and frequency of every spectral component. In normal subjects during resting conditions, the spectral analysis of heart rate variability has three major components: a very-low frequency component (0–0.03 Hz) not addressed in the present study based on short time recordings, and two additional components at LF (~0.1 Hz) and HF (~0.25 Hz). Whereas the HF component has been considered a marker of vagal modulation since its initial observation [3–8], the interpretation of the LF component as an index of sympathetic activation was controversial [7,8] but now appears to have been confirmed [3–5]. Each spectral component is presented in terms of frequency (Hz) and amplitude, which are determined by its area and measured in absolute values as milliseconds squared. The power of each component can also be expressed in normalized units (nu) obtained by dividing the power of a given component by the total power (from which the very-low-frequency component was subtracted) and multiplied by 100.

Data are presented as mean ± standard error. An analysis of variance with the Scheffé test was used to assess the differences between groups. Differences were considered significant when $p < 0.05$ was observed.

RESULTS

The mean RR interval and variance of the 75 patients studied 2 weeks after myocardial infarction were 859 ± 16 ms and 1110 ± 92 ms^2, respectively. The spectral analysis of RR variability was characterized (Figure 1) by a predominant LF (71 ± 2 nu) and a smaller HF (16 ± 1 nu). As a result, the LF/HF ratio was 10 ± 1.4. In most cases, a consistent part of the spectral power was distributed in the very-low-frequency range below 0.03 Hz.

No differences were detectable between patients with an anterior versus an inferior localization of the infarction. All these values were significantly different from those observed in a population of age-matched control groups and previously reported by our group [2,4,5].

Forty-four of the 75 patients did not present cardiovascular events during the follow-up period. These patients (Figure 2) presented a mean RR interval

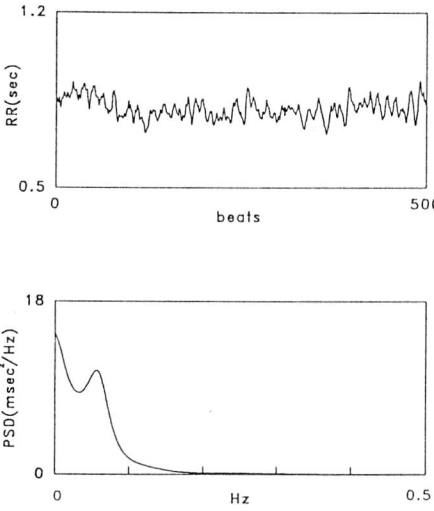

Figure 1. Spectral analysis of RR variability in a patient 2 weeks after an uncomplicated anterior myocardial infarction. The spectral profile is characterized by a predominant LF component which indicates sympathetic activation.

and variance of 836 ± 23 ms and 1126 ± 140 ms^2, respectively, during the recording performed 2 weeks after the acute event. Spectral analysis of the RR variability indicated the presence of a predominant LF (73 ± 2 nu) and a smaller HF (15 ± 1 nu), with a LF/HF ratio of 8 ± 2.

A complicated outcome was present in 31 cases. In these patients, the RR interval and variance measured 2 weeks after the acute myocardial infarction were 876 ± 26 ms and 948 ± 140 ms^2. Their spectral profile was characterized by a predominant LF (65 ± 3 nu) and a smaller HF (17 ± 2 nu), with a LF/HF ratio of 7 ± 1. As indicated in Methods, these patients were divided into three groups according to the severity of complications, which ranged from high-threshold postinfarction angina or nonsustained ventricular arrhythmias (first group, 15 patients), to re-infarction or postinfarction heart failure (second group, 8 patients), to cardiac death (third group, 8 patients).

As illustrated in Figure 3, when uncomplicated patients were compared with complicated patients divided into three groups, significant differences became evident. Whereas the mean RR interval was similar in all four groups, the RR variance was significantly reduced (384 ± 89 ms^2) in the subgroup of patients who died within the follow-up period. Moreover, this subgroup of patients was characterized by a LF component (51 ± 8 nu) and a LF/HF ratio (3 ± 1) that were smaller than in uncomplicated patients, while the HF component value was similar in all subgroups.

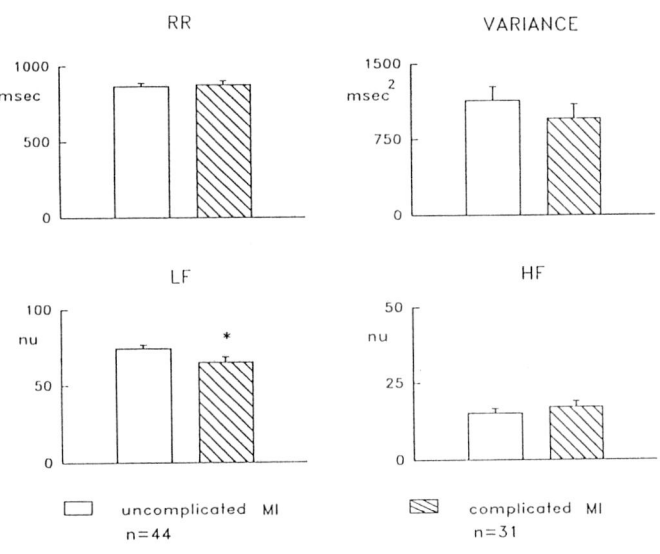

Figure 2. Analysis of RR variability in the 75 patients 2 weeks after myocardial infarction divided according to the presence or absence of complications in the follow-up period. A decreased LF characterized patients with a complicated outcome.

DISCUSSION

These data indicate that the analysis of RR variability measured on short-time ECG recordings in patients 2 weeks after an acute myocardial infarction provides relevant clinical information. A reduction in RR variance characterized the subgroup of 8 patients who died in the follow-up period. Moreover, their spectral profile exhibited a particular pattern, with the lack of a predominant LF component. These findings appear of interest in relation to their possible clinical relevance and to the methodology employed in this study.

Our study confirms previous observations obtained from 24-h Holter recordings: the reduction in time domain measures of RR variability (standard deviation or variance) characterizes patients with an increased mortality after myocardial infarction [1,9]. Also of interest is the possibility that even short-time ECG recordings collected during controlled resting conditions might provide relevant clinical information without the necessity of the time-consuming and costly analysis of 24-h recordings.

In this study we found signs of sympathetic activation and of a reduced vagal tone as indicated by the increased LF and LF/HF ratio and diminished HF component in the group of 75 patients as a whole, a finding which confirms our previous observation based on short-time [2] as well as 24-h

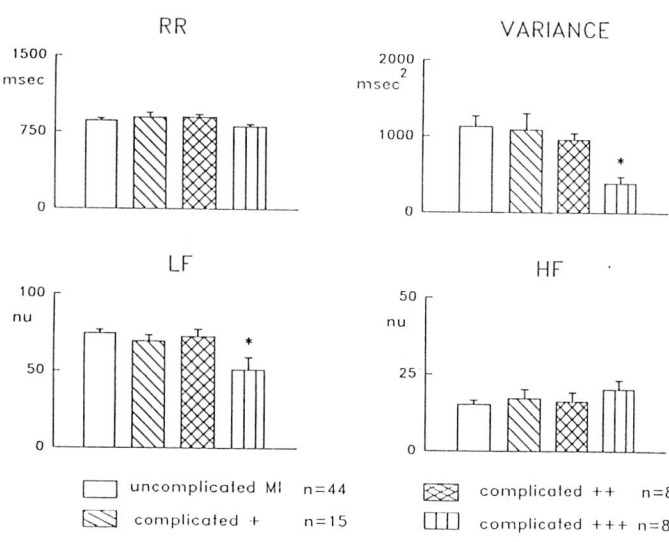

Figure 3. Analysis of RR variability 2 weeks after myocardial infarction. This group of patients was divided into four subgroups (see Methods) in relation to the presence of complication in the postinfarction period. A very reduced RR variance and a diminished LF component characterized the eight patients who suffered from cardiac death in the follow-up period.

[10] Holter recordings in the early postinfarction period. However, one of the most interesting results was the absence of an increased LF component and LF/HF ratio in the subgroup of patients who exhibited a very low RR variance and who died in the follow-up period. Both findings appear in contrast to the original interpretation of Kleiger et al. [1] and cast further doubts, in our opinion, upon the simple interpretation of equating a reduced RR variability to a specific autonomic pattern consisting of a diminished vagal tone and increased sympathetic activity [1,11].

It is worth emphasizing that even during resting controlled conditions, the spontaneous oscillations of heart period which can be quantified by RR variance or standard deviation are the result of a complex interaction between the sympathetic and vagal neural regulatory mechanisms and the sinus node. In most instances, the responsiveness of the sinus node to neural modulation is assumed to be linear. Thus, an increase in sympathetic activity must be associated with a shortening of the RR interval as well as with an increase in the 0.1-Hz rhythmical oscillations, whereas an increase in vagal activity directed to the heart must determine a lengthening of the heart period and an increase in the respiration-related sinus arrhythmias, the latter events leading to an increase in overall RR variability.

However, there is ample evidence that sympathetic and vagal neural regulatory mechanisms continuously interact at various levels, thus making too simplistic the assumption of an algebraic summation of their effects. Moreover, it is unlikely that the responsiveness of the sinus node to neural modulation will remain unmodified under different clinical conditions characterized by a persistent sympathetic activation or by left ventricular dysfunction. The possible effects of pharmacological treatment with ACE inhibitors, beta-blockers, or antiarrhythmic drugs [5,12,13] have also to be considered. Thus, in patients with a reduced heart rate variability, only a frequency domain analysis is capable of separating conditions in which the efficacy of the neural regulatory mechanisms is maintained from those in which a more complex alteration is likely to be present. The absence or marked attenuation of the LF component in a condition likely to be characterized by an increased sympathetic tone might indeed reflect a diminished responsiveness of the sinus node to sympathetic stimulation. Moreover, our findings indicate that this information can be easily extracted from short-time recordings, thus making the analysis of heart rate variability on a 10-min ECG recording one of the most interesting and clinically relevant predischarge tests in postmyocardial infarction patients. Concerning this, it is important to recall that another bedside test (the evaluation of baroreflex mechanism sensitivity) has been shown to provide relevant clinical information in postmyocardial infarction patients [14,15]. However, at variance with our approach, this latter technique, by evaluating the responsiveness of the sinus node to a pharmacologically induced pressure rise, provides information on neural mechanisms according to an open-loop stimulus-response model. The clinical value of a possible integration of the two approaches still remains to be established.

Concerning the predictive value of a reduced heart rate variability, it is important to note that Bigger et al. [16] recently analyzed the relationship of frequency domain measures of heart period variability and mortality after myocardial infarction. They found that a reduction in the entire energy of the spectrum and in the power of the different frequency bands into which they divided the spectral profile characterized patients who died within 1 year of the acute event.

Two main features, however, distinguish the above from our study. Bigger et al. [16] estimated with a fast fourier transform (FFT) algorithm the spectral density of the entire 24-h period, divided the spectral energy in four predetermined bands, and avoided using normalized units. As the power measured in preselected bands is directly correlated to the overall energy of the autospectrum, it is not unexpected that a similar negative predictive value was found for the whole power and its fractions. Moreover, by considering in a single autospectrum the entire 24-h period, the pattern of change of the LF and HF components related to their circadian variations was not detectable. For this reason and for the presence of non-stationarity of the signals which may occur in a 24-h recording, it was not surprising that most of the energy was below 0.03 and that LF and HF accounted for less than 6% of total power.

It is, however, important to recall that spectral analysis based on short-time recordings cannot provide information on the still undefined mechanisms contributing to the generation of that part of RR variability below 0.03 Hz. New approaches based on different algorithms and on long-time recordings [17,18] are now emerging although their computing robustness and clinical utility are far from being proven.

REFERENCES

1. Kleiger RE, Miller JP, Bigger JT, Moss AR, Multicenter postinfarction research group: Decreased heart rate variability and its association with increased mortality after acute myocardial infarction. Am J Cardiol 1987;59:256–62.
2. Lombardi F, Sandrone G, Pernpruner S et al. Heart rate variability as an index of sympatho-vagal interaction after myocardial infarction. Am J Cardiol 1987;60:1239–45.
3. Brovelli M, Baselli G, Cerutti S et al. Computerized analysis for an experimental validation of neurophysiological models of heart rate control. Comp Cardiol (IEEE Comput Soc) 1983;205–8.
4. Pagani M, Lombardi F, Guzzetti S et al. Power spectral analysis of heart rate and arterial pressure variabilities as a marker of sympathovagal interaction in man and conscious dog. Circ Res 1986;59:178–93.
5. Malliani A, Pagani M, Lombardi F, Cerutti S. Cardiovascular neural regulation explored in the frequency domain. Circulation 1991;84:482–92.
6. Baselli G, Cerutti S, Civardi S et al. Heart rate variability signal processing: A quantitative approach as an aid to diagnosis in cardiovascular pathologies. Int J Biomed Comp 1987;20:51–70.
7. Akselrod S, Gordon D, Ubel FA, Shannon DC, Barger AC, Cohen JR. Power spectrum analysis of heart rate fluctuations: A quantitative probe of beat-to-beat cardiovascular control. Science 1981;213:220–2.
8. Pomeranz B, Macaulay RJB, Caudill MA et al. Assessment of autonomic function in humans by heart rate spectral analysis. Am J Physiol 1985;17:H151–H3.
9. Odemuyiwa O, Malik M, Farrell T, Bashir Y, Poloniecki J, Camm J. Comparison of the predictive characteristics of heart rate variability index and left ventricular ejection fraction for all-cause mortality, arrhythmic events and sudden death after acute myocardial infarction. Am J Cardiol 1991;68:434–9.
10. Lombardi F, Sandrone G, Mortara A et al. Circadian variation of spectral indices of heart rate variability after myocardial infarction. Am Heart J 1992;123:1521–9.
11. Bigger JT, Kleiger RE, Fleiss JL, Rolnitzky LM, Steinman RC, Miller JP, and the Multicenter Post-lnfarction Research Group. Components of heart rate variability measured during healing of acute myocardial infarction. Am J Cardiol 1988;61:208–15.
12. Lombardi F, Torzillo D, Sandrone G et al. Beta-blocking effect of propafenone based on spectral analysis of heart rate variability. Am J Cardiol 1992; 70:1028–34.
13. Lombardi F, Torzillo D, Sandrone G, Dalla Vecchia L, Cappiello E. Autonomic effects of antiarrhythmic drugs and their importance. Eur Heart J 1992;13:38–43.
14. La Rovere MT, Specchia G, Mortara A, Schwartz PJ. Baroreflex sensitivity, clinical correlates, and cardiovascular mortality among patients with a first myocardial infarction. Circulation 1988;78:816–24.

15. Farrell TG, Odemuyiwa O, Bashir Y et al. Prognostic value of baroreflex sensitivity testing after acute myocardial infarction. Br Heart J 1992;67:129–37.
16. Bigger Jr JT, Fleiss JL, Steinman RC, Rolnitzky LM, Kleiger RE, Rottman JN. Frequency domain measures of heart period variability and mortality after myocardial infarction. Circulation 1992;85:164–71.
17. Saul JP, Albrecht P, Berger RD, Cohen RJ. Analysis of long term heart rate variability: methods, 1/f scaling and implications. Comp Cardiol (IEEE Comput Soc) 1988;419–22.
18. Cerutti S, Baselli G, Bianchi A et al. Chaotic characteristics of heart rate and arterial pressure variability signal in 24 hour. IEEE Proceedings, Comp Cardiol Conf 1991:705–8.

11. Signal averaged ECG

Technical principles, possibilities and limitations

ALFONS SINNAEVE & HUGO TASSIGNON

INTRODUCTION

Late potentials are low-amplitude, high-frequency signals which are continuous with the QRS complex and last a variable time into the ST segment. These signals are believed to originate in myocardial zones with slow and inhomogeneous activation patterns. In all probability, they are due to the delayed depolarization of relatively normal ventricular tissue within a diseased area [1,2]. Myocardial areas involved in the generation of late potentials may serve as the underlying anatomic substrate for malignant re-entrant ventricular arrhythmias. Hence, late potentials may be considered as hallmarks of life-threatening sustained ventricular tachycardias, and the accurate detection of these signals may be of vital interest to prevent the sudden death of some patients.

In the last decade, signal averaging techniques have been applied to high-resolution electrocardiography (HRECG) in order to estimate and subsequently analyse late potentials. These techniques of signal-averaged electrocardiography (SAECG) are noninvasive, relatively inexpensive, and easy to perform. However, rather sophisticated digital signal processing (DSP) is required, involving a computer and some mathematical algorithms. Moreover, the available commercial systems differ considerably in their technical aspects. Therefore, knowledge of the different basic principles is an essential prerequisite to differentiate late potentials from artifacts and to compare the results of systems from various companies. This chapter is addressed to physicians and is intended to be a readable essay on these basic principles.

ECG LEAD SYSTEMS

To make sure that all 'late potential' information is recorded, the heart should be examined from different directions, and therefore an orthogonal

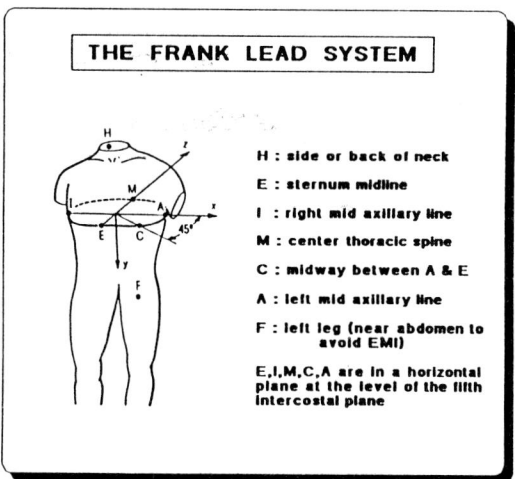

Figure 1. Diagram of the torso showing the placement of the seven electrodes for the Frank lead system. The positions A, C and F correspond respectively to V6, V4 and LL (left leg) of the standard 12-lead set.

lead system has to be used. The lead sets of such an orthogonal system have to be perpendicular and aligned with the major axes of the body. Moreover, they should preferably have equal vector sensitivity on each axis. Since the introduction by Einthoven in 1913 of the concept of the cardiac vector, many orthogonal reference frames for vector cardiography have been developed. In general, they fall into two major and divergent groups, i.e. the uncorrected and the corrected systems [3].

Corrected leads offer the advantage of a more accurate representation of the spatial distribution of ECG signals, because they take into account the shape and the inhomogeneity of the torso. Hence, these corrected leads enable a better estimate of the cardiac source of signals of interest and offer a more reproducible approach for comparing results among patients. The Frank lead system is the most popular corrected orthogonal lead system since it uses a relatively simple electrode placement. Seven electrodes are required: five placed in a horizontal plane around the thorax at the level of the fifth intercostal space, one on the head and one on the left leg (Figure 1). The appropriate gain adjustments are made by a simple resistive balancing network (Figure 2).

The *uncorrected systems* historically precede the corrected ones. Their strength lies in the fact that they are easier to apply. Most studies about late potentials have used an uncorrected bipolar XYZ lead system with only six electrodes (Figure 3). The X lead is positioned between the right and left midaxillary lines at the fourth intercostal space. The Y lead is placed on the

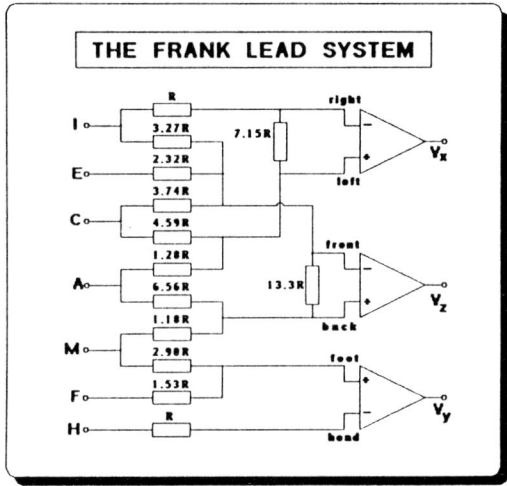

Figure 2. Resistive balancing network for the Frank lead system. R is an appropriate chosen resistance (e.g. 50 kΩ) and I, E, C, A, M, F, H represent the electrodes. V_x, V_y, V_z at the output of the three buffer amplifiers are the components of the cardiac vector.

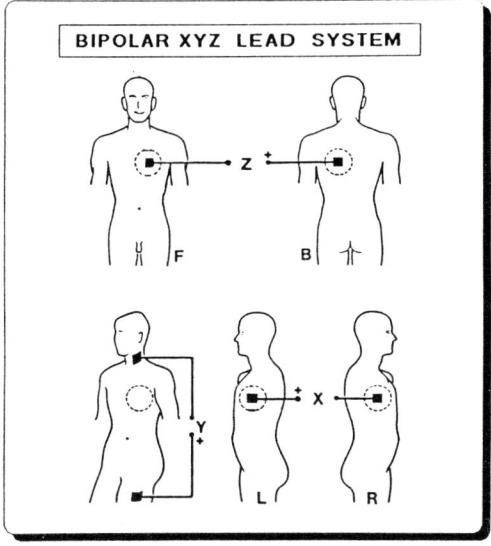

Figure 3. Placement of the six electrodes for the uncorrected bipolar XYZ lead system.

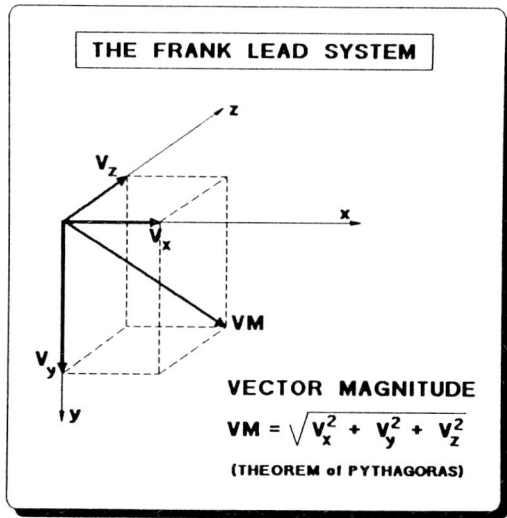

Figure 4. Definition of the spatial vector magnitude VM. For corrected leads, such as the Frank lead system, VM corresponds fairly well to the main cardiac vector.

superior aspect of the manubrium and either on the proximal left leg or left iliac crest. The frontal Z electrode is at the fourth intercostal space at the V_2 position, with the second electrode directly posterior on the left side of the vertebral column. Positive electrodes are left, inferior and anterior.

The X, Y and Z leads are commonly combined according to the theorem of Pythagoras to give a spatial vector magnitude (VM) which is a measure that sums the high-frequency information contained in all three leads (Figure 4). The results of most studies have been based upon the analysis of this vector magnitude.

If the cardiac source could be represented by a single dipole and if the X, Y, Z leads were truly orthogonal and accurately corrected, the vector magnitude would describe the complete activity of the heart. Unfortunately, these conditions are not perfectly met. It follows that the results of HRECG are lead-dependent and hence that the criteria and approaches established using one lead system may not be applicable to the other lead systems. Moreover, the accuracy of the measurement of late potentials from the vector magnitude using an automatic algorithm may be compromised; it has been shown that this approach tends to underestimate the extent of late potential activity [4].

THE NOISE PROBLEM

Cardiac late potentials cannot be detected by the well-known conventional ECG. The useful voltages in a normal ECG are typically between 30 μV and

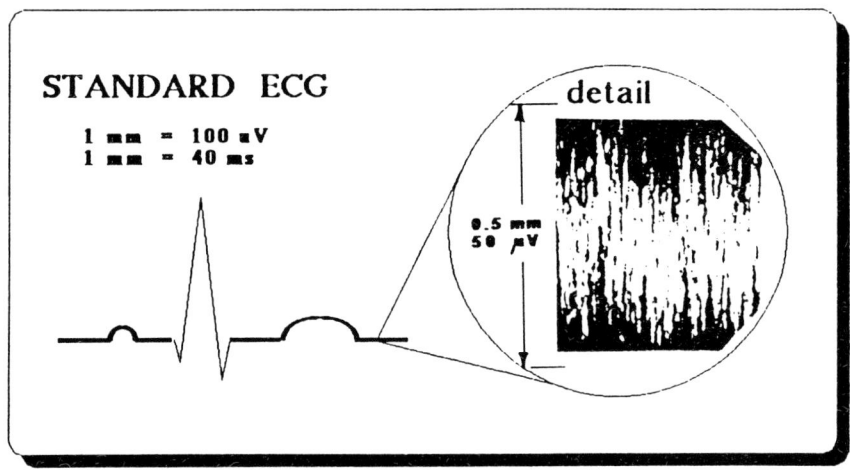

Figure 5. The standard ECG and its typical noise of ca. 40 to 50 μV which is impeding the perception of late potentials.

1500 μV (= 1.5 mV). With the standard vertical sensitivity of ECG machines of 1 mm corresponding to 100 μV, a thickness of the isoelectric line of a 0.5 mm already stands for a noise amplitude of 50 μV (Figure 5). Since late potentials typically range from about one to some tens of μV, they are normally buried in the noise of conventional ECG.

Any unwanted electrical signals, which tend to impede the perception of wanted signals, are called artifacts or noise. Since noise is usually the limiting factor in the detection of desired signals, an understanding of noise is needed to enable the evaluation of the measuring system. Figure 6 shows the many artifacts that may cause problems in electrocardiographic recording. Three primary categories of noise can be recognized: (a) motion artifacts, (b) electromagnetic interference, and (c) device noise [5].

Motion artifacts may be due to the muscles, the skin, the electrodes, and the cables. Myopotentials which can have an amplitude of several tens of μV have to be minimized by a comfortable and relaxed position of the patient in a room at a sufficiently warm temperature. Skin potentials are due to a potential difference between the outside and inside of the barrier layer (stratum granulosum). Stretching the skin may produce variations of this voltage of up to 5 mV. These motion artifacts should be reduced by abrasion of the skin with fine sandpaper (or by a 0.5 mm puncture) and by a good mechanical stabilization of the contact. Motion artifacts from the electrodes are generated by variations of the charge (and hence the voltage) in the double layer at the metal-electrolyte interface. This kind of noise should be circumvented by careful mechanical stabilization (avoid pulling on the cables!) and the use of Ag/AgCl electrodes, recessed away from the move-

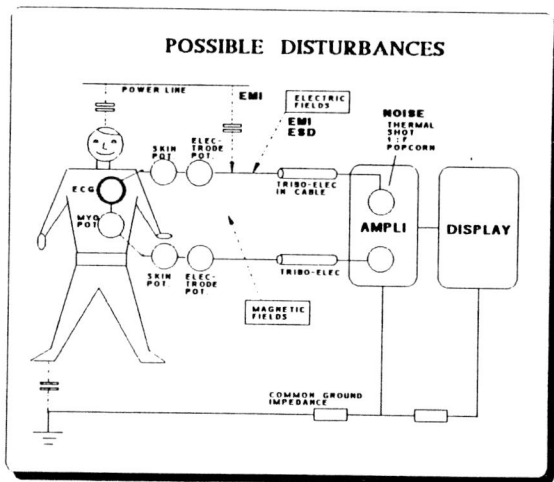

Figure 6. Survey of all possible problems in electrocardiographic recording. EMI = ElectroMagnetic Interference, ESD = ElectroStatic Discharge, AMPLI = Amplifier, pot. = potential, elec. = electricity, ECG = ElectroCardioGram.

ment at the skin by a gel sponge. Motion artifacts from the cables may originate as static voltages due to friction between the cable insulation and the metallic conductors or as piezoelectric voltages in some kinds of insulation. To get rid of these artifacts, special low-noise cables should be used, and precautions should be taken to prevent their movement (certainly don't bend them!).

Electromagnetic interference (EMI) is usually periodic and regular in form. Hence, the voltage as a function of time is predictable when the circumstances remain unchanged. These types of disturbances are mostly 'man-made' and are generated by the power-line (50 or 60 Hz) and its harmonics or by HF-transmitters such as broadcasting stations, electrosurgical units, diathermy equipment, etc. Interference can often be minimized or even eliminated by a good layout of circuit components, by adequate shielding and by careful filtering. Common ground coupling may be bypassed by grounding all units in one single point via thick wires with a very low resistance. The influence of low frequency magnetic fields will be minimized by avoiding any loops or making the surface area of loops as small as possible i.e. by twisting the wires as far as feasible and by keeping the cables close to the body. Since magnetic fields decrease rapidly with increasing distance, transformers, electric motors, ballasts of fluorescent lights, etc. should be kept away from the measurement site as far as possible. The effect of electric fields may be diminished by the use of well shielded cables and by making them as short as possible. The best way to reduce EMI caused by electric fields is to enclose the patient and the recording system in a grounded Faraday cage. Shielding the room with copper-metallized fabrics, which can be placed in the same way as ordinary wallpaper, may offer an inexpensive alternative for such a cage and may enable sensitive measurements in 'noisy' environments [6].

Voltages caused by electric fields or by a common ground impedance are for the most part of the common-mode type, and their effect is amply cancelled by the use of differential amplifiers with an excellent common-mode rejection ratio (CMRR). However, the common mode voltage may be partly converted into a differential-mode voltage if the two electrode-skin impedances are unequal. Since this differential-mode voltage appears in series with the wanted signal, it is very difficult to eliminate it. Therefore, the use of high-quality electrodes together with a careful preparation of the skin is extremely important.

Device noise is composed of randomly occurring voltages which are unrelated in phase or frequency and may sometimes be very peaky in nature. The exact magnitude of these voltages cannot be predicted at any instant of time. When a large number of samples are taken, the probability distribution of amplitudes appears to be Gaussian, and the mean value becomes zero (Figure 7). Device noise is characteristic for the physics and the materials used in the devices and can only be minimized by statistical methods, i.e. by 'signal averaging'. Johnson (or Nyquist) noise is generated by the thermal agitation of the electrons in a resistor and depends upon temperature, resistance, and bandwidth. Shot (or Schottky) noise is caused by current flowing through a junction, and its value is determined by the DC current and the bandwidth. Since the Johnson noise and the shot noise are both proportional to bandwidth, it is usually limited at 300 Hz. Flicker noise and popcorn noise are both negative indicators of semiconductor process quality. They are also called 'excess noise', and semiconductor manufacturers continue to introduce devices with better noise specifications.

TIME DOMAIN, FREQUENCY DOMAIN, AND FILTERING

The traditional way of observing signals is to view them in the time domain. The time domain is a record of what happened to a parameter (e.g. a voltage) versus time. Amplitude, slew rate, pulse duration, repetition rate, etc. are read directly from the calibrated axes of such a record. We are accustomed to observing electrical voltages with respect to time on oscilloscopes, strip chart recorders, ECG monitors, etc. However, there is still another way to represent the variation of a parameter.

The French mathematician Baron Jean-Baptiste Fourier showed that any waveform that exists in the real world can be generated by adding up a number of simple sine waves (Figure 8). These sine waves are called harmonics, because their frequencies are all integral multiples of the fundamental (i.e. the lowest) frequency. By correctly choosing the amplitude and the

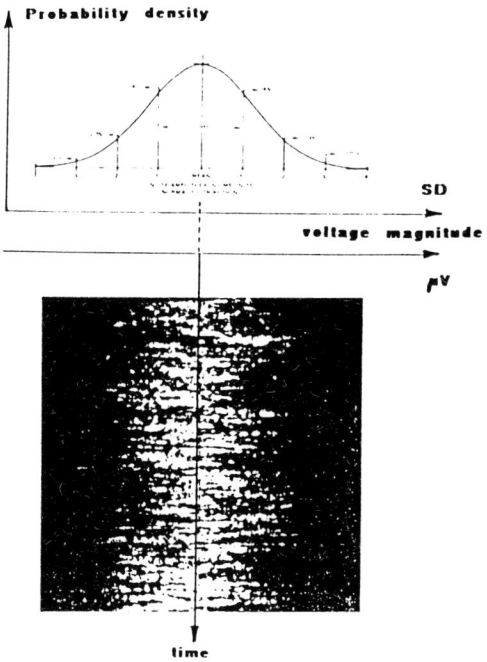

Figure 7. Bell-shaped or Gaussian amplitude distribution around a zero mean value, juxtaposed against a chart of random noise voltage versus time. σ = SD = standard deviation = equals the RMS value (effective value) of the noise.

phase of the different harmonics, every particular waveform may be reconstructed. The graphic representation of the amplitude (vertical axis) of the harmonics versus their frequency (horizontal axis) is called the frequency domain. The set of vertical lines, each having a length corresponding to the amplitude of a particular harmonic, is called a Fourier spectrum (Figure 9).

It is important to understand that no information is either lost or gained by converting from one domain to another. Both frequency and time domains are just different representations of the same phenomenon: it is like looking at the same three-dimensional graph from different angles. The two domains are mathematically correlated by the formulas of Fourier involving a lot of calculations. Therefore, the transformation has to be implemented on a digital computer using an algorithm, i.e. a prescribed set of well-defined instructions for the solution of the problem. Such an algorithm for transfor-

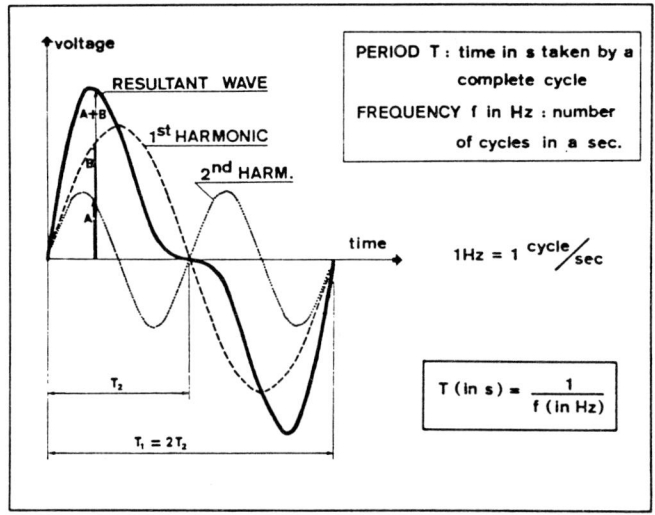

Figure 8. An illustration of the Fourier principle. Any arbitrary periodic signal may be represented by a sum of simple sine waves called harmonics.

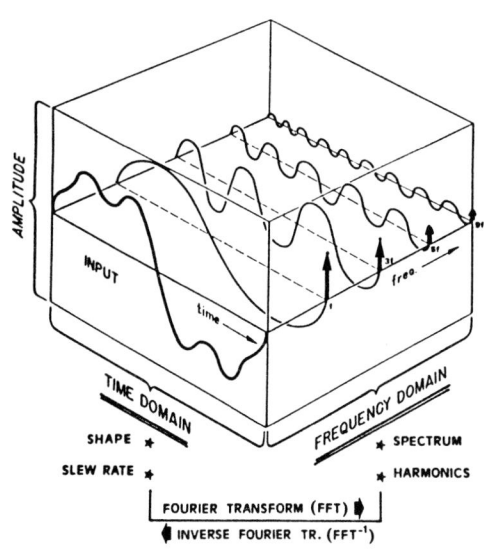

Figure 9. Graphic representation of the relationship between time domain and frequency domain of the same periodic signal.

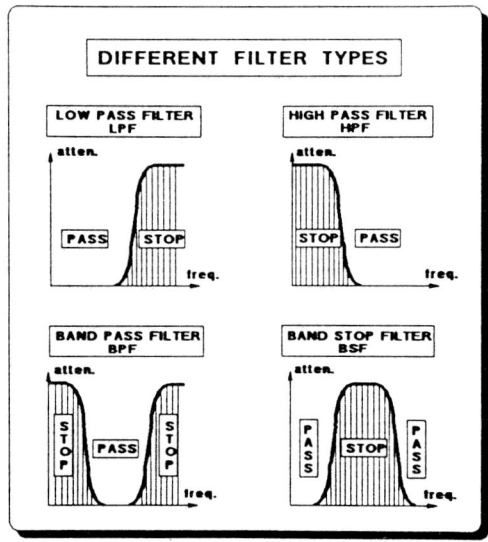

Figure 10. Various types of electronic filters are distinguished by the parts of the frequency domain they transmit or suppress.

ming data from the time domain to the frequency domain is called the Fast Fourier Transformation (FFT).

The frequency domain provides a useful tool for the understanding of electronic filtering. An electronic filter is a device that will transmit some components of the frequency spectrum of a signal within a certain designated range and suppress all other components. The band of frequencies going unattenuated through the filter is called the pass band, while the frequency components which are strongly attenuated are within the rejection band or stop band. Four basic types of filters may be distinguished (Figure 10). Low-pass filters transmit all frequency components below a certain limit called the cut-off frequency, while high-pass filters reject all components below their cut-off. Band-pass as well as band-stop filters have two cut-off frequencies and may be realized by placing a low-pass and a high-pass filter in series. A band-stop filter with an extremely narrow bandwidth, suppressing only one single frequency, is called a notch filter.

While measuring late potentials, filters are very helpful to eliminate some of the noise. In order to remove the DC offset and the very low frequencies associated with motion artifacts from the skin-electrode interface, the signals from the X, Y, and Z leads are high-pass filtered with a cut-off frequency of 0.5 Hz. Note that this cut-off frequency is too high for classical ECGs since it may result in a slight change of ST morphology. A low-pass filter which limits the upper frequency to 300 Hz, reduces the thermal device noise

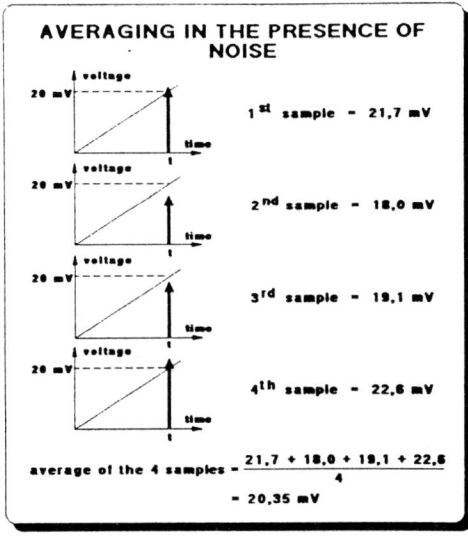

Figure 11. Illustration of the straightforward arithmetic procedure of 'ensemble-' or 'time domain averaging'.

by restricting the bandwidth and also suppresses the highest frequencies of the myopotentials. Notch filters against power line interference (50 or 60 Hz) should not be used since diagnostic information at this frequency would be lost.

THE PRINCIPLE OF ENSEMBLE AVERAGING

Linear averaging is the straightforward arithmetic procedure of adding together the results of a sequence of measurements and dividing the sum by the number of measurements. This is illustrated in Figure 11 where the magnitude of a voltage is to be measured at a fixed time t after its start. Due to noise and artifacts, the exact voltage (20 mV) is never displayed. However, the difference between the exact value and the average (or mean) is smaller than the deviations of the individual results. Obviously, the larger the number of results averaged, the less responsive is the average to individual variations.

Of course, a set or 'ensemble' of results is needed to allow the calculations of an average, hence the name ensemble averaging. Since the distinct results are measured sequentially in the time domain, this mathematical procedure is also referred as sequential averaging or time domain averaging.

Before averaging, a large number of similarly shaped beats are recorded

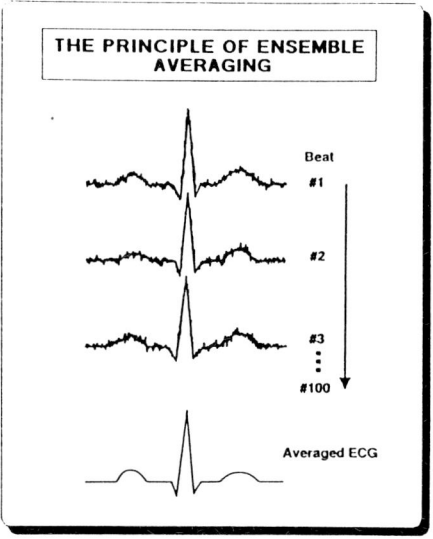

Figure 12. Signal averaging to reduce the noise of the ECG.

and accurately aligned (Figure 12). The ECG is repetitive and so are its associated late potentials. This periodic part will always be exactly the same in each time-record, and the average will be its accurate value. On the contrary, the random noise follows a Gaussian distribution, and the mean of an infinite number of samples tends toward zero. So, it is equally likely for this noise to have a positive or a negative value at any instant of time, and the random noise cancels itself as more beats are summed together. According to the theory of statistics and probability, the reduction of the random noise voltage is proportional to the square-root of the number of beats processed, i.e. the noise decreases with a factor $\sqrt{k}$ if k beats are averaged. Since the useful signal (S) remains the same while the noise (N) diminishes, the signal-to-noise ratio (S/N) will improve correspondingly. For example, a 100-beat average will improve the S/N ratio by a factor 10, while a 200-beat average results in a 14 to 1 enhancement. Generally, averaging about 100 to 200 beats is sufficient to result in a satisfactory S/N value (noise level below 0.3 to 1 µV).

Artifacts due to skeletal muscle activity or to some form of EMI are not random, and their average may be different from zero. However, since these unwanted signals are not synchronized with the waveform of interest, they are attenuated, but their decrease may be much smaller than the reduction of random noise. Therefore, it remains extremely important to suppress both interference and motion artifacts by all the means already mentioned.

PREPARING THE SIGNALS

As pointed out earlier, many calculations have to be performed in a very short time for the averaging of a large number of ECG beats. Hence, the whole procedure has to be implemented on a digital computer if the results are to be sufficiently accurate. Fortunately, with the advent of microprocessors, it is easy and inexpensive to incorporate all the needed computing power in a small instrument package. However, a digital computer is not able to deal directly with small, continuously changing voltages. So, the signals of the X, Y, and Z leads have to be prepared and adapted. This preparation is called data acquisition and includes several steps: (1) amplification, (2) sampling, and (3) quantizing.

The ECG signals from the three leads are first electronically amplified. The voltage amplification or gain of the amplifier is typically set between 1000 and 10 000. Since an absolute quantification of the late potentials in microvolt is required, the gain adjustment is only possible in fixed and calibrated steps, with an accuracy better than ± 2%. The bandwidth is usually limited at its lower end to 0.05–0.5 Hz and at its upper end to 250–300 Hz. The dynamic range of input signals for which the amplification has to be linear should not be less than ± 2.5 mV. Whereas signal averaging is not intended for arrhythmia monitoring, the amplifiers need not be protected against damage during defibrillation. On the contrary, patients should be safeguarded against electrocution by leakage currents, and therefore the equipment has to meet the requirements of international standards such as IEC 601-1 and IEC 930 [7].

A digital computer cannot handle continuous signals. Hence, a 'sampling technique' is used to measure the signal repeatedly during a very brief instant to produce a set of discrete values that is representative of the information contained in the whole (Figure 13). Since the signal is only known to the computer at discrete points in time, it is obvious that some information may be missed when the sampling frequency is too low. In particular, sharp peaks and transitions in the slope of the signal are likely to be lost (Figure 14). For the detection of late potentials, the sampling frequency is usually 1000 Hz (or 2000 Hz), making the time between two consecutive samples 1 ms (or 0.5 ms).

If a lead voltage contains components with a frequency higher than half the sampling frequency ($fs/2$), a new problem, called aliasing, may arise. A signal with a frequency above $fs/2$ may give rise to exactly the same samples as another (alias) signal with a frequency lower than $fs/2$ (Figure 15). As a consequence, some HF myopotentials or electromagnetic interference may be interpreted erroneously as late potentials. Therefore, the necessary measures are to be taken to suppress all artifacts or disturbances with frequencies above $fs/2$. In most technical applications an 'anti-aliasing' low-pass filter is used to solve such problems. If the bandwidth of the amplifier is limited to 300 Hz while the sampling frequency is at least 1000 Hz, no special filtering is required for the correct detection of late potentials.

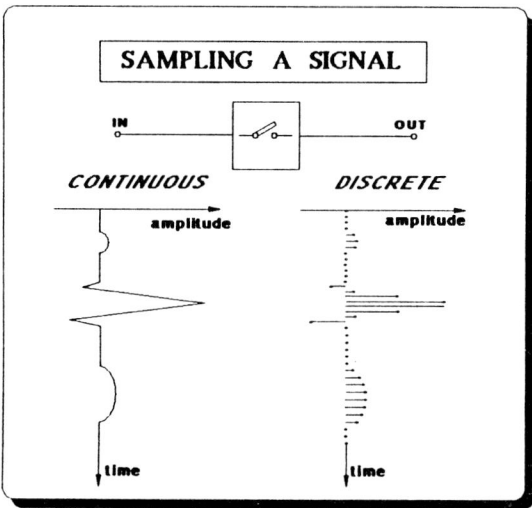

Figure 13. The sampling circuit acts as a fast switch, briefly closing at regular intervals and thus producing a set of discrete values.

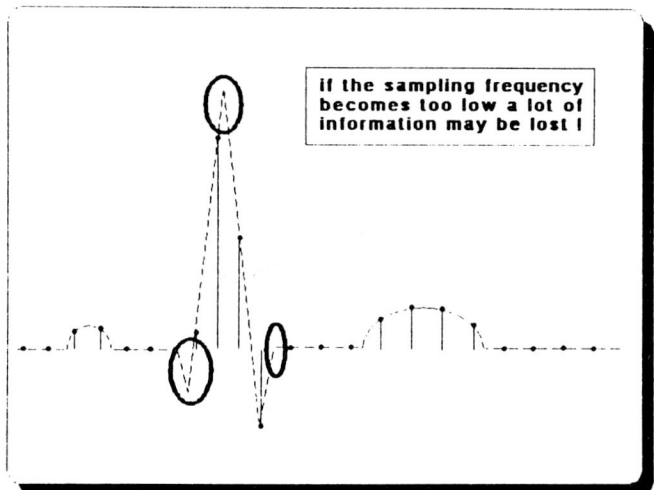

Figure 14. In order that the output samples represent the input signal without significant loss of information, the sampling rate has to be sufficiently high.

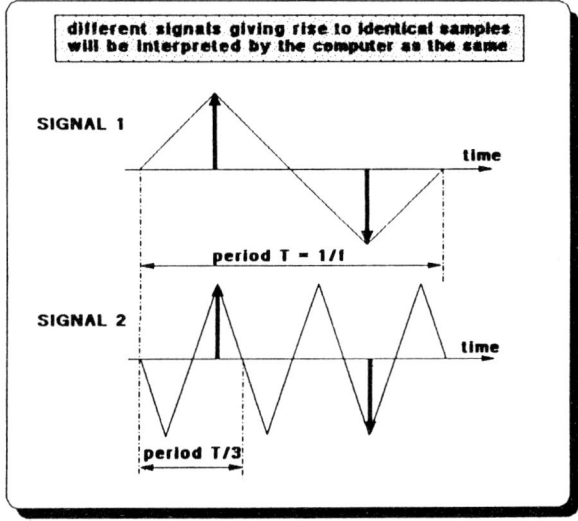

Figure 15. An elucidation of the 'aliasing problem'. The sampling rate should be at least double of the highest signal frequency.

Although discrete in time, the samples are still analog voltages, and a digital computer accepts nothing but binary numbers. The indispensable quantization is accomplished by an analog-to-digital converter (ADC) which translates a voltage to a series of binary digits or bits (i.e. 0's or 1's), as illustrated in Figure 16. The resolution, i.e., the smallest variation of input voltage which can be measured, equals the least significant bit (LSB). It depends upon the number n of bits and the full-scale input voltage (Figure 17):

$$\text{Resolution} = \frac{\text{Full-scale input voltage}}{2^n}$$

Obviously, the full-scale input voltage of the amplifier is much lower than the maximum voltage of the ADC. If, for instance, the maximum voltage of the ADC is 10 V while the gain of the amplifier is 1000 ×, the full-scale input voltage equals 10 V : 1000 = 10 mV. With a 12-bit ADC, the resolution becomes 10 mV : 2^{12} = 2.5 μV. In that case, late potentials with an amplitude smaller than 2.5 μV cannot be measured. The equipment is usually designed for a resolution better than 1 μV (or even < 0.5 μV).

BEAT SELECTION AND SYNCHRONIZATION

Before the averaging process can actually be accomplished, two remaining problems have to be solved. As pointed out before, one prerequisite is that

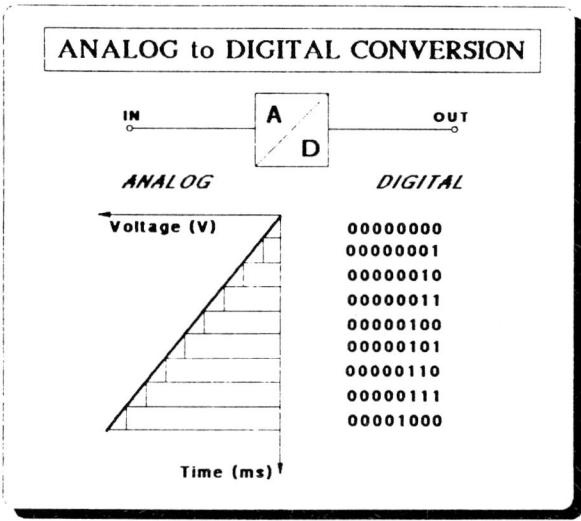

Figure 16. The A/D converter 'translates' each voltage sample into a series of 'bits' (= binary digits, i.e., 0's or 1's).

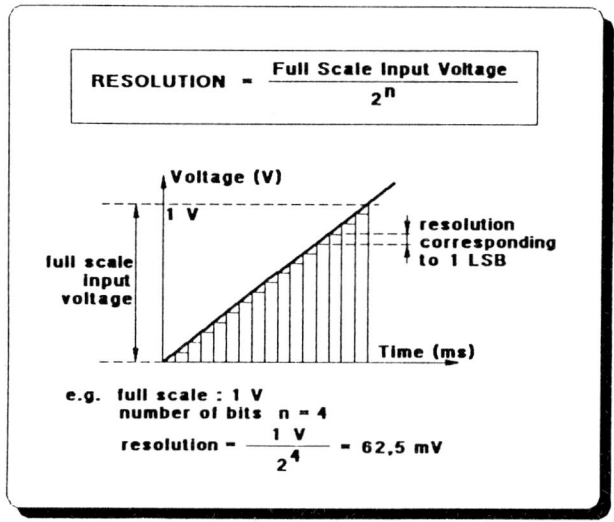

Figure 17. Resolution or smallest variation of input voltage which can be measured. (LSB = Least Significant Bit = bit on the extreme right of the row.)

the signals of interest be repetitive. Therefore, only beats of the same origin and morphology may be averaged. Usually only normally conducted beats during sinus rhythm are accepted, while ectopic beats, PVCs and aberrantly conducted beats have to be excluded.

Due to heart rate variability, the QRS complexes are not generated at precise regular intervals. However, the time domain averaging must be performed on samples taken at exactly corresponding times of the successive QRS complexes. Hence, beat alignment is a critical precondition for the averaging process. If the beats are imprecisely aligned (called "jitter"), there will be some attenuation of the high-frequency components, the very ones we are interested in! The sum of two sine waves is always zero, if they have the same frequency (f) and the same amplitude, but are shifted in time over half their period ($1/2f$). For a frequency of 300 Hz, this phenomenon will appear with a shift of 1.66 ms. It follows that the jitter, i.e. the uncertainty of the alignment, has to be smaller than about 1 ms.

Recent equipment advances take care of the beat selection as well as the beat alignment on the basis of a chosen target beat or a template. The user may opt for a specific template by visual selection of a desirable beat (e.g. a regular sinus beat) from a graphic display, but most often a template is generated automatically or half-automatically by the computer. A simple algorithm for this purpose includes the acquisition of an 8-s segment of X, Y, or Z lead data, followed by the "pre-averaging" of the beats within that segment which appear to be the most normally conducted (having the shortest QRS duration). More sophisticated algorithms are generally unpublished; nevertheless, it should be noted that even they may run into trouble in the presence of frequent PVCs (e.g. in postmyocardial infarction patients).

The first step in the process of alignment is the determination of a provisory fiducial or reference point on each incoming QRS complex. For that purpose a simple comparator may be used as a level detector (Figure 18). When the arriving complex exceeds the predetermined reference voltage, an output pulse is generated to serve as the desired hallmark. This reference point will be used for a provisional coarse lining-up of the successive complexes. Around the reference point a time-window of at least 40 ms is established (i.e. 40 samples if the sampling rate is 1 kHz).

The final alignment of each beat to the selected template is accomplished in the time domain using the sliding window technique. Starting at corresponding provisory reference points, the correlation coefficient ρ is computed between the incoming beat and the template for every sampling instant included in their windows (Figure 19). Next, the incoming beat is shifted one sampling point (i.e. 1 ms), and the correlation is computed again. By repeating this last step a few times in both directions from the provisory reference, the highest correlation coefficient may be found. This maximum value of ρ indicates the position of best alignment and thus the final fiducial point.

If the incoming beat and the template are perfectly matched and correctly

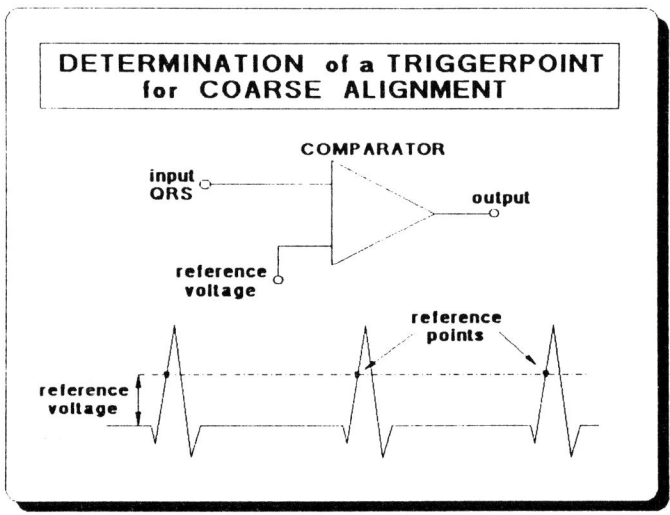

Figure 18. Determination of a provisional trigger- or reference point on each incoming QRS complex.

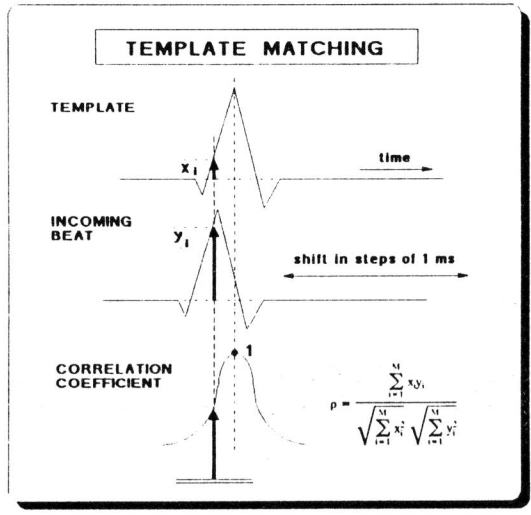

Figure 19. Final alignment of incoming beats with a sinus beat template, using the sliding window technique.

aligned, the correlation coefficient ρ should be 1. Due to noise, somewhat lower values are usually noted. However, if the maximum value of ρ is less than 0.98, the tested beat does not fit closely enough to the template and must be excluded from the averaging.

The FFT offers a somewhat alternative method of alignment. A windowed 128-ms region within the QRS of each beat is converted to the frequency domain by the FFT algorithm. The FFT of an incoming beat is compared to 21 FFTs obtained from the template, each time shifted in 1-ms increments, to find the best match. After alignment, the averaging itself is done in the time domain using 512-ms segments of unfiltered ECG from all three leads.

The length of time required to obtain a desired number of averaged beats is a function of the heart rate and how well each beat correlates with the chosen template. Excessive noise or a change in dominant rhythm or in QRS morphology will retard or even halt the averaging process.

FILTERING OF THE AVERAGED BEATS

Late potentials are due to delayed ventricular depolarizations. Hence, the high-frequency signals generated by these depolarizations should be emphasized, while all components of the ECG that reflect repolarization have to be removed as best as possible. Therefore, after signal averaging, the signal is usually band-pass filtered. To suppress the low-frequency power of the QRS complex as well as the low-frequency activity contained in the PR and ST segments, a lower cut-off frequency of 25 Hz or 40 Hz is generally chosen (some experimenters used 80 Hz as well). The remaining noise in the averaged leads is usually further cut back by limiting the bandwidth at a higher cut-off frequency of 250 Hz.

Since the averaged signals are stored in the memory of a digital computer, it is obvious that the filtering of the SAECG is performed digitally. Three basic types of digital filters are available: (1) finite impulse response (FIR) filters, (2) infinite impulse response (IIR) filters, and (3) spectral window filters. However, filters may introduce distortions of the signals of interest. The two common distortions are phase shift and ringing. The *phase shift* caused by a filter may be frequency dependent in a non-linear way, making the different components of the spectrum shift in relation to each other and resulting in a distortion of the signal morphology. A change in the shape or the duration of the signal may induce errors in the various time and amplitude measurements. *Ringing* is a damped oscillation at some higher frequency after a large amplitude signal has passed the filter, i.e. the detection of small amplitude late potentials may be impeded by the ringing after the QRS complex.

FIR filters with a good discrimination in the frequency domain demand a really large number of filter coefficients. As a consequence a relatively long computing time is needed, and the speed of the system may be too slow for

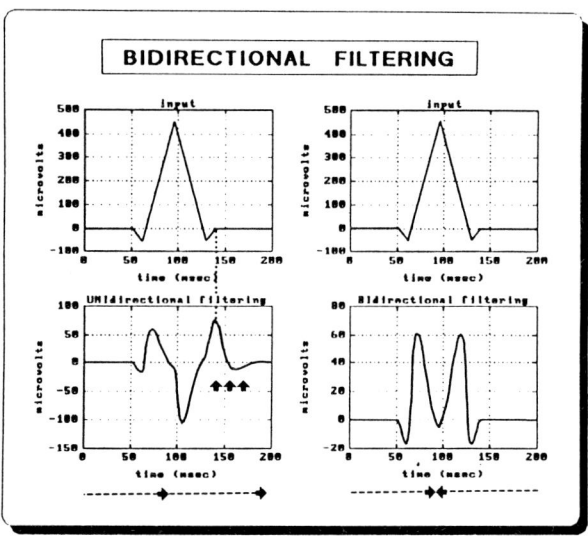

Figure 20. Comparison between unidirectional filtering (left) and bidirectional filtering (right), using a 40 to 250 Hz band-pass digital filter of the 2-pole Butterworth type. Note the 'ringing' or prolongation of the output signal after the test signal ends (arrows) in the case of unidirectional filtering.

real-time averaging. On the contrary, the time domain performance of the FIRs is excellent. The ringing at the end of the QRS, and hence the uncertainty of its endpoints, are strictly limited. Moreover, the morphology of the QRS is preserved, and accurate amplitude and time measurements are possible.

IIR filters present a fairly good discrimination in the frequency domain with a limited number of filter coefficients, resulting in a greater speed. Unfortunately, their performance in the time domain is rather poor. Ringing at the end of the QRS, causing uncertainty of the endpoint, will cause some error in the time measurement while partly masking the late potentials. Spreading of the QRS power in the direction of the filtering creates errors in the amplitude measurements. A very popular version of the IIR, avoiding the problem of ringing, is the bidirectional filter. This filter processes forward in time until 40 ms into the QRS complex. The filter is then reset and processes the signal backward in time up to the same point in the QRS complex (Figure 20) [8]. In this way the distortion caused by ringing is in the middle of the QRS complex, leaving the critical endpoints unchanged.

Spectral window filters represent a compromise since they have characteristics of both FIR and IIR. The filtering starts with an FFT to the frequency domain where a window selects the desired frequencies and suppresses the

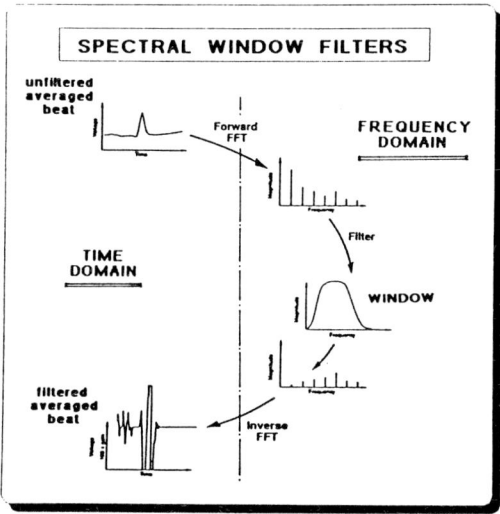

Figure 21. Digital filtering by manipulating the spectrum in the frequency domain. (FFT = Fast Fourier Transform.)

other components. An inverse FFT transforms the filtered signal back to the time domain (Figure 21). Spectral window filters have a well-defined response in the frequency domain, and their performance in the time domain is rather good. There is only a moderate ringing at the beginning and end of the QRS, so a fairly accurate estimation of its endpoints is possible. Moreover, the morphology of the QRS complex is sufficiently preserved.

TIME DOMAIN MEASUREMENTS

According to the Task Force Committee of the European Society of Cardiology (ESC), the American Heart Association (AHA) and the American College of Cardiology (ACC), the measurements should be carried out on the absolute value of the band-pass-filtered VM, which is based upon the averaged X, Y and Z leads [2]. The analysis should include the determination of three typical parameters (Figure 22): (1) the filtered QRS duration (QRSD), (2) the root mean square voltage of the terminal 40 ms of the QRS (RMS40), and (3) the duration of the low-amplitude signal, i.e. the time that the filtered QRS complex remains below 40 μV (LASD or HFLAD).

For a 40–250 Hz band-pass filter, it is assumed that a patient shows late potentials if QRSD > 114 ms, RMS40 < 20 μV, and HFLAD > 38 ms.

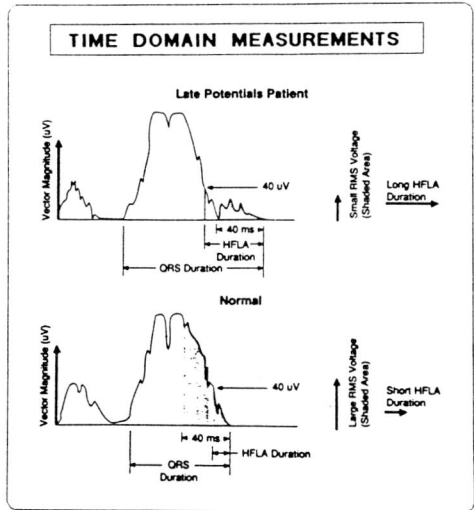

Figure 22. Time domain measurements as proposed by the 'Task Force Committee'. HFLA = High Frequency Low Amplitude Signals. RMS = Root Mean Square = effective value.

CONCLUSION

SAECG is a very attractive and relatively new field which is still undergoing investigation in order to improve its diagnostic power. However, some pitfalls have to be avoided since it is possible to create signals which could be interpreted as late potentials (e.g. ringing of a filter), and it is also easy to mask late potentials (e.g. jitter due to poor alignment). With very fast computers today at an affordable price, digital signal processing (DSP) will bring other advanced techniques, like spectrotemporal mapping and other time-frequency representations, directly to the physician. A lot of research has already been done, and some information is also available for interested readers [9].

REFERENCES

1. El-Sherif N, Gomes J, Restivo M et al. Late potentials and arrhythmogenesis. PACE 1985;5:440–62.
2. Breithardt G et al. Standards for analysis of ventricular late potentials using high resolution or signal-averaged electrocardiography. Eur Heart J 1991;12:473–80.
3. Horan L, Flowers N. The relationship between the vectorcardiogram and the actual dipole moment. In: Nelson C, Geselowitz D, editors. The theoretical basis of electrocardiology. Oxford Medical Engineering Series, 1976.
4. Lander P, Deal R, Berbari E. The analysis of ventricular late potentials using orthogonal recordings. IEEE Trans Biomed Eng 1988;35:629–39.
5. Webster J. Reducing motion artifacts and interference in biomedical recording. IEEE Trans Biomed Eng 1984;31:823–6.

6. Sinnaeve A. Flectron: an easy solution to radiated EMC problems. IEE Colloquium on EMC and Medicine, London, April 1993, pp. 11/1–11/7.
7. International Electrotechnical Committee (IEC), Geneva, Switzerland: IEC 601-1, Medical electrical equipment. Part 1: General requirements for safety, 1988; IEC 930, Guidelines for administrative, medical and nursing staff concerned with the safe use of medical electrical equipment, 1988.
8. Simson MB. Use of signals in the terminal QRS complexes to identify patients with ventricular tachycardia after myocardial infarction. Circulation 1981;64:235–42.
9. Lander P, Berbari E. Principles and signal processing techniques of the high-resolution electrocardiogram. Prog Cardiovasc Dis 1992;35:169–88.

12. Optimizing the predictive value of the signal-averaged ECG for serious arrhythmic events in the postinfarction period

NABIL EL-SHERIF

INTRODUCTION

In the last few years a number of studies have shown that the signal-averaged electrocardiogram (SAECG) can stratify patients recovering from acute myocardial infarction (MI) into high- and low-risk groups for late serious arrhythmic events [1–4]. These studies, however, have a number of limitations: (1) the definition of an abnormal SAECG was either determined empirically or was derived from relatively small study groups [1–4]; (2) the assignment of the cause of unwitnessed death to cardiac arrhythmia was done by the investigators without an independent review process; (3) the incidence of serious arrhythmic events in the first year post-MI in some studies (as high as 14% [2]) is significantly higher than the current incidence. Thus, previous study groups may not represent the current post-MI population.

The SAECG can be analyzed in a time-domain or frequency-domain mode. Both types of analysis have several limitations. Time-domain analysis is limited in the presence of intraventricular conduction defects, which many patients at risk have and which may make interpretation of the recording difficult [5]. On the other hand, some frequency-domain analysis techniques have been criticized as unreproducible [5,6]. Recently, the combined use of time- and frequency-domain variables has been suggested to improve their predictive value [7]. The present chapter briefly reviews two recent studies that were conducted with the goal of optimizing the predictive value of the SAECG for serious arrhythmic events in the post-MI period.

DEFINING THE BEST PREDICTIVE CRITERIA OF TIME-DOMAIN SAECG IN THE POST-INFARCTION PERIOD [8]

Background and methods

A substudy was conducted prospectively in conjunction with the NIH-sponsored Cardiac Arrhythmia Suppression Trial (CAST). There were 1211 patients with CAST-qualifying acute MI [9] who were recruited from 10 CAST centers. The patients were recruited without application of the ejection fraction and arrhythmia restrictions of the main CAST protocol. They were enrolled into the study 5 to 30 days post-MI. Several clinical variables, ventricular arrhythmias on Holter, left ventricular ejection fraction, and 6 SAECG parameters [the filtered QRS duration (QRSD), the root mean square voltage in the last 40 ms (RSM 40), and the duration of late potentials of $\leq 40\,\mu V$ amplitude (LPD 40) recorded at both 25 and 40 Hz high bandpass filtering] were obtained. All patients were followed for up to 1 year. The primary endpoint was an arrhythmic event defined as sustained VT and death or resuscitated cardiac arrest judged to be due to arrhythmia. All events were classified by the primary investigator and were reviewed and finally approved by the CAST Events Committee.

Results

Of the 1211 patients recruited into the study, 52 had either right or left bundle branch block and were excluded from further analysis. The remaining 1160 patients were followed for an average of $10.3 + 3.2$ months. Forty-five patients (4.3%) suffered serious arrhythmic events (42 sudden cardiac deaths judged to be due to arrhythmias, and 3 nonfatal sustained VT).

Using the Cox proportional hazards regression model [10] and controlling for the clinical variables that showed a significant difference, the SAECG parameters were found to be independently predictive of arrhythmic events. The most predictive continuous parameter was then determined using Cox regression without correcting for baseline characteristics. The filtered QRSD at 40 Hz was found to be the most predictive, with the highest chi-square value of 34.5. To determine the best cut-off value for the filtered QRSD at 40 Hz, dichotomous variables were created. A filtered QRSD of ≥ 120 ms had the highest chi-square value and, thus, provided the best predictive criterion. The combination of a filtered QRSD at 40 Hz with other dichotomized SAECG parameters did not improve the predictive value of the test. Thus, an abnormal SAECG was defined as a filtered QRSD at 40 Hz ≥ 120 ms. The incidence of an abnormal signal-averaged ECG in the study group was 12%. The positive, negative, and total predictive accuracy of a 40-Hz QRSD ≥ 120 ms was 17%, 98%, and 88%, respectively. In a further regression analysis including all clinical, Holter, and left ventricular ejection fraction variables, a QRSD-40 Hz ≥ 120 ms was the most significant predictor of arrhythmic events ($p < 0.0002$). The probability of remaining free of serious arrhythmic events during the first year postinfarction was significantly higher in patients with a normal SAECG (98%) compared with those with an abnormal record (81%; $p < 0.0001$).

COMBINED TIME- AND FREQUENCY-DOMAIN ANALYSIS OF THE SAECG IMPROVES ITS PREDICTIVE ACCURACY IN POSTINFARCTION PATIENTS [11]

Background and methods

One of the limitations of time-domain late potentials analysis of the SAECG is that partial obscuring of the late potentials may occur if the abnormal myocardial region is activated relatively early during the QRS complex. This occurs more often with anterior wall (AW) MI than inferior wall (IW) MI and may partially explain the higher incidence of false-positive abnormal recordings in patients with IWMI [12]. On the other hand, in a preliminary report a higher incidence of abnormal spectral turbulence in AWMI (36%) was found compared with IWMI (15%). This led to a high incidence of false-positive abnormal test results in patients with AWMI [13]. A study was therefore conducted to investigate the hypothesis that combined time- and frequency-domain analysis of the SAECG could improve its predictive accuracy in post-MI patients.

The study group consisted of 262 patients with acute MI who were followed prospectively for 1 year for the incidence of serious arrhythmic events. A SAECG was obtained 5 to 30 days post-MI. The time-domain criteria for an abnormal recording were those published from this laboratory and consisted of a RMS 40 amplitude at 25 Hz ≤ 25 μV plus a RMS 40 amplitude at 40 Hz ≤ 16 μV [15]. Spectral turbulence analysis of the SAECG was performed by a technique that was previously published from this laboratory. The recording could be scored between 0 and 4, and an abnormal spectral turbulence analysis was defined as a score of 3 or 4 [5]. Figure 1 illustrates the time-domain late potential analysis in the upper panel and spectrocardiograms in oblique, horizontal, and transparent views in the lower panel in a patient with AWMI showing abnormalities with both tests.

Results

Of the 262 patients, 12 had bundle branch block and were included in both time- and frequency-domain analyses. During a mean follow-up of 10.5 months, there were 17 arrhythmic events (sustained VT in 4, and arrhythmic death in 13 patients). Table 1A shows the positive predictive accuracy (PPA),

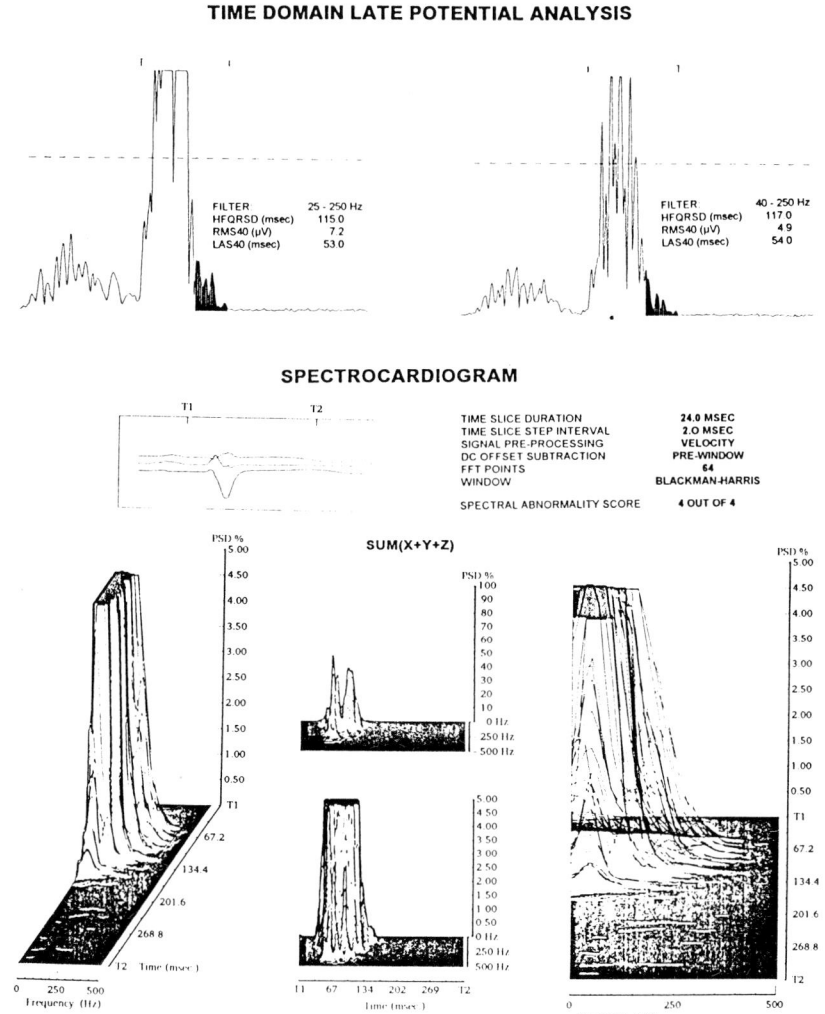

Figure 1. Time-domain plots (top) and spectral plots (bottom) of the signal-averaged electrocardiogram of a patient with anterior wall myocardial infarction. The spectrocardiogram is displayed in different views: an oblique view (left), a horizontal view at both low and high gains (middle), and a transparent view (right). Note the presence of late potentials in the time-domain plots and an abnormal spectral turbulence score of 4 in the spectral plots. The patient succumbed to a sudden arrhythmic death 4 weeks following the myocardial infarction.

Table 1. Predictive accuracy of combined time-domain and spectral turbulence analysis of the SAECG in the post-infarction period.

	PPA	NPA	TPA	OR
A. Total group (262 patients)				
TD	28%	97%	87%	12
ST	14%	96%	78%	4
TD + ST	35%*	96%	92%	12
B. First AWMI or IWMI (153 patients)				
TD	24%	96%	86%	8
ST	15%	96%	75%	5
TD + ST	40%*	96%	92%*	15*

AWMI = anterior wall myocardial infarction; IWMI = inferior wall myocardial infarction; NPA = negative predictive accuracy; OR = odds ratio; PPA = positive predictive accuracy; ST = spectral turbulence analysis; TD = time-domain analysis; TPA = total predictive accuracy.
* $p < 0.05$.

negative predictive accuracy (NPA), total predictive accuracy (TPA), and odds ratio (OR) of time-domain (TD), spectral turbulence analysis (ST), and their combination (TD + ST) in the total group of 262 patients. The NPA was high (96–97%) in all three analyses. The PPA, TPA, and OR of the time-domain analysis were higher than those of spectral turbulence analysis. On the other hand, a combination of both analyses provided a significant improvement of the PPA (35%). The TPA of the combined analysis (92%) was higher than those of the time-domain analysis and spectral turbulence alone, but the difference was not statistically significant.

Table 1B analyzes the results in 153 patients with their first AWMI or IWMI. Once again, the NPAs of all three analyses were high (96%), while the PPA, TPA, and OR of the time-domain analysis were higher than those of the spectral turbulence analysis. On the other hand, combined time-domain and spectral turbulence analyses resulted in a significant improvement of the PPA (40%), TPA (92%), and OR (15).

Table 2 analyzes the results separately in patients with their first IWMI or AWMI. In 79 patients with first IWMI, there was no significant difference in the PPAs of the time-domain and spectral turbulence analyses. However, the combined analysis resulted in a significant improvement of both the PPA and TPA. In 74 patients with first AWMI, the combined time-domain and spectral turbulence analysis resulted in a significantly higher PPA of 50% and an odds ratio of 27.

DISCUSSION

Two general approaches have been utilized to derive criteria for an abnormal time-domain SAECG. The first approach investigated 'normal' study groups to obtain 'upper limits' for the normal SAECG [14,15]. This approach has

Table 2. Predictive accuracy of combined time-domain and spectral turbulence analysis of the SAECG in patients with first inferior or anterior wall myocardial infarction.

	PPA	NPA	TPA	OR
First IWMI (79 patients)				
TD	15%	98%	85%	12
ST	13%	98%	81%	9
TD + ST	25%*	97%	94%*	12
First AWMI (74 patients)				
TD	37%	94%	88%	9
ST	17%	94%	68%	3
TD + ST	50%*	94%	91%*	27*

*$p < 0.05$.
For abbreviations, see Table 1.

been criticized because 'normal' study groups are not representative of the population with coronary artery disease. The second approach evaluated the predictive value of the SAECG criteria for patients with spontaneous and/or inducible sustained VT [16,17]. In this group of patients, the time-domain SAECG criteria reflecting the presence of late potentials (i.e. RMS 40 and/or LPD 40) were usually the most predictive. The electrophysiologic rationale for the predictive value of these criteria was that late potentials represent the slowed and disorganized conduction of localized myocardial zones that could provide the anatomic-electrophysiologic substrate for reentrant VT [18]. It does not necessarily follow that these criteria would also be predictive in the post-MI period when the majority of serious arrhythmic events are fatal ventricular tachyarrhythmias rather than nonfatal sustained VT. In the present study, time-domain SAECG indices of late potentials did not provide the best prediction criteria for serious arrhythmic events. The signal-averaged QRSD at 40 Hz high-pass filter was found to be the single best predictive criterion. The electrophysiologic rationale as to why an abnormally long signal-averaged QRSD best predicts fatal arrhythmic events in the first year post-MI is not clear. However, it is possible that this may reflect the slowed and nonhomogeneous conduction of a larger mass of ventricular myocardium. Such hearts may be more vulnerable to fast VT/VF.

In the second study in this report, it was found that the combined time-domain and spectral turbulence analysis of the SAECG significantly improves the predictive accuracy of the test, especially in patients with first AWMI. The technique of spectral turbulence analysis reflects abrupt changes in the frequency signature of the QRS wavefront velocity as it propagates throughout the ventricle around areas of abnormal conduction, which would result in a high degree of spectral turbulence [5]. Patients with first AWMI have a high incidence of abnormal spectral turbulence analysis, probably reflecting a large mass of myocardium with abnormal conduction. This results in a high incidence of false-positive results [13]. However, combining spectral turbulence analysis with time-domain criteria for late potentials in this group of patients markedly improves the positive predictive accuracy of the test to 50%.

A somewhat unexpected finding in this study is that the predictive accuracy of spectral turbulence analysis for serious arrhythmic events in post-MI patients was generally lower than that of time-domain late potentials analysis. In a previous study we have shown that spectral turbulence analysis is superior to time-domain late potentials analysis in its predictive accuracy for inducible sustained monomorphic VT [6]. However, it is possible that the criteria of spectral turbulence analysis predictive of inducible sustained VT may not necessarily apply to the prediction of serious arrhythmic events in the post-MI period. The latter are mainly due to fatal ventricular tachyarrhythmias rather than nonfatal sustained VT. Optimizing the spectral turbulence analysis criteria in post-MI patients and using it in combination with the best predictive criteria of time-domain analysis in this setting may improve further the predictive accuracy of the test.

REFERENCES

1. Kuchar D, Thorburn C, Sammel N. Prediction of serious arrhythmic events after myocardial infarction: signal-averaged electrocardiogram, Holter monitoring and radionuclide ventriculography. J Am Coll Cardiol 1987;9:531–8.
2. Gomes JA, Winters SL, Stewart D, Horowitz S, Milner M, Barreca P. A new noninvasive index to predict sustained ventricular tachycardia and sudden death in the first year after myocardial infarction: based on signal-averaged electrocardiogram, radionuclide ejection fraction and Holter monitoring. J Am Coll Cardiol 1987;10:349–57.
3. Cripps T, Bennett ED, Camm AJ, Ward DE. High gain signal-averaged electrocardiogram combined with 24 hour monitoring in patients early after myocardial infarction for bedside prediction of arrhythmic events. Br Heart J 1988;60:181–18.
4. El-Sherif N, Ursell SN, Bekheit S et al. Prognostic significance of the signal-averaged ECG depends on the time of recording in the post-infarction period. Am Heart J 1989;118:256–64.
5. Kelen GJ, Henkin R, Starr A-M, Caref EB, Bloomfield D, El-Sherif N. Spectral turbulence analysis of the signal-averaged electrocardiogram and its predictive accuracy for inducible sustained monomorphic ventricular tachycardia. Am J Cardiol 1991;67:965–75.
6. Malik M, Kulakowski P, Poloniecki J et al. Frequency versus time-domain analysis of signal-averaged electrocardiograms. I. Reproducibility of the results. J Am Coll Cardiol 1992;127–34.
7. Nogami A, Iesaka Y, Akiyama J et al. Combined use of time and frequency domain variables in signal-averaged ECG as a predictor of inducible sustained monomorphic ventricular tachycardia in myocardial infarction. Circulation 1992;86:780–9.
8. El-Sherif N, Denes P, Katz R et al. Defining the best prediction criteria of time-domain signal averaged electrocardiogram for serious arrhythmic events in the post-infarction period (abstract). Circulation 1992;86:I-525.
9. The CAST Investigators. Preliminary report. Effect of encainide and flecainide on mortality in a randomized trial of arrhythmia suppression after myocardial infarction. N Engl J Med 1989;321:406–12.
10. Cox DR. Regression models and life tables. J R Stat Soc(B) 1972;34:187–94.
11. Ahuja R, Ibrahim B, Caref EB, El-Sherif N. Combined time- and frequency-domain analysis

of the signal-averaged electrocardiogram improves its predictive accuracy in postinfarction patient (abstract). Circulation 1992;86:I-526.
12. Breithardt G, Borggrefe M. Pathophysiological mechanisms and clinical significance of ventricular late potentials. Eur Heart 1986;3:64–85.
13. Ibrahim BB, Caref EB, Kelen GJ, El-Sherif N: Spectral turbulence analysis versus late potentials analysis of the signal averaged ECG in anterior versus inferior wall myocardial infarction (abstract). Circulation 1990;84:III–355.
14. Denes P, Santarelli P, Hauser RG, Uretz EF. Quantitative analysis of the high-frequency components of the terminal portion of the body surface QRS in normal subjects and in patients with ventricular tachycardia. Circulation 1983;67:1129–38.
15. Gomes JA, Winters SL, Stewart D, Targonski A, Barreca P. Optimal bandpass filters for time-domain analysis of the signal-averaged electrocardiogram. Am J Cardiol 1987;60:1290–8.
16. Caref EB, Turitto G, Ibrahim BB, Henkin R, El-Sherif N. Role of bandpass filters in optimizing the value of the signal averaged electrocardiogram as a predictor of the results of programmed stimulation. Am J Cardiol 1989;64:16–26.
17. Simson MB. Use of signals in the terminal QRS complex to identify patients with ventricular tachycardia after myocardial infarction. Circulation 1981;64:235–42.
18. El-Sherif N, Gomes JAC, Restivo M, Mehra R. Late potentials and arrhythmogenesis. PACE 1985;8:440–62.

13. Signal-averaged analysis of the P wave: possible applications in different settings

M. ALI OTO

High-resolution ECG (HRECG) is a field in which modern computing techniques are being applied and new and more powerful data acquisition methods are used to extract information from the surface-recorded ECG. Technically, HRECG detects low-amplitude, high-frequency activity in the ECG, enabling the investigation of these microvolt level signals. The procedure includes several powerful signal processing techniques: signal averaging to decrease the level of noise that contaminates the surface ECG and high-pass filtering on the averaged data to reduce the large-amplitude, low-frequency signal content.

HRECG has been successfully used in the prediction of malignant arrhythmias and risk stratification after acute myocardial infarction (MI) based on the quantification of the microvolt level signals detected in the terminal portion of the QRS complex which are known as 'late potentials' [1]. Late potentials are thought to originate from small areas of delayed and disorganized ventricular activation. These areas appear to represent separate bundles of surviving muscle mass in the necrotic myocardium. In this regard, a high incidence of late potentials has been detected in ischemic heart disease complicated with ventricular arrhythmias.

It has been thought that depolarization heterogeneity may also take place in the arrhythmogenesis of supraventricular premature contractions and atrial tachyarrhythmias. However, high-resolution analysis of the P wave and its clinical relevance are not yet fully understood.

One of the main difficulties in the detection of inhomogenous conduction in the atria comes from the fact that the amplitude of the P wave is much lower than that of the QRS complex, and a conduction delay may not be detected in the surface recordings. Alignment is the second crucial point in the high-resolution analysis of the P wave. An R wave-triggered approach may cause alignment errors due to changes in the PR interval. On the other hand, inaccurate template matching frequently observed in P wave-triggered systems may interfere with the signal.

Although an atrial conduction delay was demonstrated in patients with atrial flutter in 1978 [2], the first report of a signal-averaged analysis of the P wave appeared 10 years later. In 1988, Engel et al. reported their experience with 17 patients with atrial fibrillation or flutter (persistent and paroxysmal) and 26 controls using HRECG techniques [3]. However, their results were inconclusive as to whether or not high-frequency analysis of the P wave is useful in predicting the paroxysms of atrial fibrillation. High-frequency P wave durations were sometimes longer than expected because of antiarrhythmic therapy. Control patients with structural heart disease and heart failure had delayed atrial activation when compared with normal individuals. These were thought to be the P wave abnormalities clinically ascribed to atrial overload and a reflection of dilatation, with longer depolarization pathways or fibrosis and delayed conductions. Chang et al., in a study of 27 patients with hypertrophic cardiomyopathy and paroxysmal atrial fibrillation (PAF) and 25 controls, were able to identify hypertrophic cardiomyopathy patients with PAF by signal-averaged P wave analysis with a sensitivity of 92% and specificity of 92% [4]. Yamada et al., when comparing the high-resolution ECG recordings obtained from 17 patients with PAF and 17 controls, found that the total duration of the P waves was longer and root mean square voltages (RMS) in the last 20 ms were lower in the former group [5]. Therefore, they claimed that the risk of PAF could be identified from body surface recordings during sinus rhythm with a sensitivity of 88% and specificity of 82%. On the other hand, Pellerin et al. reported a longer filtered P wave duration in 7 patients with PAF, and these results were also confirmed by electrophysiologic study [6]. In another study performed by the same group, it was shown that the high-resolution analysis of P wave was able to identify the intra-atrial conduction delay [7]. In a recent study, Fukunami et al. defined the atrial late potentials for the first time [8]. This study comprised 42 patients with PAF and 50 healthy controls. The authors separated the groups according to the presence of organic heart disease and compared the filtered P wave duration and RMS voltages in the last 10, 20, and 30 ms. They concluded that a filtered P wave duration over 120 ms and an RMS voltage in the last 20 ms less than 3.5 μV were convenient criteria to define the atrial late potentials with a sensitivity of 91% and specificity of 76%. Some authors attempted to increase the P wave amplitude by transesophageal recordings and found that those recordings were more sensitive in identifying the risk for PAF [9].

Recently, Stafford et al. studied 9 patients with PAF and 15 healthy controls and found that the filtered P wave duration and RMS voltages in the last quarter of the P wave were discriminative in separating the groups [10]. The filtered P wave duration was also suggested as an accurate predictor of atrial fibrillation following open heart surgery [11].

Spectral temporal mapping of the P wave in subjects with and without PAF was the target for another study. Paylos et al. demonstrated that the spectral analysis of the P wave from patients with PAF showed a significantly lower energy content on the EGG leads facing the posterior and posterolateral atrial myocardium, where zones of slow conduction and blocks have been described which could be responsible for this energy distribution [12].

I and my colleagues developed a PC-based, flexible HRECG data acquisition system for P wave analysis [13]. By this system, the signals from the X, Y, and Z leads are amplified 16,000 times in order to analyze the low-amplitude signals better. The data are digitized with 12-bit accuracy and with a sampling rate of 1000 Hz by means of an analog-to-digital converter with 1 μV bit resolution.

With this system, we performed a study to analyze the P wave in patients with PAF while in sinus rhythm in order to detect a substrate for reentrant atrial arrhythmias and to define a reliable method for determining the risk of reentrant atrial arrhythmias [13]. After having completed the recording, a template in the P wave was selected, and averaging using the minimum function was performed. At least 200 beats were averaged off-line. Simultaneous esophageal recordings were obtained in 18 patients, and averaging with a template chosen on the esophageal P wave was also performed in this group. Fourth-order Butterworth filters were employed on the signal-averaged P waves, and filtered P wave durations and RMS voltages in the last 20, 25, 30, and 40 ms of the P wave were calculated. We studied 22 patients with at least two documented paroxysms of atrial fibrillation, of whom 14 were men and 8 were women [14]. Their ages ranged between 36 and 72 years, with a mean of 57. The control group comprised 14 men and 6 women with a mean age of 51 (range 27–84). We measured the filtered P wave duration and RMS values in the last 20, 25, 30, and 40 ms by using 25–250 and 40–250 Hz filters both unidirectionally and bidirectionally. The templates were chosen in the Z and esophageal leads manually. When all the parameters were analyzed and the groups compared, we found that the P wave duration (125.6 ± 3.4 ms vs. 102.8 ± 1.3 ms in patients with PAF and controls, respectively; $p = 0.000$) and RMS voltages in the last 20 ms of the P wave (3.06 ± 0.3 μV vs. 5.66 ± 0.96 μV in patients with PAF and controls, respectively; $p = 0.000$) at 40–250 Hz bidirectional filtering were the most significant ones to discriminate the groups. We conclude that the analysis of the P wave by appropriate signal averaging techniques can be used in identifying patients at risk for PAF, and this probably may be extended to reentrant atrial tachyarrhythmias.

After having demonstrated that the SAECG analysis of the P wave could discriminate the patients at risk for the development of PAF, we performed another study to investigate the effects of the relief of left atrial wall tensions by balloon mitral valvuloplasty (BMV) in patients with mitral stenosis. It has been hypothesized that increased left atrial pressure and wall tension in mitral stenosis play a role in the development of atrial fibrillation, the most frequent arrhythmia in these patients, by causing a delayed and fragmented depolarization. Successful BMV is a typical example of acute reduction in atrial pressure and wall tension. We investigated the short-term effects of BMV on the high-frequency content of the signal-averaged P wave as a reflection of delayed and nonhomogenous depolarization in 13 patients with rheumatic mitral stenosis who underwent successful BMV. We used the same high-gain data acquisition hardware and obtained recordings before and 72 h after the procedure. The high-frequency P wave duration and RMS voltages in the last 20, 25, and 30 ms of the P wave were calculated. However, we could not demonstrate any statistically significant difference in these parameters before and after the procedure ($p > 0.05$; filtered P wave duration 116.9 ± 3.6 vs. 116.5 ± 3.1 ms, RMS voltages in the last 20 ms 9.47 ± 0.92 vs. 6.65 ± 0.82 μV before and after the procedure, respectively). Therefore, our data did not support the suggestion that the increased atrial wall tension might be related to the development of a substrate for atrial fibrillation in patients with mitral stenosis.

As described above, the signal-averaged analysis of P waves has some advantages. The smaller amplitude and the gradual change in the waveform of the P wave from the baseline create difficulties in investigating it by conventional systems analyzing the QRS complex, and investigators have been directed to develop new software for this purpose. Some authors selected the QRS complex as the template and found no difference in the filtered P wave duration between controls and PAF patients [3]. It has indeed been demonstrated that choosing the QRS complex as a reference may cause significant changes even in the same patient due to the changes in the P-R interval [8]. The authors also found that this system lowered the amplitude of the signals on the P wave (smoothing effect) due to the matching errors. Our own experience in an earlier study was also consistent with these findings, and we developed a P wave-referred system as explained above [14]. However, it should be emphasized that a surface P wave-referred system is not an ideal one. Significant alignment errors may be encountered depending on the technique used. Donnerstein et al. suggested choosing the template after filtering by a 10–300 Hz filter to reduce the alignment errors. Thus, we filtered the data before choosing the P wave reference in our study. We also evaluated the possible alignment errors in our studies. For this purpose, the esophageal recordings were used which showed clear waveforms with a higher amplitude of P waves. When the temporal relation of the beats aligned with esophageal reference was compared with those of the classical Z lead reference, we found a 1.8 ± 0.6 ms alignment error, which is acceptable for our system of 1 ms sampling rate.

On the other hand, we recognized that the way of filtering is also important as unidirectional filtering has resulted in the artificial extension of the signal (ringing effect), while it has been possible to obtain clear tracings with bidirectional filtering. We suggest using bidirectional filtering to reduce artifacts created by the recording technique itself.

In conclusion, the currently available data suggest that the SAECG analysis of P wave might be useful in evaluating patients with atrial tachyarrhythmias when the appropriate technique is used. Moreover, the application of this method may also be expanded to evaluate patients with atrial infarction as well as those with atrial pacing to detect an arrhythmogenic substrate. Further studies are needed to reach a consensus on the value of the high-resolution analysis of the P wave.

REFERENCES

1. Simson MB. Use of signals in the terminal QRS complex to identify patients with ventricular tachycardia after myocardial infarction. Circulation 1981;64:235.
2. Leier CV, Meacham JA, Schaal SF. Prolonged atrial conduction: a major predisposing factor for atrial flutter. Circulation 1978;57:213.
3. Engel TR, Vallone N, Windle J. Signal-averaged electrocardiograms in patients with atrial fibrillation or flutter. Am Heart J 1988;115:592.
4. Chang AC, Winkler JP, Fananazapir L. P wave signal averaging identifies hypertrophic cardiomyopathy patients with paroxysmal atrial fibrillation. J Am Coll Cardiol 1990;15(Suppl):191A.
5. Yamada T, Fukunami M, Ohmori M et al. Clinical significance of atrial signal-averaged electrocardiogram for detection of patients with paroxysmal atrial fibrillation during sinus rhythm. Circulation 1989;80(Suppl II):636.
6. Pellerin D, Attuel P, Davy M et al. Signal-averaged P wave analysis: a new technique for detection of patients with paroxysmal atrial arrhythmias and noninvasive evaluation of intraatrial conduction time. Correlation with Holter monitoring and electrophysiologic study (Cardiostim 1990 abstract). RBM 1990;12:142.
7. Pellerin D, Attuel P, Davy M et al. Evaluation of signal averaged P wave in patients with and without history of atrial arrhythmias. Comparison with ECG and electrophysiologic study. Eur Heart J 1991;12(Suppl):P1429.
8. Fukunami M, Yamada T, Ohmori M et al. Detection of patients at risk for paroxysmal atrial fibrillation during sinus rhythm by P wave triggered signal-averaged electrocardiogram. Circulation 1991;83:162.
9. Villani GQ, Rosi A, Gandolfini A et al. Analysis of atrial signal averaged ECG recorded by the transesophageal technique. Eur Heart J 1991;12(Suppl):P1428.
10. Stafford PJ, Turner I, Vincent R. Quantitative analysis of signal averaged P waves in idiopathic paroxysmal atrial fibrillation. Am J Cardiol 1991;68:751.
11. Zelenkofske S, Gelernt M, Wong SC, Menchevez GE, Steinberd JS. The value of P wave signal averaged ECG for predicting atrial fibrillation after open heart surgery: a prospective study. JACC 1993;21:181A.
12. Paylos JE, Cordero B, Lopez de Sa E, Saenz Dela Calzade C. Spectral temporal mapping of the P wave in subjects with paroxysmal atrial fibrillation. JACC 1993:121:181A.
13. Özin B, Oto MA, Saki C, Müderrisoğlu H, Korkmaz M, Ider Z. Analysis of signal averaged P wave identifies patients at risk for paroxysmal atrial fibrillation. Circulation 1992;86:1–131.
14. Müderrisoğlu H, Özin B, Korkmaz M, Saki C. Ider Z, Oto MA. Signal averaged analysis of the P wave. Eur JCPE 1992;2:A161.

14. Late potentials during acute myocardial ischaemia

P.E. VARDAS, F.J. PARTHENAKIS & E.G. MANIOS

INTRODUCTION

Although it is recognised that acute myocardial ischaemia can lead to ventricular arrhythmogenesis, it is not clear how often this result occurs, nor has the mechanism which produces the arrhythmogenesis been elucidated. In recent years, particular significance has been given to late potentials on the signal-averaged electrocardiogram (SAECG), which are considered to reveal a substrate for the development of ventricular arrhythmias due to reentry mechanisms [1–4].

It is thus reasonable to seek a relationship between acute myocardial ischaemia and late potentials. A positive correlation would support the view that ischaemia causes a modification of intraventricular conduction and non-homogeneous depolarisation of the ventricular myocardium, leading to the development of reentry conditions and the appearance of arrhythmias [5–9]. To date, a small number of studies have examined this relationship using the SAECG and have concluded that acute ischaemia does not cause any significant changes in either the amplitude or the duration of the terminal portion of the QRS complex [10–12]. The purpose of this study was to examine the SAECG before and after a positive exercise test in a large number of non-syncopal ischaemic patients in order to investigate the effects of ischaemia on late potentials in three distinct, selected patient groups with differing severity and prognosis.

PATIENTS AND METHODS

Study population

Four groups of individuals were studied, including a control group (Group 1) comprised of healthy individuals with an age and sex distribution similar to the other three groups. The other three groups included patients with known ischaemic heart disease and recent positive exercise test. To ensure the uniformity of these groups and to minimise the effect of multiple factors in the final statistical evaluation, all patients had to satisfy the following criteria:

1. Resting ECG in sinus rhythm with no indication of bundle branch block, QRS duration < 120 ms, no ST-T segment abnormalities. Patients with pacemakers were also excluded.
2. No medication whatsoever taken during the three days prior to the study. Any patients requiring such treatment during that period were excluded, as were any who had taken amiodarone during the month before the study.
3. Depression or the ST segment ⩾ 1.5 mm on at least two leads in a recent exercise stress test. A coronary angiography was not considered necessary, even though 68 of the 96 coronary patients had in fact undergone angiography previously.
4. For those patients with a history of infarction, this had to have occurred at least 3 months before the study.
5. Patients satisfying the above criteria were excluded if they had a history of syncope of probable cardiac origin.

All the patients were examined in the hospital after giving their informed consent to the study.

Patient groups

Group I (control group) contained 30 individuals (20 men, 10 women), aged 40–65 years (53 ± 8; mean ± SD), non-smokers with no history of arterial hypertension or diabetes mellitus. All had performed a normal exercise stress test a few days before the study, as well as 24-h Holter ECG monitoring which showed no ventricular arrhythmogenesis.

Group II consisted of 35 patients with known ischaemic heart disease (24 men, 11 women), aged 57 ± 8 years, with a recent positive exercise stress test but no history of myocardial infarction and no ventricular arrhythmias in the history or on 24-h Holter ECG monitoring.

Group III included 35 patients (28 men, 7 women), aged 53 ± 6 years, with a history of myocardial ischaemia, a recent positive exercise test and proven ventricular arrhythmogenesis.

Group IV contained 26 patients (22 men, 4 women), aged 53 ± 5 years, with a history of at least one infarction, recent positive exercise stress test and proven ventricular arrhythmogenesis (Lown II, III, IV) on 24-h Holter ECG monitoring.

Study protocol

All the individuals studied underwent a baseline 12-lead resting ECG and a SAECG, followed by a treadmill exercise test (Marquette CASE 12) and a further SAECG 2 min after the end of the test, with the patient in a reclining position. The endpoint of the treadmill test was age-adjusted target heart rate and/or ST segment depression 1.5 mm, fatigue or chest pain.

The SAECG was recorded using the Arrhythmia Research Technology 1200EPX system using Simson's methods. Electrodes were applied in standard bipolar orthogonal X, Y and Z configuration, and the three leads were recorded simultaneously. Each signal was digitalised to 16-bit accuracy with a sampling rate of 4 kHz. Averaging was based on an algorithm which selected the most representative QRS forms. Thus, ectopic beats, as well as those with excessive noise components, were excluded from the averaging process. In each case, at least 250 beats were averaged to obtain satisfactory noise reduction.

After averaging, the data were transferred for magnetic storage using a Hewlett Packard 386 IBM PC compatible computer, at a sampling rate of 1 kHz (i.e. 4:1 data compression). For analysis in the time domain, the signal was passed through a two-way band-pass filter (40–250 Hz). The three leads were combined into a graph showing the root mean square (RMS) vector magnitude ($X^2 + Y^2 + Z^2$). The parameters measured were as follows:

1. Duration of filtered QRS (QRSD).
2. The duration of the low amplitude signals (< 40 μV) of the QRS complex (LAS40).
3. RMS of QRS amplitude during the last 40 ms recorded (RMS40).

Late potentials were defined according to the following criteria:

a. QRSd > 120 ms
b. RMS40 < 25 μV
c. LAS40 > 38 ms

Late potentials were considered positive if two of these criteria were fulfilled. A noise level range not exceeding 0.3 μV was considered to be acceptable. If this was not achieved within 2 min from the end of the exercise test, the patient was excluded from the study.

Increased arrhythmogenesis, during or after exercise, was defined as a threefold increase in ventricular ectopic beats compared with the resting ECG and/or the appearance of bigeminy, couplets, non-sustained or sustained ventricular tachycardia.

Statistical analysis. Values of the SAECG parameters before and after exercise within the same group were compared using the paired *t*-test.

Table 1. Signal-averaged ECG parameters before and 2 min after exercise testing in the four groups of the study.

	Group I	Group II	Group III	Group IV
QRS-R (ms)	101 + 12	103 + 11	101 + 13	105 + 9
QRS-PE (ms)	100 + 11	103 + 12	101 + 12	112 + 12
Δ (ms)	−1	0	0	+7
p value	NS	NS	NS	< 0.05
LAS-R (ms)	29 + 11	33 + 12	30 + 11	33 + 11
LAS-PE (ms)	28 + 11	33 + 12	29 + 11	41 + 13
Δ(ms)	−1	0	−1	+8
p value	NS	NS	NS	< 0.05
RMS-RE (μV)	45 + 13	37 + 10	38 + 19	37 + 14
RMS-PE (μV)	44 + 12	36 + 11	36 + 18	35 + 16
Δ (μV)	−1	−1	−2	−2
p value	NS	NS	NS	NS

QRS-R = QRS resting; QRS-PE = QRS post-exercise; LAS-R = low amplitude signals resting; LAS-PE = low amplitude signals post-exercise; RMS-R = root mean square resting; RMS-PE = root mean square post-exercise.

RESULTS

Of the 126 individuals who initially comprised the four study groups, 18 were excluded for the following reasons:

1. Thirteen (Group I: 2, II: 5, III: 4, IV: 2) because of unacceptable noise level immediately after exercise.
2. Five because of problems during the exercise test which invalidated the subsequent evaluation. Two of these (Group II: 1, III: 1) suffered intense ischaemic pain. One (Group III) suffered supraventricular tachycardia. The other two (Group IV) experienced severe deterioration of the ventricular arrhythmogenicity.

Immediately after exercise and during the recording of the SAECG, ST segment depression persisted in 26 patients of Group II, 28 of Group III and 20 of Group IV.

The parameters calculated from the SAECG are shown in Table 1. There were no significant differences between the values before and after exercise in any group. More detailed findings from the individual groups were as follows:

Group I. Of the 30 controls, before exercise one had late potentials which disappeared after exercise. Also, after exercise in eight subjects, there was a tendency to shortening of the duration of the QRS complex and the LAS40 and a small increase in the RMS40 value.

Group II. Of the 35 patients, three (9%) had late potentials before exercise. These disappeared after exercise in one but were sustained in the other two. Another patient with normal parameters before exercise exhibited late potentials immediately after exercise, and these persisted for 20 min. None of these patients had any appreciable arrhythmogenesis. As mentioned above, another six patients of this group, all with no late potentials, were excluded from the study for the reasons described.

Group III. Of the 35 patients, five (14%) had late potentials at rest. After exercise, four patients showed no significant change, while the measured parameters were normal in the remaining one. A further two patients with normal results before exercise developed late potentials after exercise. Ventricular ectopic beats (Lown II, III) were observed in 15 patients during exercise and/or immediately afterwards. Two of these had late potentials before and immediately after exercise.

Group IV. Of the 26 patients, six (23%) experienced late potentials before exercise. The parameters were unchanged after exercise in 4, while in the remaining 2 the values showed changes tending towards normal. Another three patients had late potentials after exercise only.

All of the six patients with pre-exercise late potentials showed a worsening of arrhythmia during exercise. Three had non-sustained ventricular tachycardia. Two of the three patients with post exercise late potentials showed a worsening of arrhythmia during exercise. A further seven patients with no late potentials before or after exercise showed a worsening of arrhythmias during exercise.

As mentioned above, four patients of this group were excluded from the post-exercise measurements because of a high noise level or the appearance of dangerous ventricular arrhythmias. One of these without late potentials before exercise had ventricular flutter and was defibrillated, while two exhibited non-sustained ventricular tachycardia.

DISCUSSION

The findings of this study showed that ischaemia caused by exercise had no effect on the SAECG parameters in those ischaemic patients without a history of myocardial infarction. These results confirm the previous findings of Caref et al. [11], who also observed no changes in the SAECG after a positive exercise test, as well as those of Turitto et al. [12], who reported similar findings in patients with spontaneously developed transient myocardial ischaemia. There were, however, changes in the group of patients with a history of myocardial infarction. This should perhaps be studied further, along with the observations from certain other studies which found significant changes in the SAECG during coronary angioplasty.

It could thus be claimed that ischaemia induced by exercise or by dipyridamole administration is not severe enough to cause changes in the SAECG or the recording of late potentials. It should certainly be stressed that these assumptions must take into account the possibility that the techniques used today for the detection of late potentials might not be sufficiently accurate to locate limited ischaemic regions of the ventricular myocardium which develop slow conduction and fragmented electrical activity. Anyway, it is known from previous studies that the greater the number of sites with abnormal slow activation during endocardial mapping, the greater the chance of recording ventricular late potentials on the body surface.

It should be noted here that in our study the only patients to exhibit late potentials on the SAECG during exercise test-induced ischaemia were those who had suffered a previous myocardial infarction. This finding was probably due to the fact that the ischaemia around the infarct site covered a larger region of electrical inhomogeneity than in patients with acute ischaemia but without a history of myocardial infarction. Our results supports previous animal studies which suggest that there is a higher incidence of spontaneous ventricular tachycardia and more marked electrophysiological abnormalities when ischaemia is superimposed on a previous healed myocardial infarction.

REFERENCES

1. Breithardt G, Becker R, Seipel L, Abendroth RR, Ostermeyer J. Noninvasive detection of late potentials in man – a new marker for ventricular tachycardia. Eur Heart J 1981;2:1–11.
2. Rozanski JJ, Mortara D, Myerburg RJ, Castellanos A. Body surface detection of delayed depolarizations in patients with recurred ventricular tachycardia and left ventricular aneurysm. Circulation 1981;63:1172–8.
3. Breithardt G, Borggrefe M, Haerten K. Ventricular late potentials and inducible ventricular tachyarrhythmias as a marker for ventricular tachycardia after myocardial infarction. Eur Heart J 1986;7:127–34.
4. Breithardt G, Borggrefe M. Pathophysiological mechanisms and clinical significance of ventricular late potentials. Eur Heart J 1986;7:364–85.
5. Han J, Gael BG, Hanson CS. Reentrant beats induced in the ventricle during coronary occlusion. Am Heart J 1970;80:778–84.
6. Scherlag BJ, Helfant RH, Haft JI, Damato AN. Electrophysiology underlying ventricular arrhythmias due to coronary ligation. Am J Physiol 1970; 219:1665–71.
7. Waldo AL, Kaiser GA. Study of ventricular arrhythmias associated with acute myocardial infarction in the canine heart. Circulation 1973;47:1222–8.
8. Boineau JP, Cox JL. Slow ventricular activation in acute myocardial infarction. A source of reentrant premature ventricular contractions. Circulation 1973:48:702–3.
9. El-Sherif N, Scherlag BJ, Lazzara R. Electrode catheter recordings during malignant ventricular arrhythmias following experimental acute myocardial ischemia. Circulation 1975;51:1003–14.
10. Turitto G, Zanchi E, Risa AL et al. Lack of correlation between transient myocardial ischemia and late potentials on the signal-averaged electrocardiogram. Am J Cardiol 1990;65:290–6.
11. Caref EB, Goldberg N, Mendelson L et al. Effects of exercise on the signal-averaged electrocardiogram in coronary artery disease. Am J Cardiol 1990;66:54–8.
12. Turitto G, Caref EB, Zanchi E, Menghini F, Kelen G, El-Sherif N. Spontaneous myocardial ischemia and the signal-averaged electrocardiogram. Am J Cardiol 1991;67:676–80.

15. Radiofrequency catheter ablation in the treatment of supraventricular tachycardias

FRANK SIMONIS, ERIK ANDRIES & PEDRO BRUGADA

INTRODUCTION

Catheter ablative techniques have been used in controlling arrhythmias since the early 1980's. Initially, direct current (DC) catheter ablation was used, using a conventional defibrillator. Some 10 years ago, the first experimental studies were performed using radiofrequency energy [1,2]. Since 1987, radio frequency energy has been used in humans for the treatment of a variety of supraventricular tachycardias. Interest in its use for the treatment of ventricular arrhythmias is growing [3,4]. In this study, we describe our experience with 306 consecutive patients undergoing radiofrequency ablation for supraventricular tachycardias with special emphasis on the duration of the procedure, results, and complications.

METHODS

Patients

The patients in this study were referred to our center for electrophysiologic study and radiofrequency ablation. There were 306 patients with supraventricular tachycardia (154 men and 152 women with an age ranging from 5 to 82 years, mean 47 years). Six patients had complex congenital heart disease: three had Ebstein's disease of the tricuspid valve and a right-sided accessory pathway, one had a coarctation of the aorta with corrected transposition of the great vessels and Ebstein's disease of the tricuspid valve with two left-sided accessory pathways, one had dextroversion of the heart and a parahisian accessory pathway, and one had three congenital aneurysms of the descending thoracic aorta and a left-sided accessory pathway. Six patients had both atrioventricular (AV) nodal reentrant tachycardia and an accessory pathway.

Techniques

All patients gave informed consent to their participation in the study. The electrophysiologic study and radiofrequency ablation were performed in a single session while the patients were in a fasting unsedated state. All antiarrhythmic medications were discontinued at least 24 h before the procedure. Topical anesthesia was given with lidocaine 2%. After the catheters had been positioned, a bolus of 3000–5000 units of heparin was administered intravenously. The ablation catheter used was a 7F Mansfield catheter (Mansfield-Webster, Mansfield, MA) with a 4 mm interelectrode space. The radiofrequency device used was a HAT 200 (Dr. Osypka GmbH). The power setting ranges from 0 to 50 watts and has an automatic switch-off if the impedance rises above a critical value during the procedure, when tissue dessication or coagulum formation occurs. In that case, the ablation catheter is taken out and cleaned. Continuous unmodulated energy of 550 kHz was delivered for 30 s in the range of 30–35 watts between the tip of the ablation catheter (cathode) and a paddle placed over the left scapula (anode). The electrocardiogram was continuously monitored during the administration of radiofrequency energy. After the procedure, a 12–24 h ambulatory telemetry was carried out, and the patients were discharged from the hospital without any antiarrhythmic drugs. Acetylsalicylic acid 100 mg/day was given to all patients the first month after ablation.

Atrioventricular nodal reentrant tachycardia. In patients with AV nodal tachycardia, a 7F steerable quadripolar catheter was advanced to record bipolar electrograms in the vicinity of the AV node prior to the radiofrequency ablation. The catheter was first placed across the tricuspid annulus to record a His bundle potential and thereafter slowly drawn back so that a large atrial deflection was recorded. The target sites for fast pathway ablation have an atrial:ventricular ratio > 1 and a small (< 100 mV) or absent His bundle potential. The energy is given until the atrium to His (AH) interval prolongs by approximately 50% or when a nonconducting P wave is seen. If a sustained junctional rhythm was seen, the energy application was stopped for several seconds to assess AV conduction. Ventricular stimulation is performed after ablation to evaluate the absence of ventriculoatrial (VA) conduction. Atrial stimulation is also carried out in order to check whether or not intranodal tachycardia is still inducible and to obtain the anterograde Wenckebach cycle length and the effective refractory period of the AV conduction system. Ablation of the slow AV nodal pathway usually occurs when the ablation catheter is placed inferior to the site of recording of a His bundle potential, towards the posterior septum, while ablation of the fast AV nodal pathway is seen when locating the ablation catheter more anterior to the site of recording of a His bundle potential, towards the midseptum.

Wolff–Parkinson–White syndrome. In patients with the Wolff–Parkinson–

White syndrome, the site of ablation depends on the localization of the accessory AV pathway. In left-sided pathways, the ablation catheter is advanced through the femoral artery retrogradely to the aortic valve and left ventricle. It is then manipulated against the mitral annulus, where the energy will be applied. In right-sided and septal accessory pathways, the catheter is advanced through the femoral vein and positioned on the atrial side of the tricuspid annulus. In posteroseptal pathways, it is sometimes necessary to ablate from the left ventricle or just outside the mouth of the coronary sinus. Also in right-sided accessory pathways, a second guiding catheter placed in the right coronary artery can be used to localize the AV groove. In manifest preexcitation, mapping during sinus rhythm can reveal the correct site of ablation if (1) the earliest ventricular activation occurs as compared with the onset of the delta wave with (2) the presence of the shortest possible AV interval and (3) a discrete potential (accessory pathway?) is recorded between the atrial and ventricular activity. In concealed accessory pathways, mapping during tachycardia shows the site of ablation if (1) the earliest activation occurs and (2) the shortest possible VA interval is present and (3) an accessory pathway potential is recorded when possible (continuous activity).

Ablation of the bundle of His. In patients with chronic atrial fibrillation or atrial flutter, complete block of conduction in the His bundle was created by means of radiofrequency energy. In patients who already had a permanent pacemaker, the device was programmed in VOO mode. In all patients, a 6F catheter was advanced through the femoral vein and placed in the right ventricular apex for temporary pacing. Then the ablation catheter was introduced into the right femoral vein and manipulated across the tricuspid valve to record a His bundle electrogram, and energy was delivered at this localization. If this "right-sided approach" was not successful, the catheter was advanced to the left ventricle via a retrograde arterial approach and placed in the interventricular septum in order to obtain the largest possible His bundle potential, and radiofrequency ablation was performed at this site. This "left-sided approach" was used as first choice in the last patients who entered the study [5]. The radiofrequency ablation was considered successful if complete AV block occurred. A temporary pacing lead was left in the right ventricular apex until the implantation of a permanent VVIR pacemaker was carried out.

Ablation of atrial tachycardia and atrial flutter. Radiofrequency ablation is highly effective for the treatment of supraventricular arrhythmias related to accessory pathways or intranodal reentry. However, experience with radiofrequency ablation of atrial flutter or ectopic atrial tachycardia is more limited. In all patients with atrial tachycardia or atrial flutter, a 6F reference catheter is used which is manipulated in the high right atrium. Early potentials are used as electrophysiologic criteria for the ablation site in atrial tachycardia. In atrial flutter, a line of block was created from the inferior

Table 1. Results of radiofrequency ablation in 306 patients with supraventricular tachycardias.

	AVNT (n = 101)	AP (n = 121)	HIS (n = 70)	AT (n = 5)	AF (n = 9)
PD (min)	9–120 (mean 47)	15–420 (mean 92)	8–170 (mean 55)	20–90 (mean 56)	30–150 (mean 56)
NA	1–34 (mean 4)	1–48 (mean 10)	1–44 (mean 8)	1–14 (mean 8)	3–76 (mean 19)
RET (min)	2–65 (mean 15)	3–158 (mean 34)	3–48 (mean 19)	5–30 (mean 18)	10–105 (mean 40)
Recurrence	11 (11%)	6 (5%)	0	0	0
Redo	10	5	0	0	0
Failure	0	1	0	1 (20%)	6 (66%)
Complications	4 (AV-bl)	2 (AV-bl)	0	0	0
Success rate	99%	97%	100%	80%	34%

AVNT = atrioventricular nodal tachycardia; AP = accessory pathway; AT = atrial tachycardia; AF = atrial flutter; PD = procedure duration; NA = number of applications; RET = radiation exposure time; Redo = second ablation session; AV-bl = complete AV block.

vena cava to the coronary sinus mouth and from the coronary sinus mouth to the AV node by giving multiple applications of radiofrequency energy.

RESULTS

Atrioventricular nodal reentrant tachycardia

This group consisted of 101 patients (29 men and 72 women, aged 8–81 years) with only AV nodal reentrant tachycardia (95 patients) or with both intranodal tachycardia and an accessory AV pathway (6 patients). Radiofrequency ablation resulted in a selective block of the fast AV nodal pathway in 76 patients (75%) and of the slow AV nodal pathway in the remaining 25 (25%). The procedure duration time, the number of radiofrequency energy applications and the radiation exposure time are shown in Table 1. Ablation was successful in the first session in 90 patients; in 11 patients recurrences of intranodal tachycardia were seen. Ten other patients underwent a second procedure. One patient underwent a total of 3 ablation sessions and was finally successfully ablated. One patient is still waiting for a new attempt. In four patients complete AV block occurred, and a DDD pacemaker was implanted. Six patients presented with sinus tachycardia after the ablation procedure, with rates between 120 and 150 bpm persisting from 2 h to 4 days and disappearing spontaneously in all without any treatment. After a mean follow-up of 10 months, 100 (99%) patients are asymptomatic.

Table 2. Results of ablation of accessory pathways in relation to their localization.

	LFW	RFW	Septal	PD (min)	NA	RET (min)
Manifest preexcitation (81 patients)	45	5	31	15–240 (mean 85)	1–48 (mean 11)	3–100 (mean 34)
Concealed AP (36 patients)	21	1	14	25–420 (mean 86)	1–27 (mean 8)	5–158 (mean 31)
Multiple AP (4 patients)	3	1	6	45–360 (mean 141)	3–27 (mean 12)	10–134 (mean 47)
Total number AP (n = 127 in 121 patients)	69	7	51	15–420 (mean 92)	1–48 (mean 10)	3–158 (mean 34)

Abbreviations as in Table 1; LFW = left free wall; RFW = right free wall.

Wolff–Parkinson–White syndrome

This group of 121 patients with a total of 127 accessory pathways underwent radiofrequency ablation (69 men and 52 women, aged 7–70 years). In 81 patients, manifest preexcitation was present. A concealed accessory pathway was diagnosed in 36 patients. Four patients had multiple accessory AV pathways with a maximum of 4 in one patient. In six patients, both AV nodal tachycardia and Wolff–Parkinson–White syndrome were present, and all were successfully cured by radiofrequency energy. After a mean follow up of 8 months, in six patients the first session of radiofrequency ablation failed, or recurrences of circus movement tachycardia were observed; in another patient, a second ablation procedure was necessary because of an anatomically wide accessory pathway. In the patient with 4 pathways, 3 were successfully ablated (a posteroseptal, anteroseptal, and a left lateral one) by radio frequency energy, but a second and third procedure failed to ablate the second anteroseptal accessory pathway, and this patient is now being treated with oral flecainide. In two patients, complete AV block occurred: one patient had a parahisian accessory pathway and dextroversion of the heart, while the other patient had two septal accessory pathways. In the group of patients who showed recurrences or whose first procedure failed, five underwent a second ablation session successfully, resulting in a success rate of 97%. Table 1 shows the procedure duration, number of energy applications, and radiation exposure time; Table 2 shows these variables for the several localizations of accessory pathways.

Ablation of the His bundle

Radiofrequency ablation of the bundle of His was performed in 70 consecutive patients with atrial fibrillation (45 men and 25 women, aged 21–82 years). In the first 24 patients, the right-sided approach was used. However, in six patients it was not possible to obtain AV block after multiple (mean

Table 3. Results of ablation of the bundle of His.

	Right-sided approach (n = 26)	Left-sided approach (n = 20)	Right- and left-sided approach (n = 24)
PD (min)	24–170 (mean 73)	20–120 (mean 42)	25–105 (mean 58)
NA	1–44 (mean 9)	1–37 (mean 5)	1–33 (mean 11)
RET (min)	6–48 (mean 19)	4–45 (mean 12)	8–37 (mean 18)

Abbreviations as in Table 1.

9) applications of radiofrequency energy. For this reason, the same catheter was advanced to record a His bundle potential using a retrograde arterial approach, and AV block was created in all six patients. Subsequently, in the remaining prospective patients this left-sided approach was used as first choice, and complete AV block was achieved in all. Radiofrequency ablation of the bundle of His had a 100% success rate. Table 1 shows the procedure duration, number of applications, and radiation exposure time in the group of patients who underwent ablation of the bundle of His; Table 3 shows these variables for the different approaches used in ablation of the bundle of His.

Atrial tachycardia and atrial flutter

Five patients with ectopic atrial tachycardia underwent radiofrequency ablation (4 men, 1 woman; aged 17–75 years). In four patients it was possible to stop the atrial tachycardia and to prevent new episodes of tachycardia by radiofrequency energy, resulting in a success rate of 80%. In the group of nine patients with atrial flutter (6 men, 3 women; aged 33–76 years), the flutter was converted to sinus rhythm in only three cases, resulting in a success rate of 34%. No complications occurred in this group of patients with atrial arrhythmias. Table 1 shows the procedure duration time, radiation exposure time, and number of energy applications.

DISCUSSION

As can be observed from the reported data, radiofrequency energy can be used with a high success rate for the cure of a variety of supraventricular arrhythmias. When sufficient electrophysiologic expertise is present, success rates above 90% have been noted for a single session. However, experience with radiofrequency ablation of atrial flutter or ectopic atrial tachycardia is still limited. Especially in patients with atrial tachycardias, radiofrequency ablation seems to be a promising treatment; however, more investigation in larger patient populations is still required to make the success reproducible. A variety of factors affect the duration of the procedure, among them the presence of multiple accessory pathways or of different types of arrhythmias. However, when the more unusual patients are excluded, the duration of the procedure has remained relatively constant over time. There is certainly a learning curve for any new technique, but the duration of the procedure for radiofrequency ablation of cardiac arrhythmias cannot be expected to shorten over time. In some patients, a single catheter technique can be used with successful ablation being accomplished even within 15 min, as in one of our cases. Similarly, in rare patients, successful ablation of AV nodal tachycardia was obtained in less than 10 min. In general, however, one has to consider that radiofrequency ablation of a supraventricular arrhythmia will take 90 min. In terms of efficacy and complications, it is clear that radiofrequency ablation represents a major advance in the treatment of cardiac arrhythmias. The only other treatment which could really cure supraventricular tachycardia is surgery; however, depending upon the technique used, significant morbidity and even mortality exist. The few complications we had demonstrate the safety of our technique. Radiofrequency ablation is nowadays the therapy of first choice in the treatment of supraventricular tachycardia caused by an accessory pathway or by intranodal reentry. In patients with atrial flutter or fibrillation, ablation of the bundle of His and implantation of a VVIR pacemaker may have advantages over long-term antiarrhythmic drug treatment. Radiofrequency ablation has important advantages when compared with surgery, antitachycardia pacemakers, or long-term antiarrhythmic drug treatment.

REFERENCES

1. Huang SK, Jordan N, Graham A et al. Closed-chest catheter desiccation of atrioventricular junction using radiofrequency energy—a new method of catheter ablation (abstract). Circulation 1985;72:III-389.
2. Huang SK, Graham AR, Hoyt RH et al. Transcatheter desiccation of the canine left ventricle using radiofrequency energy: A pilot study. Am Heart J 1987;1134:43-8.
3. Huang SK. Radio-frequency catheter ablation of cardiac arrhythmias: appraisal of an evolving therapeutic modality. Am Heart J 1989;118:1317-23.
4. Gursoy S, Brugada J, Souza O, Steurer G, Andries E, Brugada P. Radiofrequency ablation of symptomatic but benign ventricular arrhythmias. PACE 1992;15:738-41.
5. Souza OF, Gursoy S, Simonis F, Steurer G, Brugada P. Ablation of atrioventricular conduction using radiofrequency energy. PACE 1992;15:1454-9.

16. Anatomical versus electrophysiological approaches for ablation of the slow pathway in patients with AV nodal reentrant tachycardia

MICHEL HAISSAGUERRE, BRUNO FISCHER,
PHILIPPE LE MÉTAYER, PIERRE JAIS, PHILIPPE EGLOFF
& JEAN-FRANÇOIS WARIN

INTRODUCTION

Different approaches have been described [1–12] for ablating the slow 'pathway' (SP) in patients with atrioventricular nodal reentrant tachycardia (AVNRT). In one approach, electrogram patterns are used to identify the ablation site [1,4], whereas in the other approach, the ablating site is selected on anatomical criteria. Both approaches appear effective, but no study (except one preliminary abstract [8]) comparing the two techniques has been published. In the following study, we analyze the results of these different techniques and investigated the prevalence of electrogram patterns and their relation to a successful outcome in a series of 164 patients.

ANATOMICAL APPROACH

This technique involves multiple unguided radiofrequency (RF) current applications in the posteroinferior interatrial septum. From the His bundle region position, the catheter is withdrawn along the tricuspid septal annulus down to the most posterior/inferior aspect of the interatrial septum adjacent to the coronary sinus ostium. However, one electrogram criterion is used by all authors to select target sites, i.e. an atrial/ventricular electrogram ratio of 0.5 or less.

One or usually two subsequent applications of RF energy are applied, and then the inducibility of AVNRT is assessed. If the tachycardia is still inducible, new RF applications are delivered at another site in a saggital or frontal plane, i.e. either at the same posterior level but more atrially by pulling back the catheter [5] or more cephalad towards the midseptum. Serial RF applications are delivered until either the noninducibility of tachycardias or the total elimination of SP conduction occurs.

The main results from published studies [2,3,5–9] are the following (see Table 1). The success rate is high (88–100%) but requires a median or mean number of 5 [9] to 20 [5] RF applications to achieve this. Fast pathway conduction is simultaneously modified in 8–13% of cases, and the prevalence of AV block is very low (0–3%). Recurrence of tachycardias is observed in 0–29% of patients, most figures being between 9 and 14% [10,11].

ELECTROPHYSIOLOGICAL APPROACHES

This technique is based on three different types of electrophysiologic criteria, retrograde SP mapping [1,2,12], spike potentials [1], and slow potentials [4].

Retrograde SP mapping

Whereas retrograde fast pathway can be nearly always mapped to guide ablation, sustained retrograde SP conduction is present in only a fraction of patients during either ventricular stimulation or atypical fast-slow tachycardia. In a study by Jazayeri et al. [12], the retrograde conduction over the SP could be identified in 24 of 106 patients. This criterion appeared an impressive marker for SP ablation, since 100% of patients were cured after a single RF application. Based on this result, the development of electrophysiologic or pharmacologic maneuvers allowing a sustained retrograde SP conduction would be of great interest.

Spike potentials

Jackman et al. were the first to demonstrate the feasibility of RF catheter ablation of the SP. Initially, these investigators used retrograde SP activation mapping and then were guided by a spike potential that is described as the SP potential or the activity of the SP atrial insertion.

During sinus rhythm, dual potentials were recorded in the posteroseptal region around or within the coronary sinus ostium. The first, a small atrial potential, was followed by a large second potential 10–40 ms later. During fast-slow AVNRT, the large SP potential preceded the smaller atrial potential. An atrial extrastimulus during fast-slow tachycardia advanced the timing of atrial activation without altering the SP potential. The target site for SP ablation was selected by the recording of the largest, sharpest and latest second potential during sinus rhythm [1].

In 80 patients, Jackman et al. eliminated AVNRT (SP in 78, fast pathway in 2) using a median of two RF pulses. No clinical recurrence of AVNRT was observed. The present experience (personal communication) of those authors includes 137 patients with a 100% success rate and a recurrence rate of 2%.

Table 1. Literature review.

Authors	Number of patients	Approach	Success rate (%)	Median or mean number of RF applications	Recurrence rate	Number of AV blocks	Modification of fast pathway (%)
Jazayeri et al.							
[2]	27	Anatomical	89	7	0	0	
[12]	82	Anatomical	93	5			13
Kay et al.							
[3]	34	Anatomical	88	10	3 (10%)	0	13
Langberg et al.							
[6]	28	Anatomical	96	7	1 (3%)	1	
Wathen et al.							
[5]	25	Anatomical	96	20	1/15 (4%)	0	8
Interian et al.							
[7]	7	Anatomical	100	7	2/7 (29%)		43
Wang et al.							
[9]	211	Anatomical	96	5	2/211 (1%)	3	11
Jazayeri et al.							
[2]	8	Retrograde	100	1	0		0
[12]	24	SP mapping	100	1	0		0
Jackman et al.							
[1]	80	Spike potential	100	2	1 (3%)	1	3
	137	Spike potential	100	1	3 (2%)	1	
Haissaguerre et al.							
[4]	64	Slow potential	100	2	0	0	8
	163	Slow potential	99	2	6 (3.6%)	0	

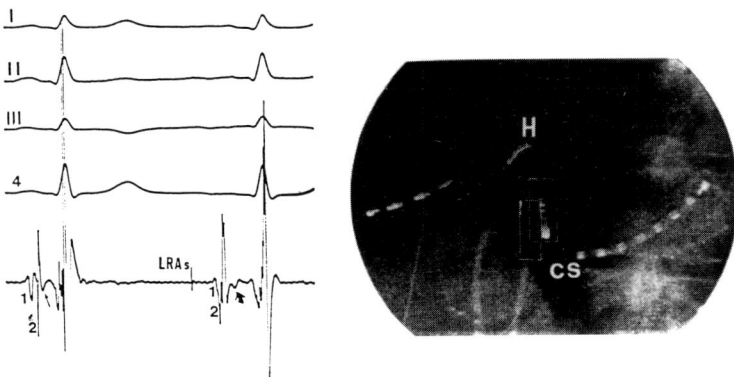

Figure 1. Radiogram shows in a left anterior oblique 60° view the usual recording site of slow potentials (top) and spike potentials (bottom) marked in two frames. The spike potential region lies more posteriorly than the slow potential region, but both overlap considerably. On the left are recordings of double potentials (1, 2) during sinus rhythm. In fact, the end of spike potential 2 is prolonged by a slow potential (arrow); this becomes evident (large arrow) with lateral atrial pacing stimulation (LRA stimulus). Note that LRA produces a fusion of potentials 1 and 2, thus shortening the double potential sequence (see [13]).

Slow potentials

Slow potentials were defined as a low-amplitude activity (0.05–0.5 mV) recordable in most humans along a band from the His bundle to the mid- and posterior part of the septum near the tricuspid annulus. The recording region of slow potentials was globally more anterior than that of the spike potentials, but both overlapped considerably (Figure 1). Slow potentials were better separated from preceding atrial electrograms at the mid-septum than at the posterior septum where they prolonged (or even were included on) the end of the atrial electrogram. Of note was the fact that atrial electrograms were often slurred and fractionated particularly in close proximity to the AV annulus (suggested by a low A/V electrogram ratio). Besides high gain amplification, atrial pacing maneuvers were mandatory to reveal slow potentials. Indeed, their most specific pattern (Figures 2–5) was their response to increasing atrial rates which resulted in: (a) a separation from preceding atrial electrograms (themselves unaltered by pacing rate), (b) a decline in amplitude and slope, and (c) an increase in duration until frequently any consistent activity disappeared. However, in some patients, a microactivity persisted, particularly during the first half of diastole in tachycardia, which probably represented the ultimate step in the rate disintegration of slow potentials (Figure 3). Significantly, stimulation could reverse the polarity of potentials. Only atrial pacing made it possible to reveal either slow potentials concealed within the atrial potential (Figures 1, 2) or slow potentials mimicking a sharp (Figures 3, 4) atrial potential (particularly in the form of multicomponent atrial potentials which nearly always included slow potentials). We have previously shown that slow potentials do not represent atrial repolarization or hisian activities [4]. Lastly, at the mid-septum, slow potentials with a significant His bundle potential could be recorded. Although atrial pacing separated them from preceding atrial electrograms, the potentials remained unaltered before the QRS complex occurring at the second half of the diastole at long AH intervals. We believe these potentials represent the activity of the compact AV node (Figure 5). The first ablation site selected was that showing a prominent slow potential in the posteroseptal region. The absence of a significant (>0.1 mV) His bundle potential was checked by atrial pacing prolonging the AV interval. Using a RF generator HAT 200, energy (20–40 W) was applied for 90 s during sinus rhythm or atrial pacing (when junctional rhythm occurred). If AVNRT was still inducible, energy was applied at posteroseptal contiguous sites showing similar recordings, then at more anterior sites.

Our experience now includes 164 patients. The fast pathway was deliberately or inadvertently ablated in eight. One high-degree AV block occurred during deliberate ablation of the fast pathway. Ablation of the SP was achieved in 154 (99%) and failed in two. In these two young patients, we judged during the ablation procedure the risk of AV block to be too high and stopped the session. SP was ablated/modified using an overall median of two RF pulses (1 pulse in 40% of patients). The time required for the therapeutic component was 41 ± 38 min, and fluoroscopic time was 14 ± 14 min. Isolated echo beats remained inducible in 64 patients and not inducible in 90. During a follow-up period of 1–33 months, 6 patients (3.6%) suffered a clinical recurrence of tachycardias 1–8 weeks alter ablation. Five of them had inducible echo beats just after ablation (8% of the 64 patients) whereas one had no echo beat (1% of the 90 patients).

We reviewed the electrograms recorded at successful SP ablation sites. Depending on their response to right lateral atrial pacing, two types of electrogram were differentiated; slow potentials and 'ordinary' atrial potentials defined as either simple or complex (either fractionated or multiple) potentials which were not deteriorated by pacing. Four electrogram combinations were present at successful sites (Figure 6): (1) both slow potentials and complex atrial potentials in 59%; (2) slow potentials and only simple atrial potentials in 23%; (3) no slow potential but complex atrial potentials in 15%; (4) neither slow potential nor complex atrial potentials in 3%. Therefore, slow potentials were present in 82% and complex atrial potentials in 74% of successful sites, their combination being the electrogram which best predicted a successful ablation. It is noteworthy that the complex atrial potential was 'a double potential' in 34% and 50% of electrograms in electro-

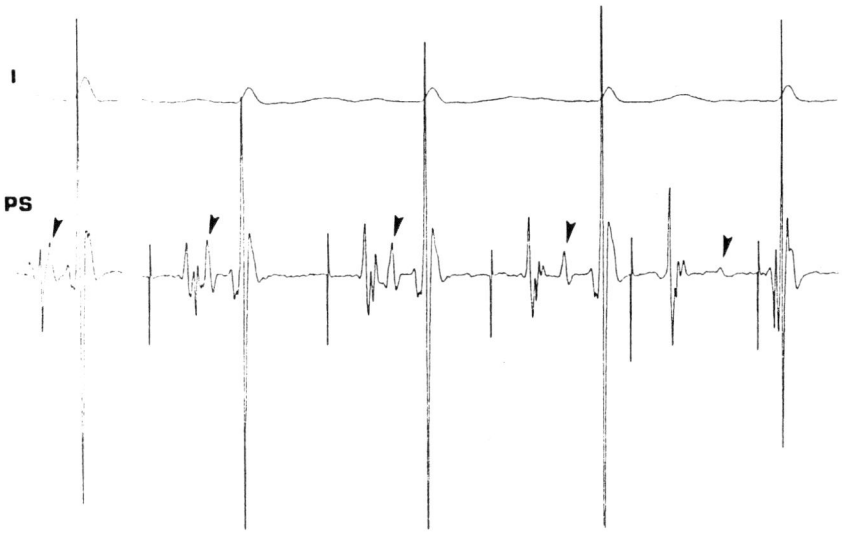

Figure 2. Simultaneous recordings of a double potential and a slow potential marked by an arrow at the posteroseptal (PS) region. During sinus rhythm, the slow potential can be confused with a terminal atrial potential. Atrial pacing separates and then attenuates the slow potential in contrast with the preceding atrial potentials.

gram combinations 1 and 3, respectively, whereas fractionated or multiple atrial electrograms were observed in other cases.

WHICH APPROACH IS BETTER?

Analysis of the current published data shows a similar success rate with both approaches. However, more RF pulses are required using the anatomical approach to achieve SP ablation (5–24 vs. 1–2). In contrast, SP can be ablated with only one RF lesion in almost half of the cases, using either spike or slow potential recordings, which argues against the need for a critical amount of tissue to be destroyed to prevent reentry. Yet, whatever the approach, the number of incidences of AV block appears not to vary. Furthermore, a high rate of AVNRT recurrence has been reported in some preliminary studies using the anatomical approach (9–14%), unlike what is observed in electrophysiologically guided ablation (2–4%). Hypothetically, this may be due to a lesser accuracy in targeting the SP. The Ann Arbor group has recently presented a preliminary study comparing prospectively both approaches for ablating the SP [8]. Both approaches were comparable in efficacy and duration, but there were significantly more 'complex' atrial

Approaches for slow-pathway ablation 151

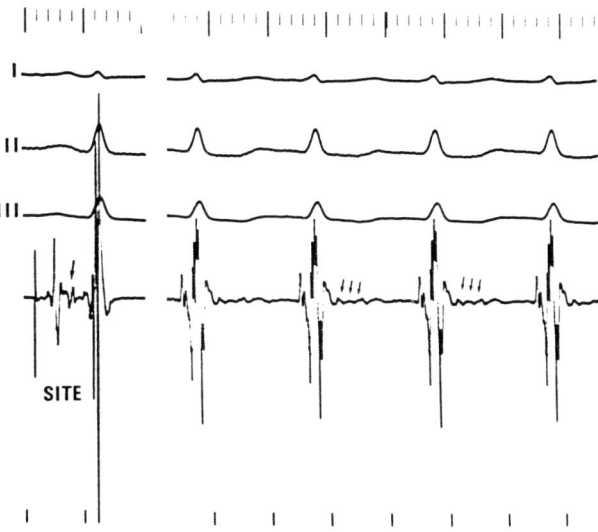

Figure 3. Slow potential at a posteroseptal site. During tachycardia, recording at this site shows a microactivity during the first half of diastole, probably representing a remnant of slow potential. RF energy delivered at this site interrupted tachycardia within 2 s by elimination of the slow pathway conduction.

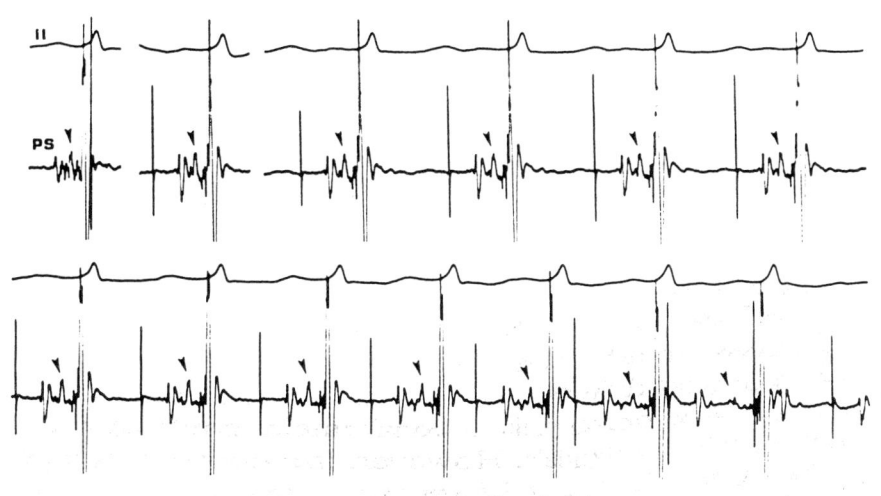

Figure 4. The first complex at the posteroseptal (PS) region appears 'nonspecifically' as a prolonged multicomponent atrial potential. As usual with this type of activity, atrial pacing shows that the terminal potential is considerably influenced by the atrial rate, thus defining a slow potential (arrow).

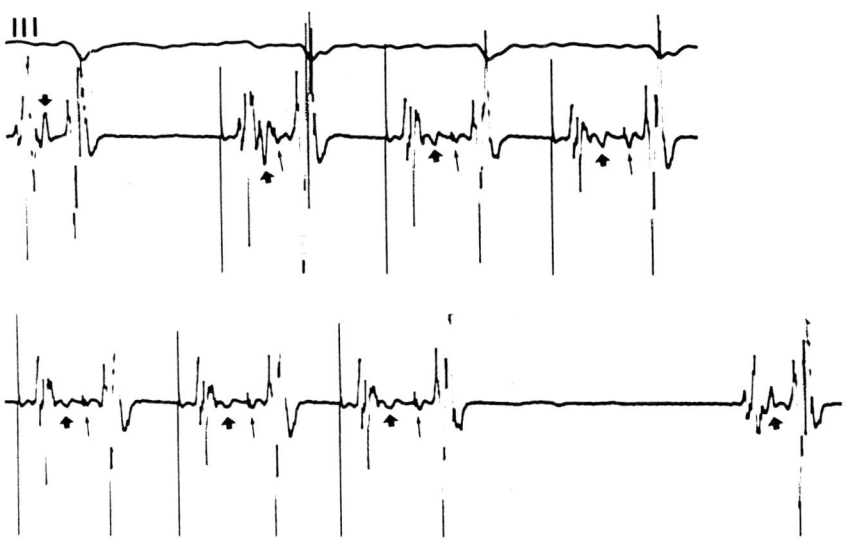

Figure 5. Recordings of slow potentials at the mid-septal region (two continuous ECG bands). Atrial pacing discloses two slow potentials. The first one progressively alters with atrial rate. The second is very slightly altered, and a spike synchronous with the His bundle activity is superimposed on it. We think this latter type of slow potential represents the activity of the compact AV node, whereas the first one is probably related to the transitional zone [14].

electrograms in successful target sites versus unsuccessful ones. This confirms the superiority of electrogram mapping on the anatomically defined target to guide SP ablation, as also demonstrated in a recent article [15].

The common point in the electrophysiologic approaches is the use of multicomponent electrograms. In fact, two types of components ('ordinary' atrial potentials and slow potentials) are to be differentiated, and this requires two study conditions, high gain amplification (50–100 mm/mV) and atrial pacing techniques. In our experience, slow potentials are present in 82% and multiple or fractionated atrial potentials in 74% of successful ablation sites, with their combination being the most predictive electrogram. The likelihood of successful SP ablation is very low in the absence of such potentials. In fact, these different potentials reflect significant functional and anatomical differences. The main electrophysiologic difference is the sensitivity of slow potentials to atrial rate in contrast with preceding (simple or complex) atrial potentials. However, if a double atrial potential is present, the site (but not the rate) of the spontaneous or stimulated atrial pacemaker considerably influences its activation sequence and morphology [4, 13], strongly suggesting that each atrial potential is activated via dissociated atrial pathways, possibly nodal inputs. The first potential is strictly correlated to the anteroseptal atrial activity, whereas the second potential has a complex relationship with the

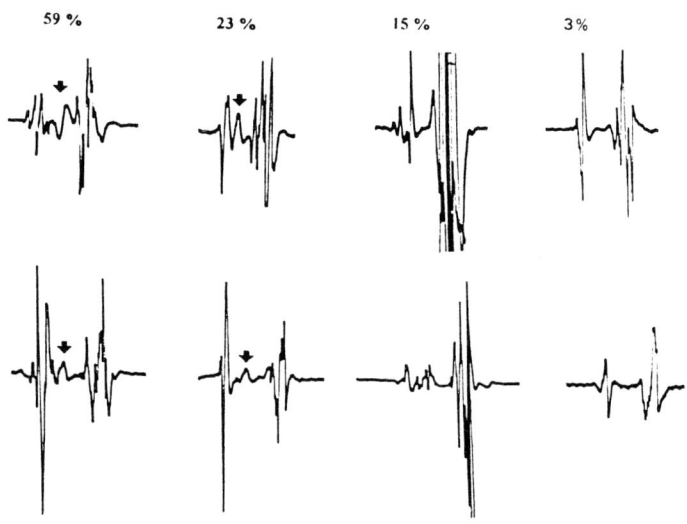

Fig. 6. Prevalence of electrograms recorded at a successful SP ablation site. Two different electrograms are shown in each group. The most frequent electrogram (59%) combines complex (fractionated or multiple) ordinary atrial potential and slow (arrow) potentials. The second group (23%) shows slow potentials and simple atrial potential. The third group (15%) shows no slow potential but complex atrial potential. In only 3% of successful sites were neither slow potentials nor complex atrial potentials recorded.

proximal coronary sinus region, suggesting that more than one (posteroinferior) pathway influences its activation [13].

Our interpretation of the electrophysiologic data recorded before successful SP ablation is the following. Complex atrial potentials reflect the *multiple atrial* fibers passing near or inputting to the transitional zone of the AV node, with the double potential being a particular form reflecting the merging of clearly differentiated inputs. Histologically, a recent study by De Bakker et al. demonstrated that slow potentials originate in subendocardially located transitional fibers [14]. Therefore, slow potentials represent a step downstream in the AV transmission, i.e. the activity of *transitional* fibers, and more anteriorly probably the activity of the compact AV node. Therefore, the recording of both complex atrial and slow potentials reflect the activity of both atrial myocardial inputs and the transitional zone. Still unclear is whether the slow pathway originates at the posteroinferior atrial inputs or the transitional zone or whether it involves the junction of both tissues. The recordings of complex atrial and slow potentials at most successful SP ablation sites support the latter hypothesis.

REFERENCES

1. Jackman WM, Beckman KJ, McClelland JH et al. Treatment of supraventricular tachycardia due to atrioventricular nodal reentry by radiofrequency catheter ablation of slow-pathway conduction. N Engl J Med 1992;327:313–8.
2. Jazayeri MR, Hempe SL, Sra JE et al. Selective transcatheter ablation of the fast and slow pathways using radiofrequency energy in patients with atrioventricular nodal reentrant tachycardia. Circulation 1992;85:1318–28.
3. Kay GN, Epstein AE, Dailey SM, Plumb VJ. Selective radiofrequency ablation of the slow pathway for the treatment of AV reentrant tachycardia. Evidence for involvement of perinodal myocardium within the reentrant circuit. Circulation 1992;85:1675–88.
4. Haissaguerre M, Gaita F, Fischer B et al. Elimination of atrioventricular nodal reentrant tachycardia using discrete slow potentials to guide application of radiofrequency energy. Circulation 1992;85:2162–75.
5. Wathen M, Natale A, Wolfe K, Yee R, Newman D, Klein G. An anatomically guided approach to atrioventricular node slow pathway ablation. Am J Cardiol 1992;70:886–9.
6. Langberg JJ, Leon A, Borganelli M et al. A randomized, prospective comparison of anterior and posterior approaches to radiofrequency catheter ablation of atrioventricular nodal reentry tachycardia. Circulation 1993;87:1551–6.
7. Interian A, Cox MM, Jimenez RA et al. A shared pathway in atrioventricular nodal reentrant tachycardia and atrial flutter: implications for pathophysiology and therapy. Am J Cardiol 1993;71:297–303.
8. Kalbfleisch SJ, Humel JD, Williamson B et al. A randomized comparison of anatomic and electrogram mapping approaches to ablation of the slow pathway of atrioventricular nodal reentrant tachycardia. PACE 1993;16:II857.
9. Wang C, Yeh S, Wen M. Radiofrequency ablation therapy using interior approach in a large group of consecutive patients with AV node reentry. PACE 1993;16:II857.
10. Baker JH, Plumb VJ, Epstein AE, Kay GN. Selective ablation of the slow AV nodal pathway: predictors of recurrent AV nodal reentrant tachycardia. Circulation 1992;86:I-521.
11. Li Hg, Stites HW, Zardini M et al. Elimination of slow pathway conduction predicts long-term success after radiofrequency AV node modification. PACE 1993;16:II856.
12. Jazayeri MR, Sra JS, Akhtar M et al. Transcatheter modification of the atrioventricular node using radiofrequency energy. Herz 1992;3:143–50.
13. Haissaguerre M, Fischer B, Le Métayer P, Egloff P, Warin JF. Double potentials recorded during sinus rhythm in the triangle of Koch. Evidence for functional dissociation from pacing of various right atrial sites. PACE 1993;16:III101.
14. DeBakker JMT, Van Hemel NM, Coronel R, Opthof T, Tasseron S, Defauw JJ. Slow potentials in the AV-junctional area; electrophysiologic and histologic correlation. PACE 1993;16:II1102.
15. McGuire MA, Bourke JP, Robotin MC et al. High resolution mapping of Koch's triangle using sixty electrodes in humans with AV functional reentrant tachycardia. Circulation 1993;88:2315–28.

PART TWO

Pacing

17. Cardiac pacing in Europe in 1992: a new survey

GIORGIO A. FERUGLIO

Many surveys on cardiac pacing in Europe were carried out and presented in conjunction with major international events in the last 25 years [1–8]. They provided considerable information on pacing epidemiology and changes in practice patterns over the years, due to the evolving technology and improved understanding of cardiac arrhythmias.

This 1992 survey, presented at the VI European Symposium on Cardiac Pacing (Ostend, June 6/9, 1993), is the ninth in a series and differs from the previous ones since the core data were derived from the national registers operating in 15 countries by using the European Pacemaker Registration Card [9]. The card, designed by the European Working Group on Cardiac Pacing in the early 1980s, provides a mechanism by which a central database can be operated in each country and that is compatible with all other countries in Europe. At present, the European Pacemaker Registration System has a database of over 500 000 registered pacemakers, the world's largest collection of patient-related pacing information.[1]

For the last 10 years, half of the nearly 280 000 pacemakers used in the world each year are being implanted in Europe (Figure 1). Data collected by the National Registration Centers in 2204 implanting hospitals in 15 countries (Table 1; Figure 2) show that the average continental implantation rate has increased further during 1992, reaching 292 primary implants per million inhabitants. However, this implantation rate is still low compared with that of the USA [10] (Table 2) and varies considerably from country to country, being over 400/M in Germany (W), France, and Belgium and below 150/M in Poland and Yugoslavia.

The ratio between total first implants and replacements was 4.23 in 1992.

---

[1] Contributing National Registers: Austria, K. Steinbach; Belgium, H. Ector; Czech Republic, P. Kamaryt; Denmark, E. Simonsen; France, M. Salvador-Mazenq, G. Pioger; Germany, W. Irnich; Greece, P.E. Vardas; Italy, G.A. Feruglio, L. Prelli; The Netherlands, C. Hooijschuur; Poland, M. Pythkowsky; Portugal, J. Correia da Cuhna; Spain, J. Silvestre; Sweden, R. Nordlander; United Kingdom, A.K. Rickards; Yugoslavia, D. Velimirovic.

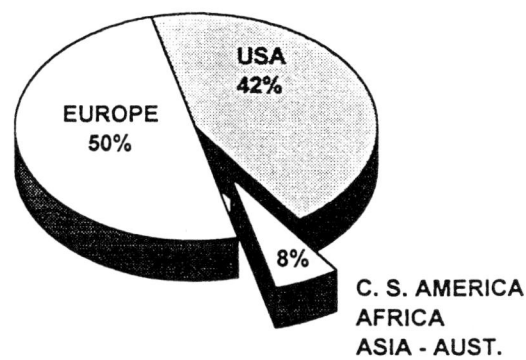

Figure 1. Of the nearly 280 000 pacemakers (PMs) used in the world in 1992, half were implanted in Europe.

Table 1. Pacing activities in the contributing countries in 1992.

	Population (× 1000)	Total PM used	First implants	Implantation rate	Implanting centres	Database registry
A	7 800	2 926	2 342	300	49	31 023
B	9 830	6 769	5 898	600	200	58 913
CZ	9 980	4 127	3 016	302	31	4 127
DK	5 132	1 808	1 545	301	11	14 424
D/W	62 000	33 300	28 300	456	815	99 100
D/E	16 000	9 000	5 950	372	65	3 538
E	39 000	9 597	7 678	235	145	9 300
F[a]	55 813	29 500	23 750	425	260	42 000
GR	10 042	3 200	2 690	267	50	2 919
I	57 200	19 500	15 650	274	256	96 044
NL	15 022	4 652	3 489	232	115	42 000
P	10 387	2 300	1 760	170	18	1 760
PL	37 799	5 193	4 383	132	43	5 193
S	8 564	3 491	2 854	328	45	3 491
UK[b]	55 487	8 722	7 264	218	80	97 378
YU[c]	10 337	435	348	32	21	435
Total	410 393	144 520	116 917	292	2204	511 645

[a]1990
[b]1991
[c]Serbia and Montenegro
D/W = West Germany; D/E = East Germany; PM = pacemaker.

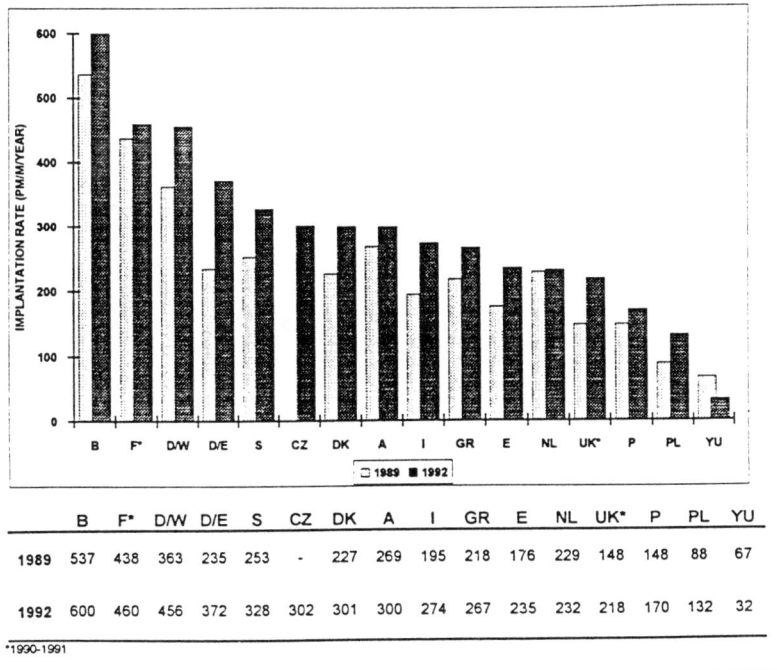

Figure 2. Compared with the 1989 survey, implantation rates have increased in practically all countries.

Table 2. Trend in primary PM implantation rate in the last 15 years in Europe and USA.

Year	Implants per million population	
	Europe	USA
1979	136	309
1981	190	518
1985	206	374
1989	224	359
1992	292	–

On average, men were paced more frequently than women (54% vs. 46%); however, in some countries (Germany, Poland) women prevailed. The patient's mean age at first implant was over 70 years in all countries, reaching a maximum of 75.1 years in Italy (Figure 3). However, the prevalence of the elderly in the various countries does not seem to affect the implantation rate substantially. Among other demographic and socioeconomic factors, only the number of implanting hospitals per million inhabitants yields some statistically significant correlation with reference to the number of first implants (Table 1; Figure 4).

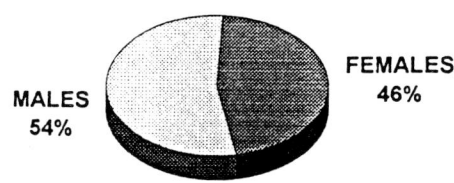

	FRANCE	57.8 / 42.2	GERMANY E	47.3 / 52.7
	ITALY	57.3 / 42.7	POLAND	49.1 / 50.9

	A	DK	D/W	D/E	E	GR	I	TOT.
MEAN AGE (YEARS)	74.2	73.9	73.9	72.5	70.9	73.2	75.1	**73.7**

Figure 3. Gender and age of patients at first implant.

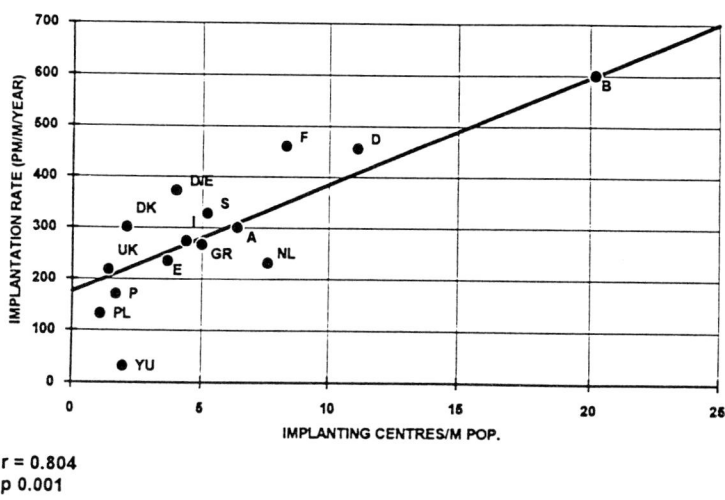

Figure 4. Among various demographic and socioeconomic parameters, the number of implanting centers per million population yielded a statistically significant correlation with reference to the number of first implants.

Table 3. Clinical indications for pacing (%).

	A	B	DK	E	F[a]	GR	I	NL	PL	UK[a]	YU
No. of implants	2342	6769	1808	9597	29 500	3200	19 500	4652	5193	8722	435
Not reported, unspecified, uncoded	8.5	24.1	2.7	23.6	0	51.1	7.6	19.5		19.1	2.3
B1, syncope	42.2	36.4	41.5	31.9	47	27.1	39.3		48	37.9	40.0
B2, dizzy spells	23.2	15.6	25.1	24.9	18	16.3	21.7	73.5		27.0	48.1
B3, bradycardia	13.8	15.2	24.4	7.1	20	3.3	13.6			7.9	9.4
C1, tachycardia	0.4	0.8	1.8	0.5	N.A.	0.4	0.7	1.3	N.A.	1.1	0
D1, prophylactic	1.3	1.8	1.4	2.2	4	0.1	4.2	0		2.5	0
D2, heart failure	9.0	4.1	2.7	8.8	7	1.5	11.9	5.7		4.1	0.2
D3, cerebral dysfunction	1.6	2.0	0.5	0.6	2	0.2	1.0	0		0.4	0

[a] 1990–1991.

Among the clinical indications for pacing, syncope was the leading cause (up to 47% and 48% of cases in France and Poland; Table 3), followed by dizzy spells, bradycardia and heart failure, in that order.

According to the pre-pacing ECG (Table 4), AV block (all degrees) was the major indication in most countries (up to 48% and 77% of cases in France and Yugoslavia), followed by atrial rhythm disturbances (up to 62% in Germany). In half of the countries, atrial rhythm disorders were more prevalent than AV block; however, in Spain and Yugoslavia such indications for permanent pacing led to less than 30% of referrals.

Supraventricular and ventricular tachycardia as indications for pacemaker implantation remained well below 1% in almost all countries (Table 4).

With regard to etiology (Table 5), fibrosis and ischemic damage of the conducting tissue were considered the most frequent causes; among the others, carotid sinus syndrome (up to 4.5% in Austria), post-AMI AV block (up to 3.3% in Denmark), surgery and congenital heart disease (up to 2.1% and 1.3%, respectively, in the UK) are noteworthy.

Preferences regarding device types and pacing modes continue to change (Table 6). The VOO and nonprogrammable VVI pacemakers were no longer used in 1992. Single chamber pacing with a standard programmable generator was the most frequent system to be implanted (in over 60% of cases in Spain, Greece, and the UK). Dual-chamber pacing was used in up to 47% of cases in Belgium, although in most countries it remained between 15% and 30%. VDD pacing with a single-pass lead was reported in up to 7% of cases in Italy.

Rate-adaptive pacing continued to expand and was employed in up to 30% of cases of single chamber pacing (Sweden) and 18% of dual chamber pacing (Belgium) (Figure 5). Activity sensors were the most commonly utilized (in up to 90% of cases in Sweden), followed by breathing and QT interval sensors (Table 7).

Table 4. Pre-pacing ECG indications (%)

	A	B	DK	D/W	D/E	E	F[a]	GR	I	NL	PL	S	UK[a]	YU
No. of implants	2342	6769	1808	28 300	5950	9597	29 500	3200	19 500	4652	5193	2854	8722	435
C1-7, AV block (all degrees)	33.3	32.1	46.5	37.8	38.1	46.6	47.8	29.0	47.3	35.9	46.2	52	45.5	76.7
D-11, BBB	2.7	2.3	1.5	0	0	5.5	7.4	11.0	7.8	2.9	0	0	4.1	5.5
E1-6, F2, atrial rhythm disturbances	49.0	46.3	35.4	62.2	61.9	24.3	35.9	53.0	37.8	43.3	53.8	43	33.9	17.9
F1, G1-3 supraventricular and/or ventricular tachycardia	0.8	0.6	1.2	0	0	0.4	N.A.	0	0.6	0.2	0	0	0.6	0.2

[a] 1990–1991.
BBB = bundle branch block.

Table 5. Etiology (%).

	A	B	DK	E	F[a]	GR	I	NL	UK[a]	YU
No. of implants	2342	6769	1808	9597	29 500	3200	19 500	4652	8722	435
A1-2, unspecified	20.0	48.9	7.9	32.7	33.3	24.2	20.7	32.3	33.3	17.2
B1, unknown	42.1	18.5	73.9	26.6	14	59.2	11.8	52.2	33.4	67.1
B2, fibrosis	2.3	14.4	1.4	22.3	33.3	6.5	44.5		18.5	3.9
C1, ischemia	20.7	6.6	7.7	6.4	5.3	3.0	8.5	8.4	5.1	5.5
C2, post-AMI	2.7	2.1	3.3	1.0	1.7	0.6	3.0		2.1	1.4
D1, congenital	0.2	0.3	0.7	0.5		0.1	0.3	0.6	1.2	0.4
E1-2, surgical	1.0	1.1	1.5	1.8	0.7	0.6	0.9	3.8	2.1	0.7
E3, fulguration	0.5	0.6	1.8	0.5		0.3	0.2		0.7	1.6
F1, carotid sinus syndrome	4.5	2.9	0.2	2.3	2.2	4.0	3.4	0.5	1.2	0.9
G1, cardiomyopathy	2.6	2.4	0.7	3.7	4.6	0.5	4.1		0.9	0.4
G2, myocarditis	0.5	0.1	0.1	0.1		0.1	0.1	2.2	0.1	0.4
G3, valv. h. dis.	2.2	2.0	0.6	2.0	2.8	0.8	2.5		1.7	0.2

[a] 1990–1991.

In Tables 8 and 9, different modes of pacing in AV block and in sinoatrial disease, as reported by the national registers, are presented. The major differences among countries are recorded with reference to the use of dual chamber pacing in AV block (from 7% in Yugoslavia to 21% in Spain and 54% in Belgium); similar disparities occur in the treatment of sinoatrial disease (17% in Spain, 41% in Belgium and Italy).

With regard to pulse generator replacement, impending battery depletion detected during follow-up was the most common cause (in up to 85% of cases in Austria); premature battery depletion was responsible in up to 3.7% of cases in Germany (W). Elective replacements prompted by causes such as local complications, need for a change of pacing mode, and device recall were reported in up to 25% of all generator replacements in Germany (W), while major electronic failure occurred in as low as 0.7% of cases in Austria (Table 10).

A variety of indications for electrode replacement were reported. Infection and ulceration were the most frequent causes (8.3% and 9.3% in Denmark and Belgium, respectively), followed by displacement, exit block, and insulation breakage, in that order (Table 11).

With reference to the manufacturers' market shares, considering the five major participants in each country (Figure 6), it would appear that a single manufacturer occupies most of the market in one-third of the countries.

In conclusion, the results of this ninth survey of cardiac pacing in Europe show a persisting and even more remarkable diversification of implantation rates, indications, pacing modes, preferences regarding device type, and complications among the various countries. The volume of pacemaker usage

Table 6. Hardware and modes of pacing (% of primary implants)

	A	B	DK	D/W	D/E	E	F[a]	GR	I	NL	S	UK[a]	YU
No. of implants	2342	6769	1808	28 300	5950	9597	29 500	3200	19 500	4652	2854	8722	435
AAI, P, M	0.9	0.27	4.6	3.0[b]	3.0[c]	1.6	1.3	0.1	1.0	[d]	3	0.6	3.4
AAIR	0.3	0.22	6.7			1.6	0.6	0.07	0.6	[d]	3	0.6	3.4
VVI, P, M	55.4	27.3	34.9	71.2[b]	67.5[c]	63.0	54.2	62.48	58.8	[d]	40	65.6	54.2
VVIR	11.8	25.2	31.5	0	0	13.8	11.0	20.07	7.6	[d]	27	5.8	27.3
VDD, P, M	0	0	0			0.9	0	2.26	7.0		0	0.5	0
DDD, M	27.3	29.3	11.8	25.8[b]	29.5[c]	12.7	26.5	9.11	20.4	68.9	18	19.5	6.2
DDDR	4.2	17.7	10.4	0	0	6.4	6.3	5.17	3.2	15.5	9	1.9	1.6
Antitachy	0	0	0	0	0	0	0	0.03	0.04	10.5	0	0	0.2

[a] 1990–1991.
[b] RR' = 23.2%.
[c] RR = 17%.
[d] AAI + VVI = 40.6%; AIR + VVIR = 24.9%; others = 3.4%.

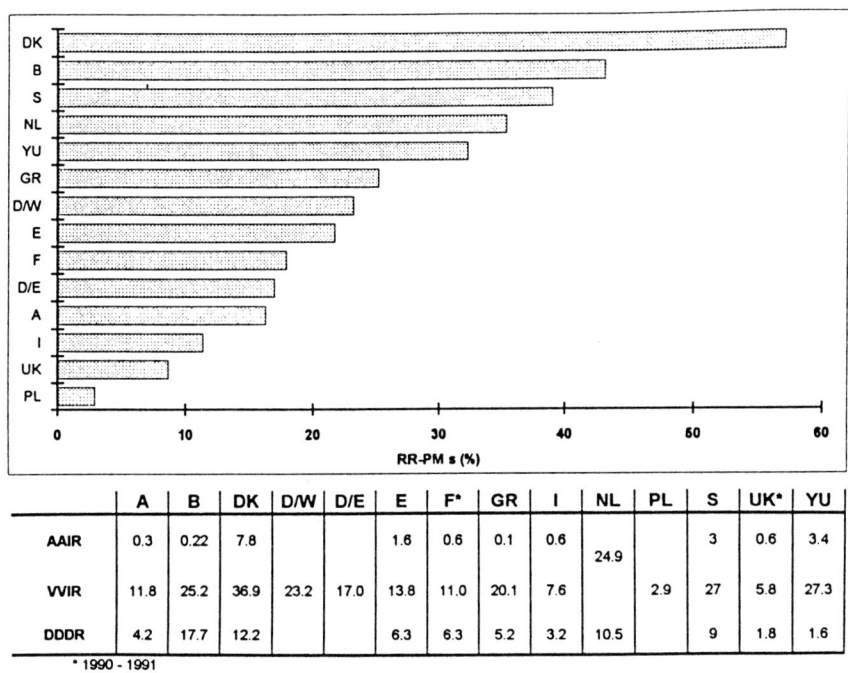

Figure 5. Rate-adaptive pacing in the various countries: percentage of total PMs used.

	A	B	DK	D/W	D/E	E	F*	GR	I	NL	PL	S	UK*	YU
AAIR	0.3	0.22	7.8			1.6	0.6	0.1	0.6	24.9		3	0.6	3.4
VVIR	11.8	25.2	36.9	23.2	17.0	13.8	11.0	20.1	7.6		2.9	27	5.8	27.3
DDDR	4.2	17.7	12.2			6.3	6.3	5.2	3.2	10.5		9	1.8	1.6

* 1990 - 1991

Table 7. Rate-adaptive sensors used.

	B[a]	GR	PL	S	YU
Activity	78.5	85.0	100	90	38
Breathing	14.7	7.0	0	3	19.4
QR interval	6.3	8.0	0	7	29.8
QT + activity	0.5	0	0	0	6.7
MV + activity	0	0	0	0	5.9

[a]1991.

Table 8. Pacing modes in AV block (RR included).

	A	B[a]	E	I	NL	S	YU
Single chamber, atrial	0.3	0.1	0	0	0	0	7.7
Single chamber, ventricular	62.2	45.6	79.2	75.2	62.2	65	85.5
Dual chamber	37.8	54.3	20.8	24.8	37.8	35	6.8

[a]1991.

Table 9. Pacing modes in sick sinus syndrome (SSS) (RR included).

	A	B[a]	E	I	NL	S	YU
Single chamber, atrial	1.8	0.86	4.9	6.6	9.3	25	0
Single chamber, ventricular	77.6	57.86	77.6	51.8	70.1	56	100
Dual chamber	20.6	41.28	17.4	41.6	20.6	19	0

[a]1991.

Table 10. Causes for generator explantation (%).

	A	B	D/W	I
B1, elective	3.3	4.0		
			16.7	10.8
B0, B2-8, syst. change	4.4	6.3		
C1-4, local complications	3.3	2.7	8.7	7.2
D1-5, failure, minor	3.1	0.7		
			8.6	6.7
E1-7, failure, major	0.7	2.1		
F2, premature battery depletion	0.7	1.6	3.7	4.2

Table 11. Causes for electrode explantation.

	A	B	DK
A1-2, unspecified, uncoded	80.1	54.9	20.4
B1, elective	0	11.7	13.9
B2, displacement	7.0	3.7	13.0
B3, exit block	4.4	6.8	18.5
B4, electromyogr. inh.	0.4	0.6	
B5, extracardiac stimulation	0.4	0.6	1.8
B6, perforation	0.4	0	0.9
B7, undersensing	0.7	3.7	5.6
C1, infection, ulceration	4.1	9.3	8.3
D1, connector failure	0	0.6	0
D2, insulation break	0.7	2.5	14.8
D3, conductor break	1.8	5.6	2.9

is still increasing in Europe and represents 50% of all pacemakers in the world. Nevertheless, some countries, mostly the same ones as in earlier surveys, are lagging behind, exhibiting implantation rates below 200/M. Correlations with demographic and socioeconomic parameters confirm that the number of implanting hospitals per million inhabitants is the major determinant of the implanting rate in each country.

Although the new approach in this survey, based on data collected by means of the European Pacemaker Registration Card and the National Registers, has yielded very up-to-date statistics and provided a basis for median calculations, it will be necessary in future surveys to solicit infor-

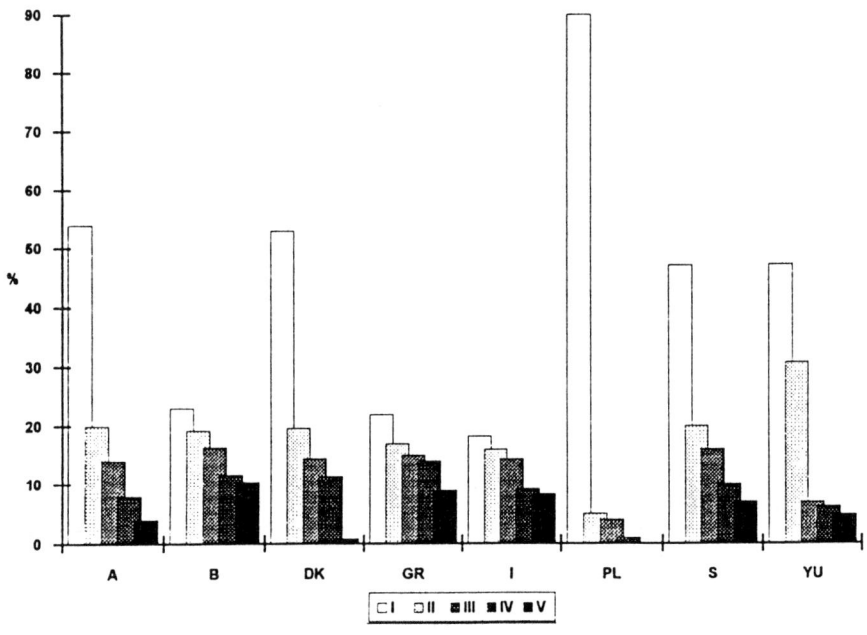

Figure 6. Manufacturers' market shares: in one-third of the countries a single manufacturer occupies most of the PM market.

mation also from individual implanting centers in order to characterize typical practices and opinion-related issues better.

REFERENCES

1. Survey on the long-term stimulation techniques all over the world. Symposium sur les Pacemakers, Monaco 17-19 September 1970. An Cardiol Ageiol 1971;20:285.
2. Thalen HJTh, editor. World survey on cardiac stimulation. Cardiac Pacing: Proceedings of the IV International Symposium, Groningen, April 17-19, 1973. Assen: Van Gorcum, 1973:41.
3. Watanabe Y, editor. World survey on long-term follow-up of cardiac pacing. Cardiac Pacing: Proceedings of the V International Symposium, Tokyo, March 14-18, 1976. Excerpta Medica, Amsterdam, 1977:555.
4. Meer C, editor. World survey on cardiac pacing. Cardiac Pacing, State of the Art 1979: Proceedings of the VI World Symposium on Cardiac Pacing, Montreal, October 2-5, 1979. Montreal, 1979:Section 41.
5. Feruglio GA, Steinbach K. Cardiac pacing in Europe after two decades: a comprehensive survey. In: Feruglio GA, editor. Cardiac Pacing, Electrophysiology and Pacemaker Technology. Padua: Piccin Medical Books, 1982:1-13.

6. Feruglio GA, Steinbach K. Pacing in the world today. Proceedings of the VIIth World Symposium on Cardiac Pacing. Darmstadt: Steinkopff Verlag, 1983:953–67.
7. Feruglio GA, Rickards AK, Steinbach K et al. Cardiac pacing in the world: state of the art in 1986. Proceedings of the VIIIth World Symposium on Cardiac Pacing and Electrophysiology. Tel Aviv: R & L Creative Communications, 1987:563.
8. The 1989 world survey on cardiac pacing. Proceedings of the IXth World Symposium on Cardiac Pacing and Electrophysiology, Washington DC, May 1991. PACE 1991;14:2073–6.
9. Rickards AK. The European Pacemaker Registration Card. Stimulation, June 6, 1988:7–10.
10. Bernstein AD, Parsonnet V. Survey of cardiac pacing in the U.S. in 1989. Am J Cardiol 1992;69:331–8.

18. The myocardium-electrode interface at the cellular level

MAX SCHALDACH

INTRODUCTION

The role of the stimulation electrode as an actuator, as well as a sensor, has been recognized to be the most important component of the artificial pacing system. An electrode with a high sensitivity to detect intracardiac signals and a low threshold to avoid loss of capture, suppress electrochemical reactions, and improve energy conservation must be developed with the highest priority. Current efforts to reach this goal utilize the multidisciplinary areas of physics, electrochemistry, materials, physiology, and neurocardiology. Using the electrode to appropriately monitor the autonomic balance, by monitoring the resulting artificial excitation in the neural status of the myocardium is a new concept which is gaining attention. Methods thus far employed prevent the loss of capture in monitoring the evoked response by using advanced electronic signal processing and detecting inotropic response as an indicator of cardiovascular needs, therefore serving as a control signal for the reestablishment of the chronotropic response [1]. Historically, many approaches have been reported [2,3], but the prerequisite of an appropriate black box performance with a matched frequency performance of the sensing interface is not yet available. The myocardium/electrode interface will be of primary concern in understanding the transport of electrical charges across the boundary into the living tissue as well as in understanding the observed evoked response at the cellular level. The neural control mechanism to be extracted from the behavior of the evoked action potential during the repolarization phase will provide a significant step toward the development of an integrated sensor-controlled neuromodulator to adjust the afferent sympathetic/parasympathetic balance by afferent stimulation or efferent triggering of the heart at the effector level. The method of evoked potential recognition by means of detecting the integrated response of the excited cells around the stimulation electrode will be supplemented by the detection principle of measuring the impedance of the electrode-blood-tissue interface to monitor the inotropic state as previously described [4]. Impedance changes caused by changes in contractility are the result of an inotropic adjustment. The stimulation electrode as a sensor has proven its clinical value in many aspects, thereby providing a new concept of electrotherapy of the heart in which the implanted device becomes a part of the autonomic nervous system (ANS). Thus, access to the flow of cardiac ANS information opens new avenues for cardiac electrotherapy, including control of chronotropic pacing therapy in response to physiological demand; monitoring acute imbalance between sympathetic and parasympathetic tone to trigger and control arrhythmia suppression therapies [5] and using the ANS signal to modulate Ventricular Assist Systems, including cardiac myoplasty preparations, which would further protect the myocardium from acute stress.

EVOKED POTENTIAL

A practical value of the evoked response was first mentioned by Auerbach and Furman [6]. The autodiagnostic pacemaker (ADP) monitored the cardiac response evoked by a stimulus at the electrode serving the stimulation as well as detection. The ability of the ADP to detect 'failure to capture' as well as 'failure to sense' made it valuable and important for the safety of patients with pacemakers. Several devices have also been proposed or are already under clinical investigation which use the evoked response as a suitable signal for rate adaptation [7] or the diagnosis of early cardiac transplant rejection [8]. All of these devices, however, require a reliable system for the detection of the ventricular evoked response. Usually, this is achieved by using two electrodes, one for pacing and one for sensing [9]. During the past two decades, many attempts have been made to pace and then to detect the evoked response using the same electrode as an actuator as well as a sensor. All attempts have failed due to a physical phenomenon of the electrode/myocardium interface, electrode polarization. After a pulse is applied to a metal electrode in contact with an electrolyte, the interface is charged like a capacitor due to the different charge transport mechanisms in the two phases. This charge leads to a slowly, nearly exponentially decaying after-potential. Consequently, the evoked response, which occurs within approximately 30 to 350 ms after the stimulation, is superimposed on an offset of 10 mV or more, even if the output connections are short-circuited directly after the pacing pulse (autoshort). This results in an overload of the sensing amplifiers or at least a distortion of the evoked potential. Several electronic measures have been developed to deal with this offset, e.g., Delle-Vedove et al. [10] proposed using a logarithmic amplifier, which provides a linearization of the polarization artifact and can detect non-linearities. However, this method turned out to be unreliable due to the unjustified assumption of an exponential decay of the polarization artifact. Another approach which used a biphasic pacing pulse and adapted the amplitude of the second phase to discharge the phase boundary after each pulse [11] required approximately 100% more battery energy as a single-phase stimulator, which was unsuitable for implantable devices. Even highly sophisticated algorithms using triphasic stimulus waveforms were unable to completely avoid the polarization artifacts [12] since a part of the stimulus charge is transferred to ions, resulting in an irreversible exchange current. There has been no satisfactory electronic solution to suppress the polarization artifact. The design of a new pacing electrode must, therefore, ensure a legible polarization.

ELECTRODE MYOCARDIUM INTERFACE

An interface between a metal and an electrolyte is characterized by two different charge transport mechanisms, the electronic conduction in the solid phase and the ionic transport in the solution phase. If a voltage is applied between these two phases, ions are driven to the interface and form a layer, which is separated from the metal by a multilayer of adsorbed water molecules, resulting in the so-called Helmholtz double layer. This structure is equivalent to a capacitor with water as the dielectric. By driving a current across this interface, e.g., during a pacing pulse, it is charged according to the following equation:

$$U = \frac{1}{C_H} \int_0^T I(t)\, dt = \frac{1}{C_H} Qst \qquad (1)$$

where U is the voltage drop across the Helmholtz layer, C_H the capacity of the Helmholtz double layer, $I(t)$ the displacement current, i.e., the overall current minus losses due to chemical reactions, T the pulse width, and Qst, the total charge at the interface. At the end of the pacing pulse, the lead remains charged, resulting in a voltage drop U across the Helmholtz double layer according to Equation 1, which is called the polarization artifact voltage. There are two possibilities to reduce this artifact voltage: (1) the charge Qst can be reduced, e.g., by lowering the pulse voltage or by the conventional method (applying a charge balancing pulse subsequent to the pacing pulse); or (2) by an increase in the capacity of the Helmholtz double layer C_H which will have the same effect on the artifact voltage. At higher electrode potentials, additional effects must be considered, such as chemical reactions, i.e., reduction of H^+ ions resulting in an exchange current and an imbalance in the ionic environment at the interface. The charged reaction products cannot be recharged by a subsequent correcting pulse because they drift away from the interface, obeying a diffusion limited transport law. Thus, the only way to avoid this contribution to the polarization artifact is to avoid these reactions, i.e., to use low threshold electrodes. As a result, two requirements must be met to achieve a pacing lead with a low polarization artifact. First, its threshold voltage should be minimized to avoid chemical reactions at the interface and the resulting diffusion problems, as well as to lower Qst.

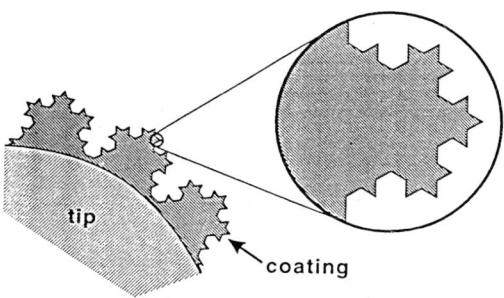

Figure 1. Diagrammatic representation of fractally coated leads showing fractal geometry.

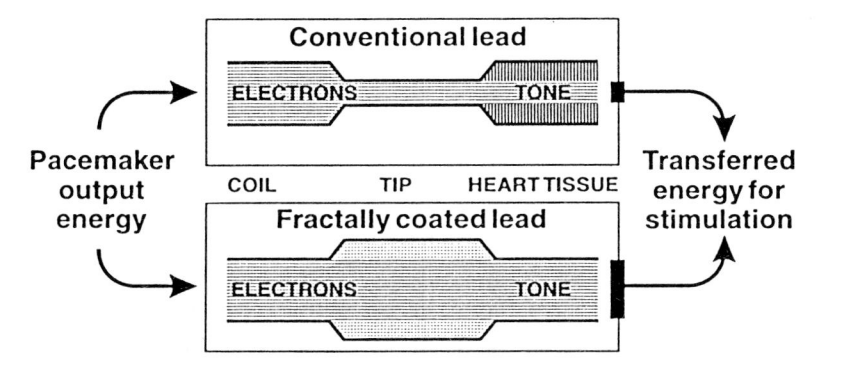

Figure 2. Diagrammatic representation of fractally coated leads showing improvement in lead tip energy transfer.

Secondly, C_H should be maximized, since according to Equation 1, a higher C_H threshold voltage is lowered by increasing C_H. Consequently, both requirements can be combined, and electrodes with high C_H should provide a low polarization artifact as well as a low stimulation threshold. Thus far, the limited frequency response of the smooth surface restricts the effective use of metal electrodes. In the past, many different technical approaches were undertaken to overcome some of the restricted interface performances by developing electrode materials or geometric configurations to reduce the electrochemical behavior of the stimulation electrode known as polarization [13,14]. The introduction of porous electrodes, such as titanium nitride and iridium as the coating material with a fractal surface structure (as shown diagrammatically in Figure 1), which provides an electrochemically active surface area with a Helmholtz double-layer capacity of up to 50 000 µF/cm², has resulted in a unique detection and stimulation (Figure 2) performance

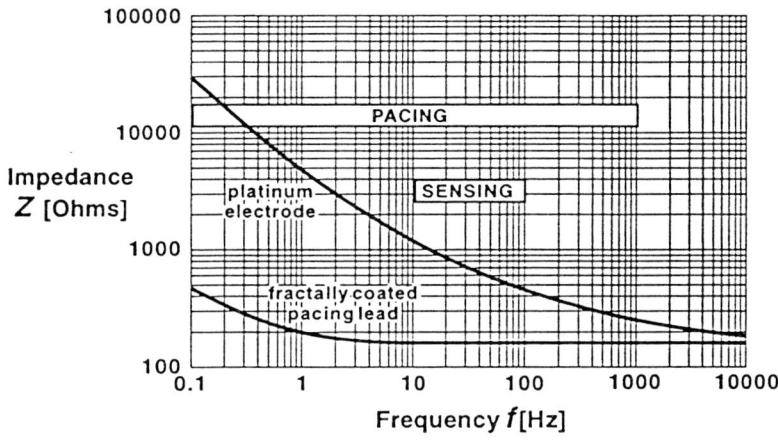

Figure 3. Impedance spectrum of fractally coated pacing lead compared with a smooth platinum lead.

[15]. It should be noted that the clinical success of electrodes with significantly reduced polarization behavior should be credited to Lewin et al. [16]. Although the results of sintered tantalum and carbon gave evidence of the necessity to tailor the interface capacity to the spectral requirements in detection and stimulation, the clinically significant breakthrough in the reliable detection of the repolarization phase of the ventricular evoked response was possible as a result of the introduction of the fractal surface structure (Figure 1) of titanium nitride and iridium [15]. Figure 3 shows the impedance spectrum of a fractally coated electrode and a smooth platinum electrode. Electrode impedance was measured as a function of sinusoidal voltages with different frequencies. The results clearly indicate that smooth platinum electrodes have cut-off frequencies 1000 times larger than the fractally coated electrodes [17]. The Helmholtz capacity (C_H) can be calculated from the impedance spectrum according to the following equation, assuming that the lead resistance of the sample is smaller than its Faraday impedance;

$$C_H = \frac{1}{2 \cdot \pi \cdot f_g \cdot R_C} \qquad (2)$$

where f_g marks the cut-off frequency, and R_c is the sum of the lead and contact resistance, which is equivalent to the high frequency impedance of the sample. By reducing the cut off frequency, the fractally coated electrodes have a significantly higher Helmholtz capacity, and as noted earlier, this ensures a negligible polarization artifact and low stimulation threshold. Thus, the development of fractally coated leads allows a better documentation of

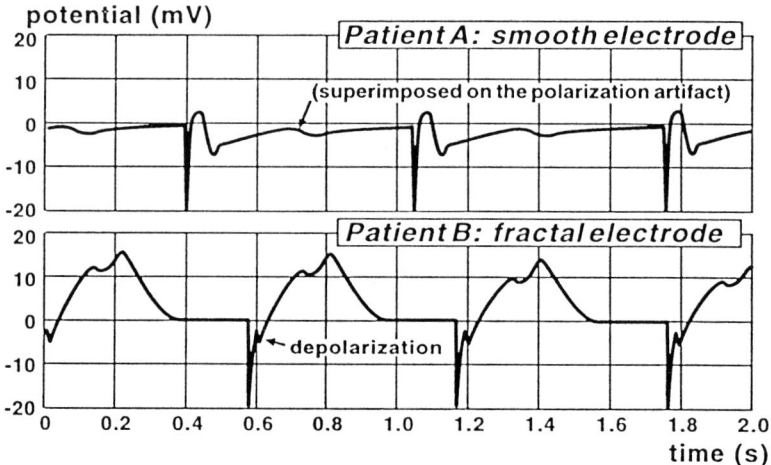

Figure 4. (a) Output signal of uncoated elgiloy electrode for above-threshold stimulation (90 ppm, 2.0 V) showing a ventricular evoked potential superimposed on the polarization artifact. (b) Output of a TiN-coated electrode with fractal surface structure for above-threshold stimulation (115 ppm, 0.3 V) showing no polarization artifact and an undistorted evoked potential.

the evoked response at the electrode-myocardial cell level and, by virtue of the lower stimulation threshold afforded by these leads, significantly improves pacemaker longevity by decreasing battery consumption.

EVOKED RESPONSE RECOGNITION FOR AUTOMATIC AMPLITUDE ADJUSTMENT

The majority of the volume of an implanted pacemaker is occupied by its energy source, the battery. Reducing the energy consumption of the pacemaker implant allows a reduction in the size of the pacemaker or, more importantly, an increase in its longevity. As described above, the low pacing threshold obtained with fractal surface electrodes are a major milestone towards this goal. However, an additional solution for minimizing battery consumption would be a technique whereby the pacemaker automatically adjusted its pacing output by measuring the capture threshold. Automatic output adjustment requires a method for confirming ventricular capture. This can be elegantly achieved by measurement of the evoked response. In this context, the superior sensing properties and low polarization artifact of fractal coated leads allow the evoked response to be accurately identified using the same electrode for stimulation and sensing (see Figure 4). Sensing the evoked

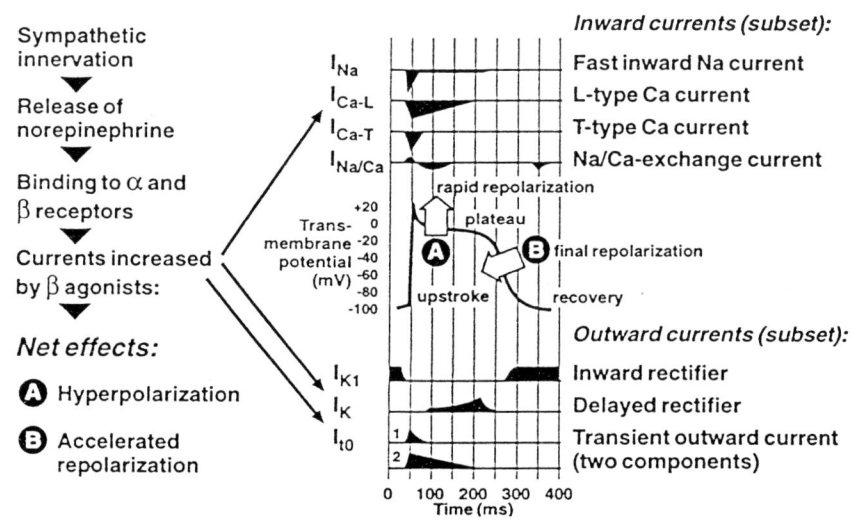

Figure 5. Autonomic receptor modulation of cellular action potential repolarization.

potential is similar to sensing of an intrinsic electrical potential. Following autoshort and blanking, the sensed signal is amplified, filtered, and compared to a threshold voltage. A threshold crossing during the 'capture recognition window' (a programmable window of sensing after the ventricular pace) sends a logic signal to the capture recognition logic for further processing. Capture loss is identified as four consecutive paces without a corresponding threshold crossing within the capture recognition window. When capture loss is identified an amplitude adjustment algorithm based on several yes or no assessments of capture loss and output amplitude voltage is activated and results in an optimized adjustment of the output voltage.

AUTONOMIC RECEPTOR MODULATION OF THE CELLULAR ACTION POTENTIAL

An essential understanding of the autonomic receptor modulation of the action potential, the currents contributing to it in the cardiac myocytes, and the effects of autonomic stimulation on repolarization is important since these complex areas not only influence the normal rhythm of the heart but also have important implications with respect to the development of arrhythmias. Figure 5 shows the autonomic receptor modulation of repolarization by sympathetic innervation. Inward ion currents carried by Na^+ and Ca^{2+} depolarize the cell during the upstroke of the action potential and, to the extent that they persist following the upstroke, influence the action potential duration by opposing the repolarizing effects of outward current. The fast inward sodium current, I_{Na}, depolarizes the cell membrane, activates the voltage-dependent repolarizing currents, and inactivates itself when repolarization begins. However, the most important contributor of inward current during the action potential plateau is the calcium current, I_{Ca-L}, which is activated at relatively depolarized potentials, flows through L-type Ca^{2+} channels, and is relatively large and long-lasting. The T-type calcium current is of shorter duration and contributes to impulse initiation rather than to the duration of repolarization. Currents carried by the K^+ ions are the major outward determinants and include the transient outward current, I_{to}, and the delayed rectifier, I_K, and inward rectifier, I_{K1}, currents. Sympathetic innervation supplies the atria and ventricles with the neurotransmitter norepinephrine. The agonist exerts α- and β-adrenergic actions by binding to α and β receptors. Beta-agonists activate the adenylate cyclase-cAMP messenger system via the GTP regulatory protein G_s. The result is activation of cAMP-dependent protein kinase and phosphorylation of Ca^{2+} channels such that current carried by the L-type Ca^{2+} channels increases. Other ionic effects of agonists include; stimulation of the Na/K pump, resulting in membrane hyperpolarization, and an increase in the delayed rectifier (I_K) and transient outward (I_{to}) currents. The net result is to hyperpolarize the membrane and accelerate repolarization. Finally, through the increases induced in Ca^{2+} current and in free intracellular Ca^{2+}, delayed and early after-depolarizations can be induced. Hence, the net effect of β-adrenergic stimulation is to accelerate repolarization and facilitate mechanisms (such as after-depolarizations, delayed after-depolarizations and automaticity) that might induce arrhythmias [18]. The myocardium/electrode interface is of great importance in understanding the transport of electrical charges across the boundary into the living tissue, as well as to provide a more thorough understanding of the observed evoked response at the cellular level, since the evoked potential as measured by the pacemaker electrode can be thought of as a superimposition of the cellular action potentials, as shown in Figure 6. The evoked potential measured in this way is probably a reflection of the superimposed cellular action potentials from the first few layers of the endocardium. However, it is unclear whether the evoked potential reflects information from cellular levels deeper than these first few layers of excitable muscle tissue. The evoked potential response to increasing exercise as measured by a fractally coated pacemaker electrode shows similar responses to that described by Rosen et al. [18] in the autonomic receptor modulation of repolarization at the cellular level. Figure 7 shows evoked potentials measured with unipolar, nonpolarizable, iridum-coated electrodes. Figure 7a clearly shows the hyperpolarization (at 200 ms in the plateau phase) and accelerated repolarization occurring during the final repolarization phase (250–300 ms) caused by the increased inotropic influence during exercise, while Figure 7b describe the frequency dependency on the evoked potential as a result of increased chronotropic influence [19]. Thus, the neural control mechanism to be extracted

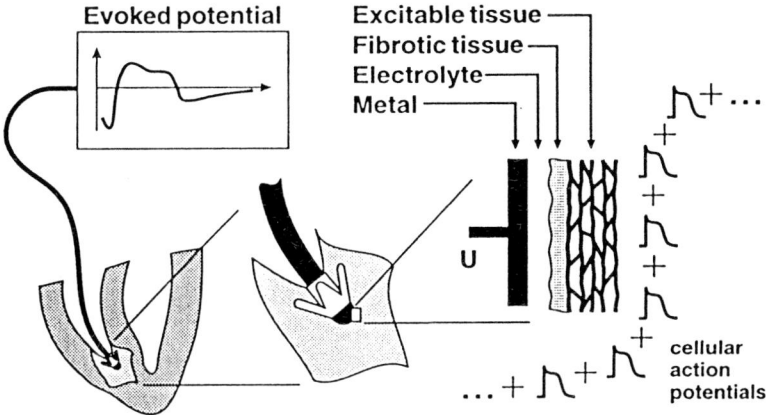

Figure 6. Diagrammatic representation of the evoked potential as a superimposition of cellular action potentials.

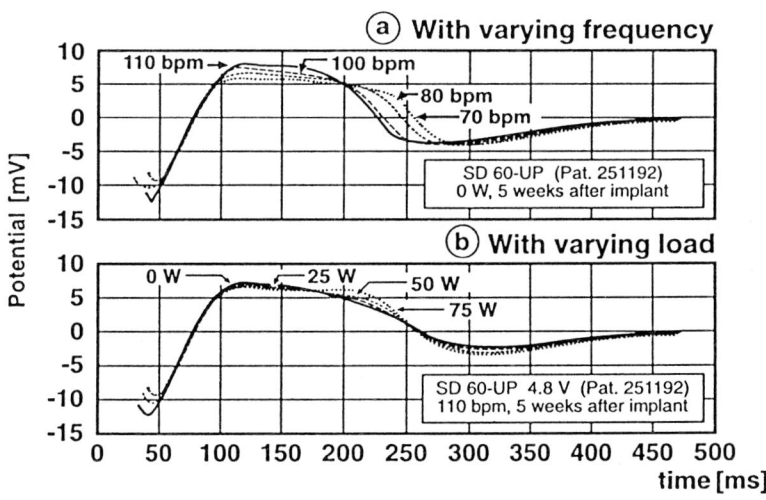

Figure 7. (a) Evoked potential during different levels of exercise, measured with a unipolar, nonpolarizable, iridium-coated electrode. (b) Evoked potential during different pacing frequency, measured with a unipolar, nonpolarizable, iridium-coated electrode.

from the behavior of the evoked action potential during the repolarization will provide a significant step towards the development of an integrated sensor-controlled neuromodulator to adjust the afferent sympathetic/parasympathetic balance by afferent stimulation or efferent triggering of the heart at the effector level.

INTRACARDIAC IMPEDANCE AS A MONITOR OF CHANGING INOTROPIC STATE

The pacemaker electrode serves two functions: as an actuator to conduct electrical energy from the pulse generator to the myocardium and as a sensor to detect intracardiac potentials. Sensing the evoked potential, as described above, can be supplemented by measurement of the impedance signal derived from the electrode-blood-tissue interface, since this signal has been linked to the inotropic status of the heart. The stimulation electrode as an intracardiac impedance sensor provides a new concept of electrotherapy of the heart in which the implanted device becomes part of the ANS [20]. Two intracardiac impedance measurement methods have been established, multipolar and unipolar. While multipolar impedance plethysmography has been used to determine changes in left ventricular volume [21], this is not applicable in the right ventricle due to its odd geometrical shape [22]. Since the normal pacemaker electrode position is in the right ventricle, it is more favorable to measure the intracardiac impedance using a unipolar electrode against the pacemaker housing as a counter-electrode. This method has, moreover, the advantage that the stimulating electrode serves at the same time as a sensor. A numerical model of the human cardiovascular system has been developed [23] for stimulating the short-term regulatory processes that adapt the cardiac output of the heart to changing circulatory demands. This model represents a way to illustrate the influence of changing ANS stimulation on the intracardiac impedance waveform. Figure 8 represents a block diagram of the model. Only the physiological subsystems and relationships directly or indirectly contributing to chronotropic or inotropic regular are controlled. The circulation is represented by a few segments only and is affected by the following: changes in preload and afterload, effects of physical exercise and temperature, and effects of orthostatic changes. The major vessels of the systemic and pulmonary circulation are considered to be compartments with elastic walls that develop a certain pressure p for a given volume V, dependent on the compliance C and the unstressed volume V_0. The flow between two compartments depends upon the pressure gradient and the flow resistance between the compartments. Finally, the net inflow of each compartment equals the volume change dV/dt. These relationships applied for each (circulatory) compartment form a set of first-order differential equations. This simple representation describes the circulation sufficiently for stimulating the load conditions for heart filling and ejection. Since the impedance signal

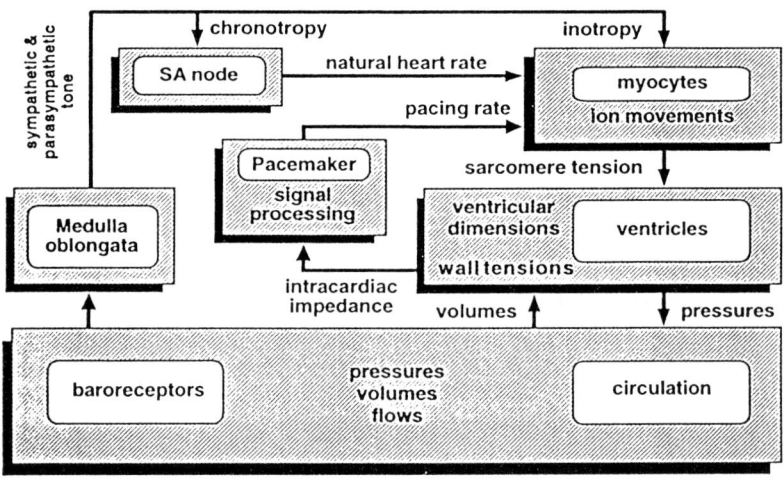

Figure 8. Block diagram of heart and circulation model.

measured by the pacemaker is determined mainly by the geometrical changes of the ventricles during myocardial contraction (Figure 9), the mechanical action is considered in more detail. The evaluation is based on a geometrical hypothesis which allows us to calculate the relationships between ventricular volumes, ventricular dimensions, resulting wall stress, and via a modified Laplace law, the ventricular pressures. Changes of the contractile status of the heart resulting from adrenergic influences on the cardiac myocyte alter the contraction pattern and thus are mapped in the time course of the intracardiac impedance. Most important of these is the intracellular Ca^{2+} concentration, which determines force of contraction and results from the dynamics of uptake, storage, and release by the sarcoplasmic reticulum (Figure 10). When the sympathetic activity is increased, a neurotransmitter, norepinephrine, is released which exerts α- and β-adrenergic actions. Via a second messenger system (cyclic AMP), the Ca^{2+} dynamics are influenced in a way that the typical inotropic effects (higher peak tension, higher rate of rise in tension, and accelerated relaxation) occur (Figure 11). Since the control aspects of heart function are of special interest, the ANS is included in the simulation. The ANS-controlled adjustment of the heartbeat is considered a closed-loop system, with mean arterial blood pressure (MABP) being the controlled quantity [24]. For this reason, the model contains a procedure simulating the baroreceptor reflex. Symbolic control variables representing the sympathetic and parasympathetic tone are calculated as a function of MABP and influence the heart rate (chronotropy), AV conduction time (dromotropy), and ventricular contraction (inotropy). The results of simulations performed with this model demonstrate that a realistic system

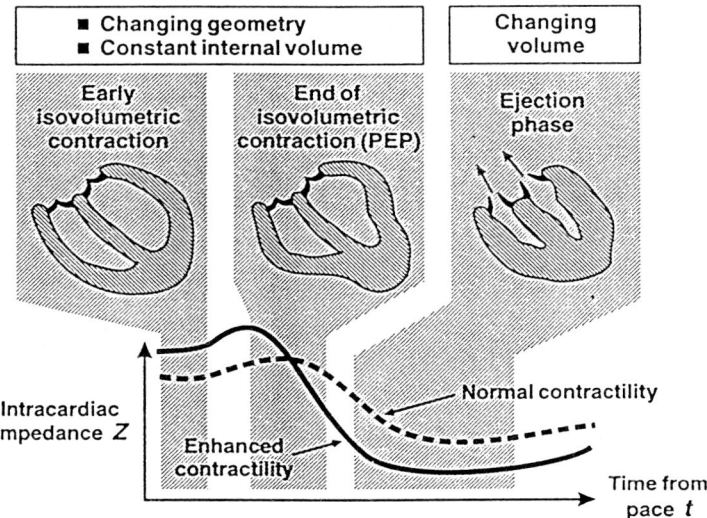

Figure 9. Intracardiac impedance waveform during contraction, showing the effects of normal and enhanced contractility.

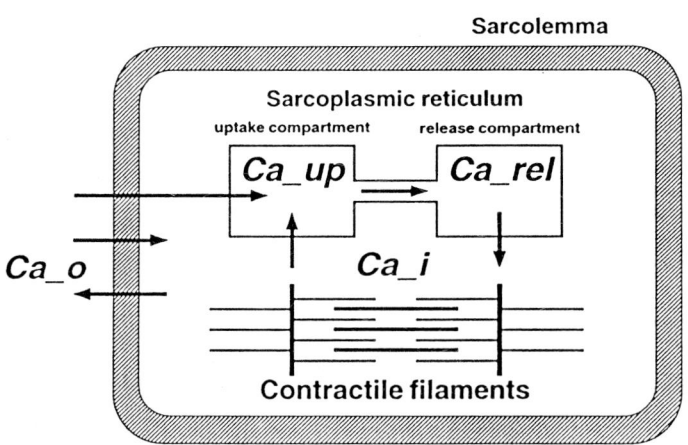

Figure 10. Model of Ca-dynamics in the myocyte.

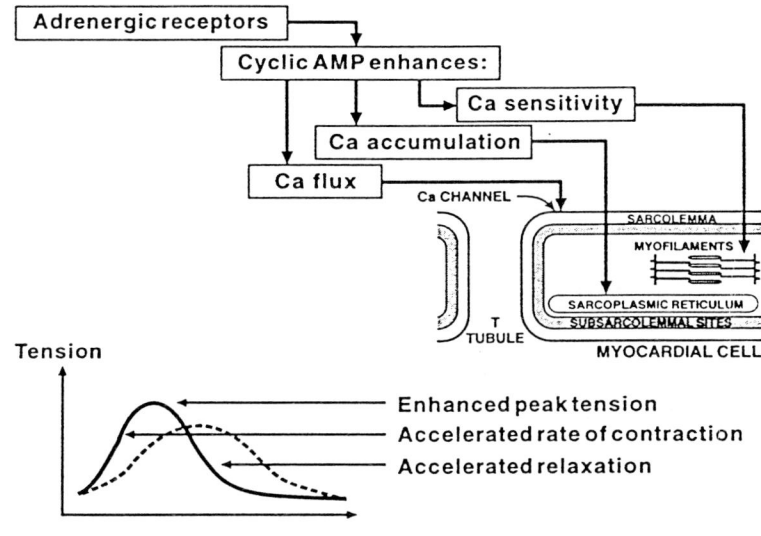

Figure 11. Adrenergic effects on contractility and wall tension.

behavior can be approximated in many aspects. Figure 12 shows the measured time courses of left ventricular wall tension and thickness (from Mirsky [25] left) compared to simulated tensions of the left ventricular wall, septum, and right ventricular free wall (right). Further simulation of this model provides evidence that the intracardiac unipolar impedance signal is mainly modulated by ventricular wall tension and wall thickness time courses (Figure 13). These parameters depend directly on the inotropic state, so the measured impedance signal contains ANS information that allows the determination of the appropriate pacing frequency and the re-establishment of closed-loop control.

CLOSED-LOOP ANS-CONTROLLED RATE-ADAPTIVE PACING SYSTEM

The aim of today's pacemaker technology is to maintain a high quality of life and physical performance of the patient. When the natural sinus rhythm is absent, a series of sensors with complex microelectronic control circuits meets the need for rate-adaptive pacemaker systems while preserving AV synchrony. Only a closed-loop control mechanism has the potential to restore the natural regulation, however. Intracardiac impedance measurement allows monitoring of the contractile status of the heart, which depends mainly on the sympathetic drive. The ANS-rate-controlled pacemaker, which uses the stimulating electrode at the same time as the measuring electrode, is of special clinical advantage (Figure 14). There are different strategies for the

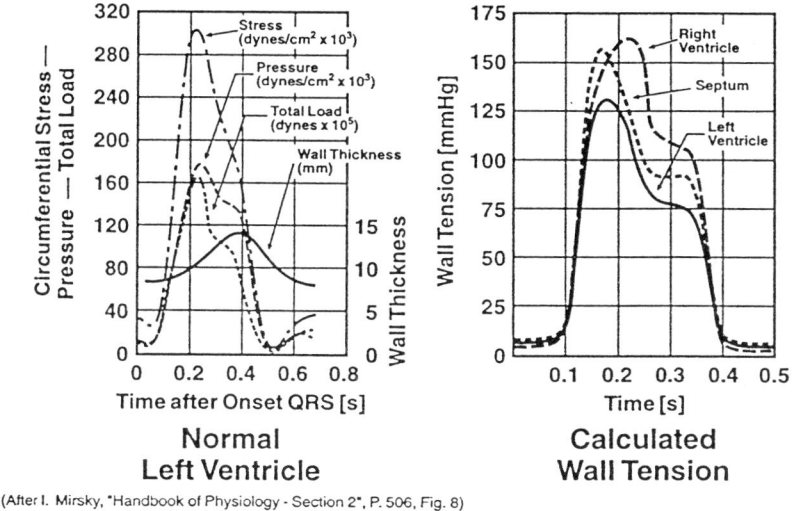

Figure 12. Comparison of measured and simulated parameters: (left) measured left ventricular wall stress (tension), thickness, pressure, and total load: (right) simulated wall tension of left ventricular wall, septum, and right ventricular free wall.

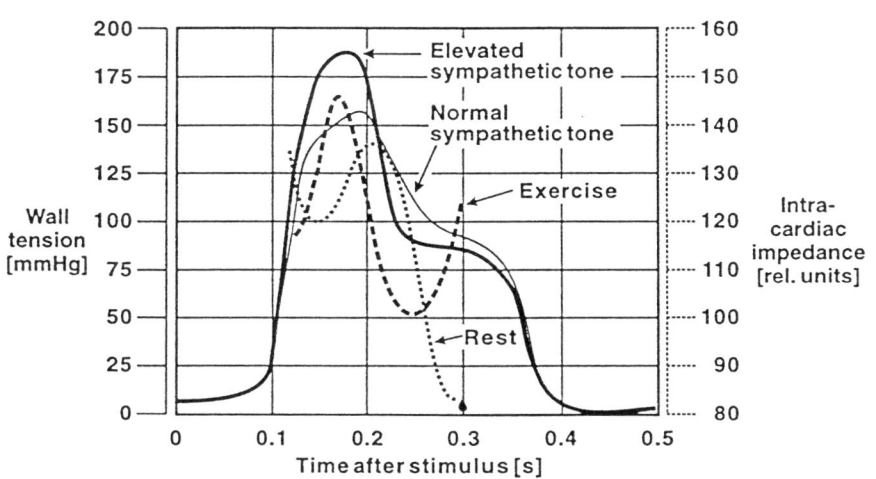

Figure 13. Simulated wall tension of the right ventricle and intracardiac impedance during normal and elevated sympathetic tone.

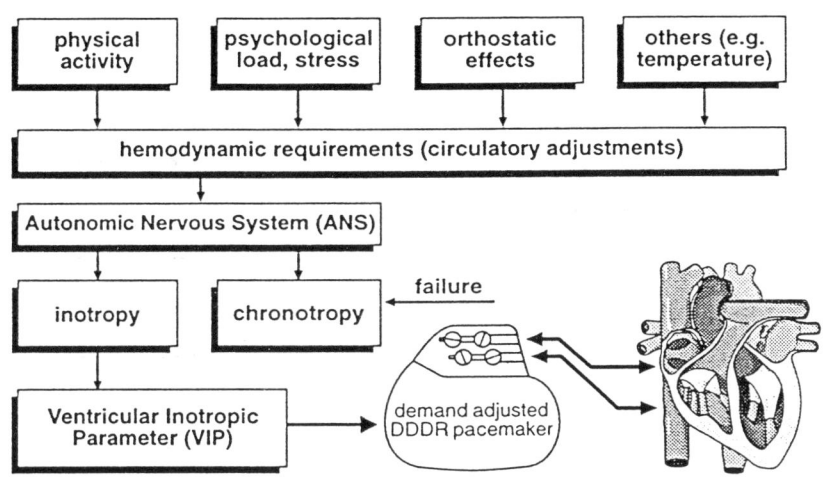

Figure 14. Block diagram showing the concept of an ANS-rate-controlled pacemaker.

adaptation of rate to meet the hemodynamic requirements. The most attractive and realistic approach presented is the ANS-controlled, closed-loop pacing system. In patients with chronotropic incompetence, only part of the entire rate control system is defective, usually the sinus node as the autonomous timer or the atrioventricular region as the most vulnerable conductive mechanism. All other parts of the system, including the sensors, the afferent pathway, the central controlling circuits, the efferent vagal and sympathetic neural pathway to the heart with all their interactions and peripherally acting modulators, as well as the working myocardium itself, are still functioning. The main difficulty is to define a measurable ANS-dependent controlling parameter. Using neurocardiological knowledge from anatomy, physiology, biophysics, and molecular biology, it is clear that such a coordinated parameter, reflecting the autonomic neural activity, can be extracted only from the myocardium, i.e., the effector level. The myocardial contractile performance was used for this purpose. Measurement was accomplished by the impedance method using the stimulation electrode as the measuring electrode [1,4]. The ventricular inotropic parameter (VIP) has been identified as an ANS-dependent value, and a special detection algorithm, regional effective slope quantity (RQ), with high ANS sensitivity has been developed. A simplified block diagram of an ANS-rate-controlled dual chamber pacemaker is shown in Figure 15. The complete pacemaker circuitry is assembled in hybrid technology, establishing the connections between the monolithic integrated circuits (CMOS technology) and passive components. It must be emphasized that this pacing system offers a unique opportunity to monitor the autonomic efferent signals of the heart.

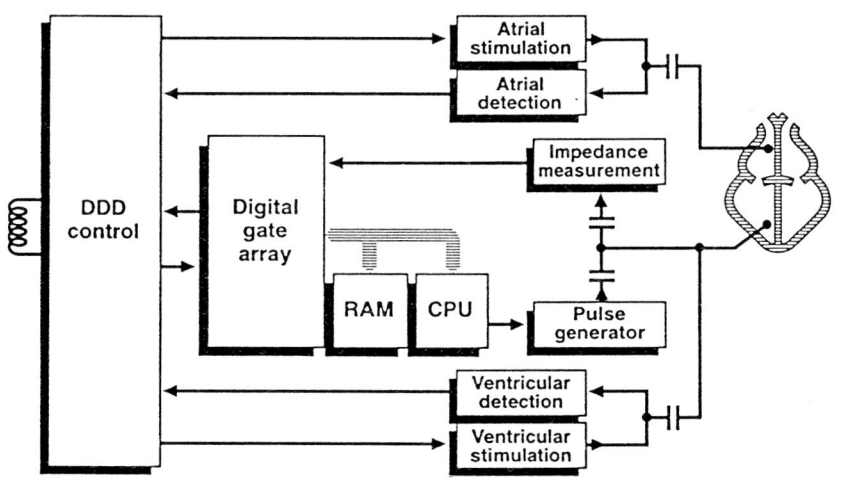

Figure 15. Simplified block diagram of an ANS-controlled dual chamber (DDDR) pacemaker.

ANS-CONTROLLED ELECTROTHERAPY

The importance of the autonomic nervous system in the genesis of cardiac arrhythmias, particularly at the time of acute myocardial ischemia, has become progressively evident from the experimental and clinical observations of many authors [26,27]. It has been shown that within a few seconds of myocardial ischemia, cardiac sympathetic excitation and vagal depressor reflexes take place. The intensity of an increase in the sympathetic activity correlates with a reduction of the ventricular fibrillation threshold and an increase of coronary vasoconstriction. At the same time, the excitation of cardiac sympathetic afferents can also selectively inhibit the activity of efferent cardiac vagal fibers, facilitating the occurrence of a dangerous tachycardia. The afferent limb of cardiac sympathetic reflexes is dependent, to a major extent, upon an intact left stellate ganglion. Activation of vagal afferents seems to be more prominent in the subendocardium of the left ventricular inferior wall, resulting in more pronounced depressor responses with inferior subendocardial ischemia. Myocardial infarction produces areas of mainly sympathetic or vagal denervation. In the latter case, it will increase the vulnerability of the heart to arrhythmia and fibrillation during acute, painful, or silent ischemia episodes. Different rational approaches have been offered for the prevention of malignant arrhythmia in coronary patients by the interruption of sympathetic activity or stimulation of the vagal influences to the heart, including left stellectomy and efferent electrostimulation of the vagal nerve. These nontraditional methods have provided a certain alternative to drugs, but have obvious limitations. The ANS-controlled pacemaker,

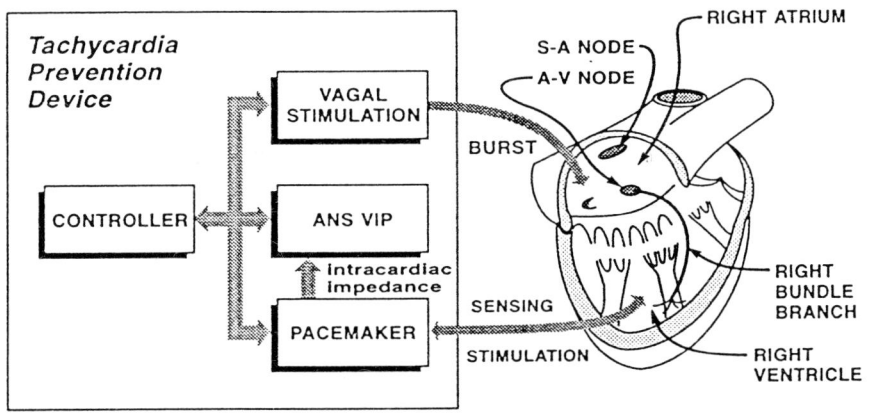

Figure 16. Block diagram showing the concept of a tachycardia-prevention device using vagal stimulation.

which serves as the regulator of autonomic tone, establishing the neural equilibrium and thereby providing a more flexible tachyarrhythmia prevention, is a new method [28]. A block diagram of such a system is shown in Figure 16. A standard pacing lead in the ventricle monitors the autonomic balance, and in the early stage of sympathetic hyperactivity, prior to the onset of tachyrhythmia, it applies bursts of electrical stimuli to the afferent vagus nerve endings at the endocardium of the right atrium during the refractory period for the working myocardium. Preliminary results demonstrate a high antiarrhythmic efficiency of this pacing system, while a coronary protective effect may also be expected [28].

EPICARDIAL ELECTROGRAM DETECTION OF ACUTE ALLOGRAFT REJECTION IN CARDIAC TRANSPLANT PATIENTS

Epicardial electrograms obtained from intraoperatively implanted pacemakers with telemetric capabilities and ventricular epimyocardial screw-in electrodes have been used to evaluate the potential of detecting acute allograft rejection from intracardiac ECG parameters. Preliminary work with such a system has employed wide-bandwidth electrodes to monitor epicardial electrograms. These electrodes allow high-resolution signals to be telemetered to a computer for further digital processing using signal averaging, beat detection, and classification techniques to yield epicardial depolarization (QRS voltage) and repolarization (T wave voltage) parameters. The results show that a reduction in the amplitude of the evoked T wave was found to

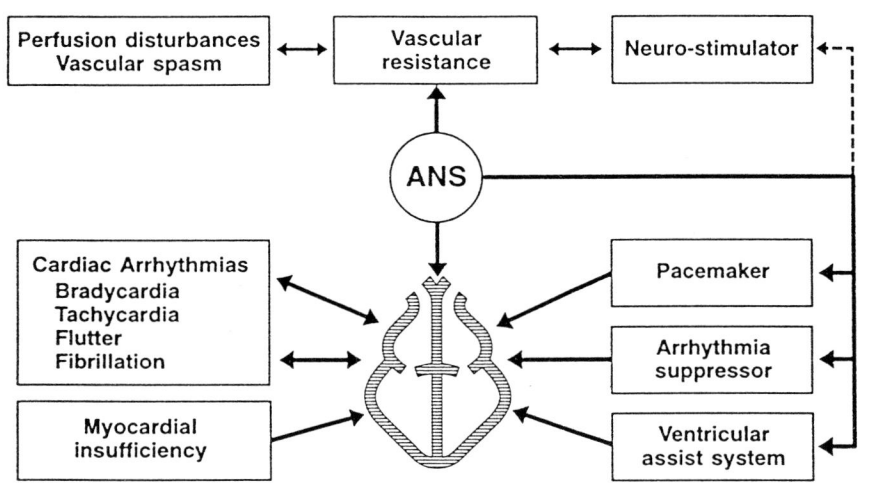

Figure 17. New concepts in the electrotherapy of the heart.

correlate with biopsy evidence of rejection [29]. This technique offers many advantages since it is noninvasive and easily accessible using simple ventricular pacing devices and could be used to monitor the transplant patient much more frequently than can be achieved by the endocardial biopsy method, making it very cost effective for monitoring patients after cardiac transplantation.

CONCLUSIONS

The refinement of the electrode-myocardium interface by the use of new fractally coated electrodes has significantly improved the detection of intracardiac signals. Thus, the electrodes have allowed not only stimulation but access to a variety of sensory information. Access to the flow of cardiac ANS information by way of these new electrodes opens new avenues for cardiac electrotherapies. where the electrode becomes both the actuator and the sensor. Figure 17 depicts many of these therapies, some of which have been discussed above. On the left are rhythm, myocardial performance, and perfusion disturbances. On the right are the therapies improved through the use of cardiac ANS information. The ANS signal can be used to control chronotropic pacing therapy in response to physiological demand. The early detection of an acute imbalance between the sympathetic and parasympathetic tone can be used to trigger and control arrhythmia suppression therapies. The ANS signal can also be used to modulate ventricular assist systems, including cardiac myoplasty preparations, which would further protect the myocardium from acute stress. Circulatory disorders triggered by pain can also be controlled by neurostimulation to block painful sensory stimuli either by a volitional act or automatic triggering. The neurostimulator effects the corrective therapy by providing an epidural neurostimulation to block nociception and, thus, disrupts the conditions leading to the emergence of angina.

REFERENCES

1. Pichlmaier AM, Braile D, Ebner E et al. Automatic nervous system controlled closed loop cardiac pacing. PACE 1992;15:1787–91.
2. Chirife R. The pre-ejection period: an ideal physiologic variable for closed-loop rate-responsive pacing. PACE 1987;10:425–31.
3. Schaldach M. Automatic adjustment of pacing parameters based on intracardiac impedance measurements. PACE 1990;13:1702–10.
4. Schaldach M, Hutten H. Intracardiac impedance to determine sympathetic activity in rate responsive pacing. PACE 1992;15:1778–86.
5. Kulbertus HE, Franck G. Neurocardiology. Mount Kisco, NY: Futura Publishing, 1988.
6. Auerbach AA, Furman S. The autodiagnostic pacemaker. PACE 1979;2:58–68.
7. Rickards AF, Norman J. Relationship between QT interval and heart rate: new design of a physiologically adaptive cardiac pacemaker. Br Heart J 1981;45:56–61.
8. Grace AA, Newell SA, Cary NRB et al. Diagnosis of early cardiac transplant rejection by fall in evoked T wave amplitude measured using an externalized QT driven rate responsive pacemaker. PACE 1991;14:1024–31.
9. Callaghan F, Vollman W, Livingston A et al. The ventricular depolarization gradient: effects of exercise, pacing rate, epinephrine, and intrinsic heart rate control on the right ventricular evoked response. PACE 1989;12:1115–30.
10. Delle-Vedove D, Lallemand Y, Hubert O. Procede et dispositif de detection de la response du coeur à une impulsion electrique de stimulation. French Patent # 8216034, 1982.
11. Schaldach M, Boheim G, Edelhäuser R. Ein Beitrag zur Erkennung evozierter Potential. Biomed Technik 1988;33:343–4.
12. Curtis AB, Vance F, Miller K. Automatic reduction of stimulus polarization artifact for accurate evaluation of ventricular evoked responses. PACE 1991;14:526–37.
13. MacCarter DJ, Lundberg KM, Corstjens JPM. Porous electrodes: concept, technology and results. PACE 1983;6:427–35.
14. Hirshorn MS, Holley LK, Skalsky M et al. Characteristics of advanced porous and textured surface pacemaker electrodes. PACE 1983;6:525–36.
15. Schaldach M. Bolz A, Breme J et al. Acute and long term sensing and pacing performance of pacemaker leads having TiN electrode tips. In: Antonioli GE, editor. Pacemaker leads. Amsterdam: Elsevier, 1991:441–50.
16. Lewin G, Myers H, Parsonnet U. A non-polarizing electrode for physiological stimulation. Trans Am Soc Artif Int Organs 1967;13:345–9.
17. Schaldach M. The stimulating electrode. Electrotherapy of the heart. Berlin: Springer-Verlag, 1992:145–168.
18. Rosen MR, Jeck CD, Steinberg SF. Autonomic modulation of cellular repolarization and of the electrocardiographic QT interval. J Cardiovasc Electrophysiol 1992;3:487–99.
19. Bolz A, Hubmann M, Hardt R, Riedmüller J, Schaldach M. Low polarization pacing lead for detecting the ventricular evoked response. Med Prog Technol 1993 (in print).
20. Schaldach M. Cardiac control parameters. Electrotherapy of the heart. Berlin: Springer-Verlag, 1992:105–43.

21. Baan J, van der Velde ET, Steendijk P, Koops J. Calibration and application of the conductance catheter for ventricular volume measurement. Automedica 1989;11:357–65.
22. Czegledy FP, Aebischer NM, Tamari A, Tortolani A. A new mathematical model for right ventricular geometry. Proc 12th Ann Intern Conf IEEE. Eng Med Biol 1990;1813–95.
23. Urbaszek A, Hutten H, Schaldach M. A heart and circulation model with emphasis on short-term regulation. Proc 14th Ann Intern Conf IEEE. Eng Med Biol 1992;429–30.
24. Schaldach M. Control aspects of cardiac output adjustment. Electrotherapy of the heart. Berlin: Springer-Verlag, 1992:73–86.
25. Mirsky I. Elastic properties of the myocardium: a quantitative approach with physiological and clinical application. In: Berne RM, Sperelakis N, Geiger SR, editors. Handbook of physiology, section 2: The cardiovascular system. Bethesda, MD: American Physiological Society, 1979.
26. Schwartz PJ, Stone HL. Effects of unilateral stellectomy upon cardiac performance during exercise in dogs. Circ Res 1979;44:637–45.
27. Verrier RL. Neurogenic aspect of cardiac arrhythmias. In: El-Sherif N, Samet P, editors. Cardiac pacing and electrophysiology. Philadelphia: W.B. Saunders, 1991:77–92.
28. Schaldach M. Reestablishment of physiological regulation. A challenge to technology. Electrotherapy of the heart. Berlin: Springer-Verlag, 1992:209–14.
29. Schreier G, Auer T, Hutten H, Schaldach M, Iberer F, Tsceliessnigg KH. Epicardial electrogram recordings for detection of acute allograft rejection in cardiac transplant recipients. To be presented at the Proc 15th Ann Intern Conf IEEE. Eng Med Biol 1993.

19. The myocardium-electrode interface at the macro level

W. IRNICH

INTRODUCTION

'The physiologic electrode is a device that provides an interface between living tissue and a machine – for example, between the patient and a diagnostic or therapeutic instrument' [1]. The following paragraphs will be restricted to the electrode's contact with the myocardial wall and to the attached sensing amplifier, whether used as a diagnostic tool (catheterization) or for therapeutic purposes (synchronization of antitachy- or antibradycardia devices). When discussing the requirements for electrodes and amplifiers, it must be clear for which purpose they are to be used. If, for instance, the heart rate will only be derived from the registration procedure or if spontaneous activity may be present or not, then the amplifier can be confined to special features. Therefore, our goal will be to describe the myocardium-electrode interface under the aspect of recording heart signals from its surface undistorted, so that even the fastest intrinsic deflection will be faithfully reproduced and the slowest T wave can be detected.

GENESIS OF HEART SIGNALS

To study the phenomena that produce heart signals, we must simplify a rather complex system as follows. One or two electrodes (if bipolar) are adjacent to a rugged trabeculated myocardial wall, which is partially surrounded by blood [2]. We neglect all of these irregularities and consider a system consisting of a very small electrode (almost a dot) in a homogeneous medium in the vicinity of excitable myocardium, with the large reference electrode lying at infinity. Figure 1 depicts the abstraction of this electrode-myocardium system in which a layer of myocardium is partially excited; the excitation is moving towards the electrode from left to right. Between fully excited and nonexcited myocardium, we must assume a diffuse zone in which a probability of fibers being excited varies from zero at the right to 100% at

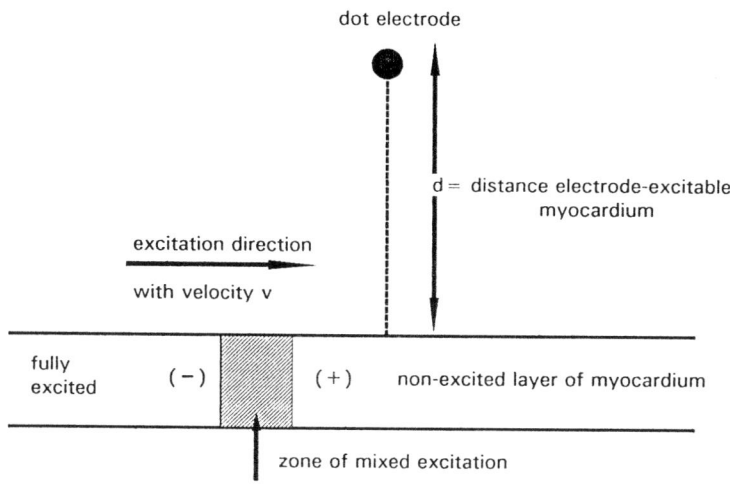

Figure 1. Abstraction of the electrode-myocardium interface: a dot electrode with distance d to a two-dimensional homogeneous layer of excitable tissue.

the left boundary. The thickness of this diffuse zone is about 1–2 mm. Figure 2 depicts the distribution of the charge around the diffuse zone in more detail. The extracellular space has a negative charge left of the diffuse zone, due to the sudden influx of sodium ions. The intracellular space, at least for a few milliseconds, has a positive charge. Together with the charge of the nonexcited region to the right of the diffuse zone, a quadrupole seems to be the result of the charge distribution. However, as the membrane of the nonexcited portion possesses a high impedance, the transversal dipole of the nonexcited right side and the intracellular longitudinal dipole are not capable of producing a current field throughout the body.

The potential field produced by the two dipoles can be derived according to the classical theory of electrophysics. The field of both dipoles is thought to be linearly superimposed, which means that both can be discussed independently.

Figure 3 illustrates how the potential at the electrode is generated by the moving dipole. The charge closest to the electrode will determine the polarity and the value of the potential, which increases with decreasing distance. When the positive pole is closest to the electrode, the potential is at its maximum. This may change rapidly as the negative pole comes closest, and therefore, the electrode assumes its minimum potential. The negative portion of the curve must be a mirror image of the positive one. This typical structure is called intrinsic deflection.

In Figure 4 a transverse dipole is assumed, formed by the negative charge of the extracellular and the positive charge of the intracellular space. This

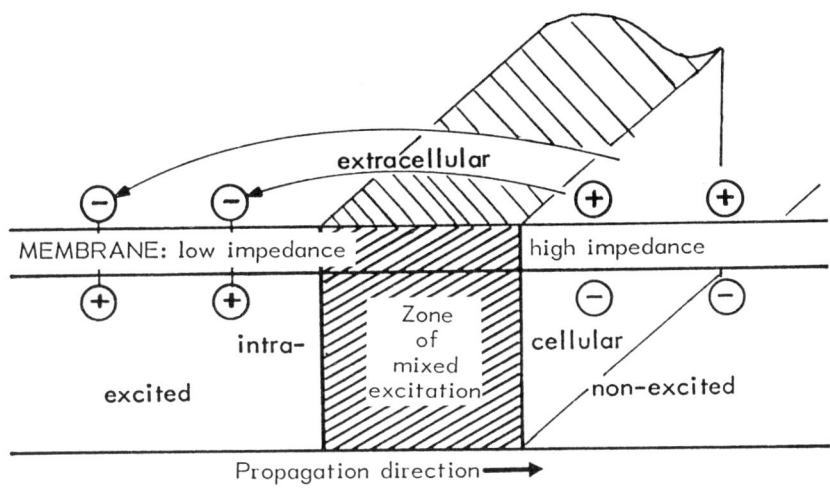

Figure 2. The diffuse zone of mixed excitation forms a two-dimensional dipole layer with positive charges in the extracellular space at the front side (excitation from left to right).

dipole is smaller than the longitudinal dipole because of a smaller dipole axis. However, if an excitation is conducted along the endocardial wall by the Purkinje system, an excitation wave starts transversely to the Purkinje excitation, moving from the inside to the outside of the ventricular myocardium. This excitation will add a transverse component to the longitudinal dipole. This means that a difference in signal structure exists between normally conducted atrial and ventricular excitations. Only if a ventricular ectopic excitation is conducted via the myocardium is the signal mechanism comparable in both the atrium and the ventricle.

Figure 4 derives the potential of an electrode with a moving transverse dipole. The potential is always negative and symmetric with respect to point B. Real heart signals are always a mixture of signals 3 and 4.

UNIPOLAR MEASUREMENTS

If unipolar electrograms are derived from the endocardium with a high-ohm oscilloscope connected to the electrode as in Figure 5, signals are obtained that are very similar to our hypothetical signals when compared to the portion with the downstroke structure.

Figure 6a–e shows that there is always a larger negative than positive amplitude if the myocardium is not injured. If injured, there is the well-known structure of injury with a positive amplitude (Figure 6f).

The velocity of the moving excitation wave is important for the typical

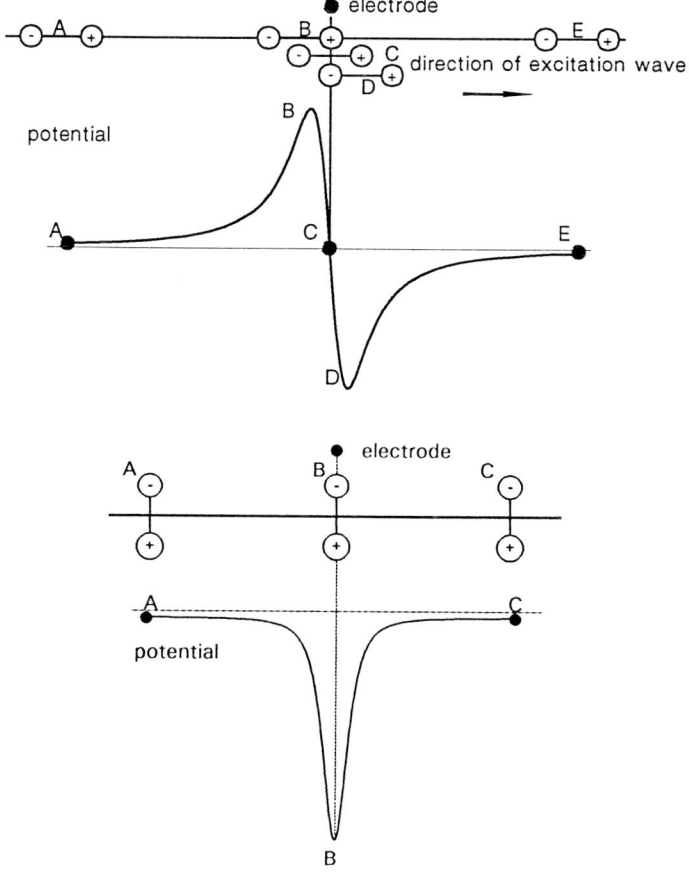

Figure 3. Potentials due to uniformly moving dipoles: (a) a biphasic signal is generated by the longitudinal dipole; (b) a monophasic negative signal is generated by a transverse dipole.

structure of the electrogram. The change from the positive to the negative peak is an expression of how fast the dipole position B is changed to D in Figure 3. Therefore, the dipole distance and the velocity of excitation will determine the time between both peaks. Figure 7 demonstrates that the decay time increases with decreasing velocity. As this structure will determine the high-frequency content of heart signals, we can conclude that the higher the frequency is, the faster the excitation velocity. Thus, it is inconceivable that atrial electrograms could have a higher-frequency content [1,6] if the excitation velocity is the same or even slower in the atrium than in the ventricle due to the lack of Purkinje fibers.

Our considerations have assumed an electrode of negligible size so far.

Myocardium-electrode interface at the macro level 193

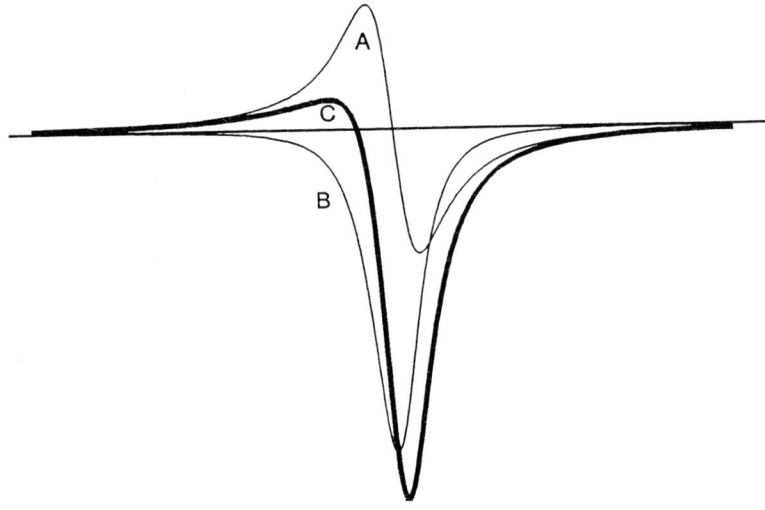

Figure 4. Composition of the dipole potentials of a longitudinal (A) and transverse (B) dipole yielding the signal mixture (C) typical for ventricular electrograms.

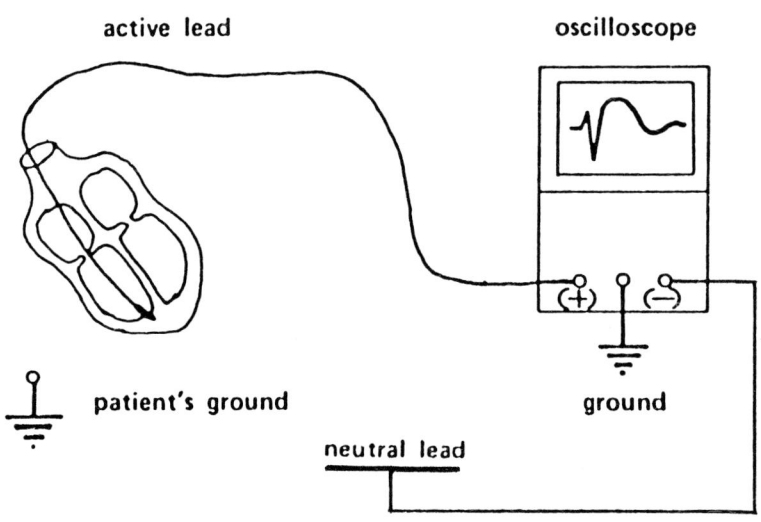

Figure 5. Measuring procedure to derive unipolar electrograms as seen by a pacemaker. The positive input of the oscilloscope is connected to the electrode in contact with the myocardial wall; the negative one is attached to a large-area electrode far away from the heart. The position of the neutral electrode of the differential oscilloscope is without influence and, thus, uncritical (from [2] with permission).

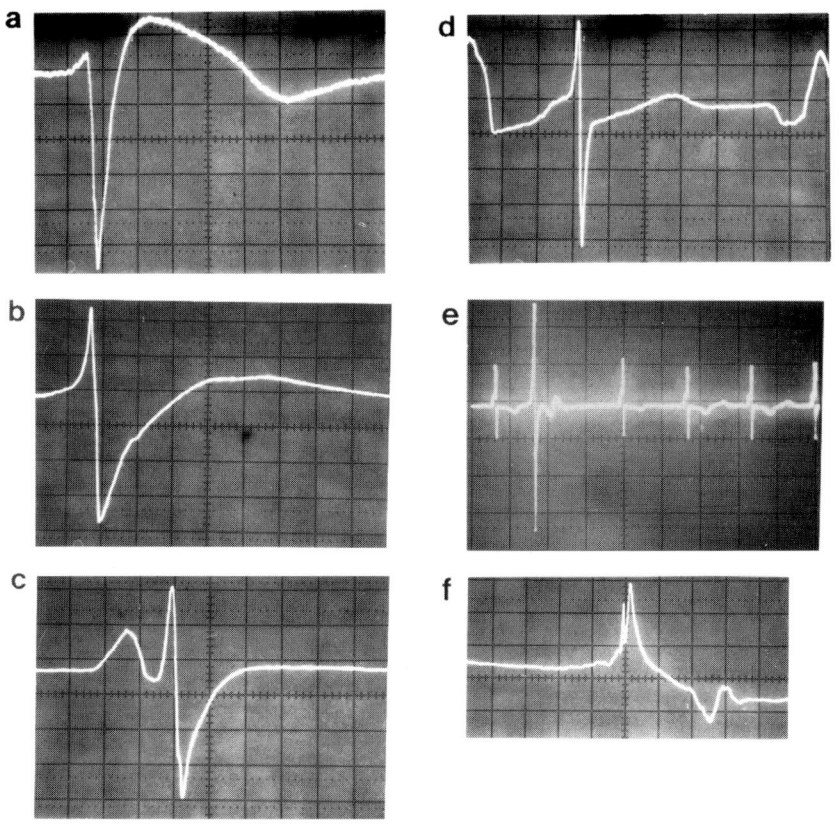

Figure 6. Registered unipolar intracardiac electrograms: (a) acute ventricular electrogram, monophasic (2 mV, 50 ms/div); (b) acute ventricular electrogram, biphasic (5 mV, 20 ms/div); (c) chronic ventricular electrogram, biphasic, 5 years (2 mV, 20 ms/div); (d) acute atrial electrograms, biphasic, signals right and left of ventricular origin (1 mV, 50 ms/div); (e) acute ventricular electrograms, 5 sinus beats, 1 ectopic beat (5 mV, 50 ms/div); (f) acute atrial electrogram after hurting the wall (1 mV, 50 ms/div) (from [2] with permission).

Let us now demonstrate its influence. A metallic electrode with a conductivity much higher than the tissue must have the same potential over all of its surface. This is achieved by averaging the potential over the entire surface. The result can be shown if two point-electrodes are assumed at a distance corresponding to the extreme ends of the real electrode. Averaging in this case results in the arithmetic mean of both potentials. Figure 8 demonstrates two essential features of larger electrodes:

1. The peak-to-peak amplitude is reduced.

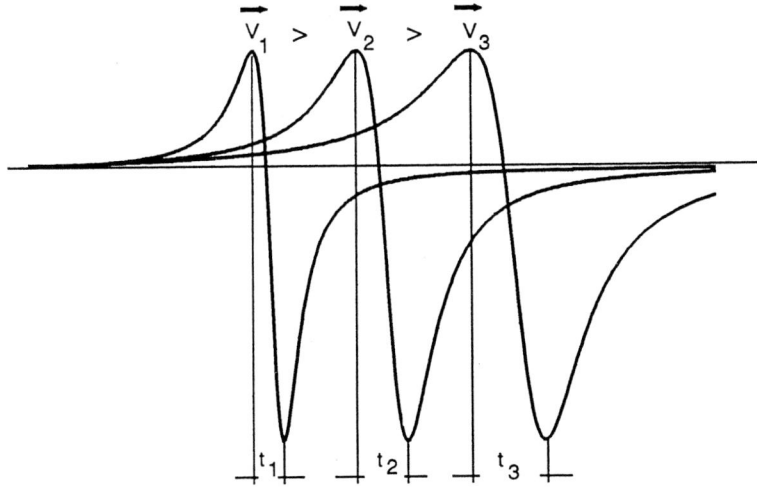

Figure 7. Correlation between excitation velocity and decay time of the intrinsic deflection: the higher the velocity, the faster the decay time and the higher the frequency content of the signal.

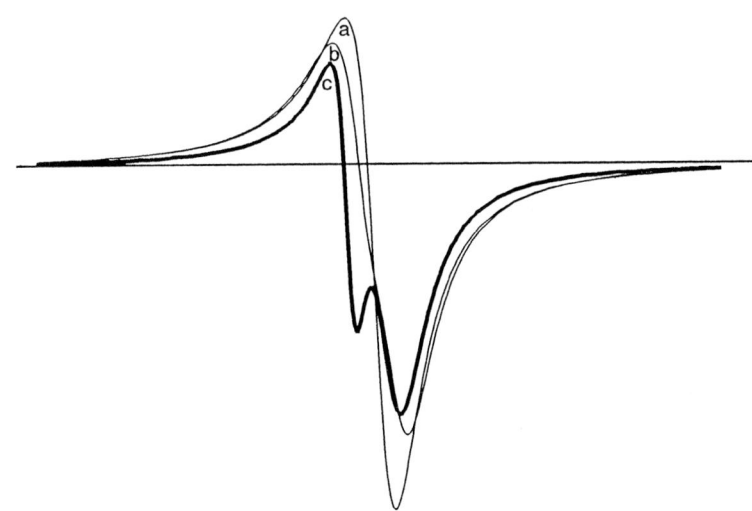

Figure 8. Influence of electrode size on signal structure: signal (a) with a point electrode, signal (b) with two closely spaced electrodes, signal (c) with widely spaced electrodes. The averaging process reduces the amplitude, increases decay time, and can introduce notches (fractionated electrograms).

2. The decay time is prolonged, which means that the frequency content of a large area electrode is lower than that of a smaller one.

BIPOLAR MEASUREMENTS

With the aid of the following formula, the signal form of an ideal bipolar electrode system can be readily calculated as the difference of both electrode potentials:

$$V_{bipolar} = V_1 - V_2$$

with V_1 = potential of the electrode connected to the positive input, and V_2 = potential of the other electrode.

In this context, ideal means that the two electrodes of equal size have equal contact to the same myocardium and are in close vicinity to each other. These conditions are not always fulfilled in reality, as the size of the second electrode is normally larger in pacing leads, and it is not always equally pressed to the myocardial wall, but sometimes floats in the bloodstream. Therefore, the bipolar electrograms, in reality, are placed between an ideal bipolar electrogram and a unipolar one. A bipolar system derives its signal from two different sites within the potential field of a moving excitation wave, comparable to a differential amplifier. Peak potentials are created under each electrode at different times corresponding to their distance. From this, it follows that the zero-peak amplitude is normally smaller than that of a unipolar system, whereas the peak-to-peak amplitude of a bipolar signal is always biphasic and larger than that of a unipolar signal (this is only valid for the near field potential). Figure 9 shows that biphasic signals for narrow electrode distances have a nearly differentiating effect. The slope is increased, the rise time can be shorter, and the slow-moving, far-field signals are suppressed.

The bipolar electrogram is largely dependent upon the direction of the excitation wave. The signs of the electrograms shown in Figure 9 are inverted if the excitation wave first crosses the electrode connected to the negative input. If there is an angle of less than 90° between the excitation front plane and the axis of the two electrodes, the distance between the electrodes effective for the formation of the bipolar electrogram is shortened, thereby reducing the amplitude of the signal. This is very typical for a derivation which is proportional to the electric field. A rough estimation of the field strength is given by the quotient of voltage divided by the distance between both electrodes.

To summarize the main difference between unipolar and bipolar derivation, one can state that a unipolar electrode yields a voltage which is nearly equal to the potential at the contact site. Ideal bipolar electrodes offer a voltage which is proportional to the electric field of the contact area. Unipolar leads offer the possibility of measuring the instant of excitation and

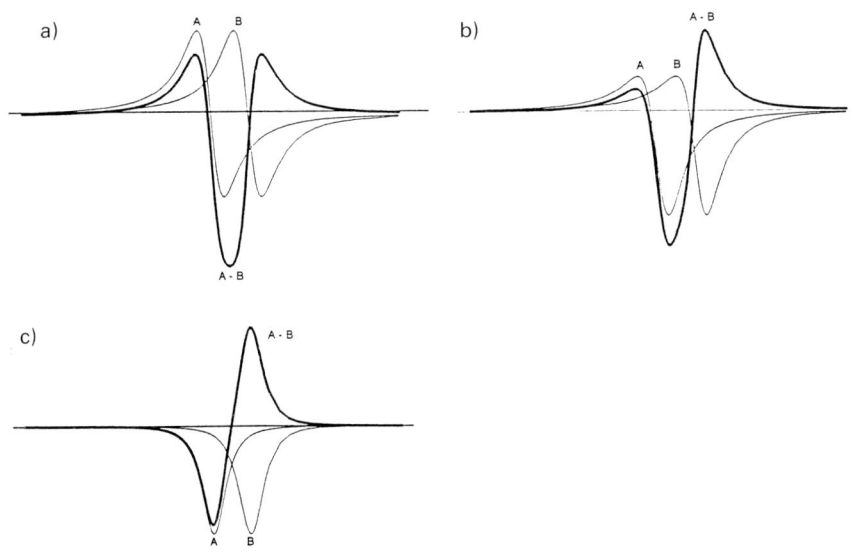

Figure 9. Bipolar electrograms according to the formula $V_{bipolar} = V_A - V_B$: (a) the biphasic signal produces an asymmetric bipolar signal; (b) the monophasic signal produces a symmetric bipolar signal but with positive upstroke; (c) mixture of monophasic and biphasic signals. Except in signal (b) the zero-peak amplitude of the bipolar signal is always larger than that of the unipolar ones.

provide a rough estimate of the excitation velocity. Bipolar leads, in contrast, can give an indication of the wave direction.

T WAVE MEASUREMENTS

The repolarization process is not only slower, but also not as well organized as depolarization. Depending on the site of the electrode, the large muscle mass of the left ventricle determines predominantly the T wave and is, therefore, a far-field signal for every right ventricular or atrial lead. This is the reason why bipolar leads are not suited for T wave detection.

CHARACRETISTICS OF HEART SIGNALS

There is a relationship between the decay or rise time and the frequency content of a signal according to Küpfmüller's Law:

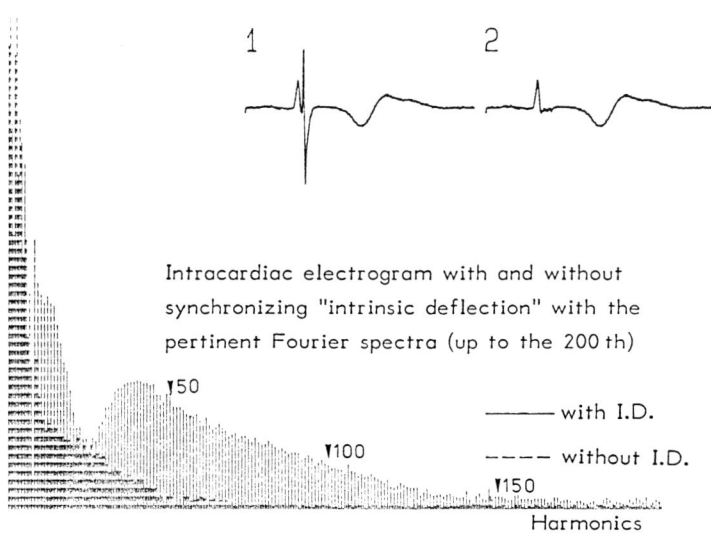

Figure 10. Fourier's analysis of a unipolar ventricular intracardiac electrogram (1) with intrinsic deflection and (2) without intrinsic deflection (blanked out artificially). The difference in both spectra characterize the frequency content of the intrinsic deflection lying between 25 and 200 Hz.

$$f = \frac{1}{2t}$$

where f = highest frequency within a signal, and t = decay or rise time.

To avoid evident distortion of the signal of more than 10%, the upper cut-off frequency of a low pass should be twice that of the frequency content [5] which means that the upper cut-off frequency of pacemaker filters should reach at least 1/2 ms = 500 Hz, to avoid the attenuation of heart signals of small-area electrodes with a very fast intrinsic deflection. The cut-off frequency must be even higher (700 Hz), if bipolar faithful derivation is desired.

Today's pacemakers have sensing circuits with cut-off frequencies of no more than 50–70 Hz [3], which may dampen heart signals noticeably. This prejudiced filtering may explain some of the poor results with small-area electrodes in the past.

Figure 10 shows the Fourier analysis of a unipolar right ventricular heart signal. It is correct that the main frequency content lies below 50 Hz [3,4,6–8]. However, if we want to know which portion of the spectrum represents the intrinsic deflection, we have to mask this structure. Figure 10 demonstrates the differences between both signals with and without the intrinsic deflection: the spectrum between 25 and 200 Hz is mainly produced by the intrinsic deflection. This result contradicts to what is claimed in literature [3,4,6,8] and what is realized in today's pacemakers. On the other hand, the lower portion is necessary if T waves are to be recognized.

The lower cut-off frequency of a band-pass suitable for endo- or epicardial electrograms is always a compromise between the signal structure wanted and possible artefacts. These artefacts can be produced by the movement of the heart itself or by respiration. They are caused by polarization voltages at both electrodes which do not cancel completely, even if the metal is manufactured of the same material. This is due to the fact that polarization is influenced by various factors such as surrounding material (blood or tissue) contact pressure, electrode size, temperature (if one electrode is subcutaneous, the other within the heart) etc. The difference in polarization of both electrodes, which is normally a DC voltage, is modulated by the artefacts, so that a shift in the baseline is produced. Therefore, the rule applies: The lower cut-off frequency should be as high as possible to avoid baseline shift due to artefacts. If the T wave is analysed for timing reasons, a lower cut-off of 5 Hz is adequate. However, if the morphology of the wave is desired with more detail, a variable lower frequency setting between 0.1 and 5 Hz would be preferable in order to find individually the compromise between desired signal and unwanted low-frequency noise.

In a similar way, the question can be answered of which sampling rate is necessary to have an intrinsic deflection recorded without noticeable distortion. Figure 11 indicates that a decay time of 1.9 ms requires at least a sampling rate of 600 Hz to reproduce the signal without great distortion. Sampled at 240 Hz, the amplitude and decay time of the intrinsic deflection are no longer faithfully reproduced.

INTERFACE IMPEDANCE

The last but not least important viewpoint is the matching of the electrode interface impedance to that of the connected amplifier. Once again, depending upon the purpose of the recording, one has to consider the higher or the lower portion of the frequency-related impedance. If the intrinsic deflection is the main structure of interest, as is the case in antitachy- and antibradycardia devices, the impedance around 100 Hz should be taken as reference. According to our investigation, the intrinsic deflection impedance ranges between 500 Ω for non-polarizable electrodes and 3 kΩ for polished platinum. To achieve a distortion of less than 10%, an amplifier input resistance of 60 kΩ or better is advisable. If, however, T waves are of interest, with electrode impedances of up to 20 kΩ, the input resistance of the amplifier should reach 200 kΩ or even more.

To conclude, it is too often said that electrodes should have a beneficial influence on heart signal derivation and that large electrodes perform better than small ones. This is not true. With correct matching of the impedances, all

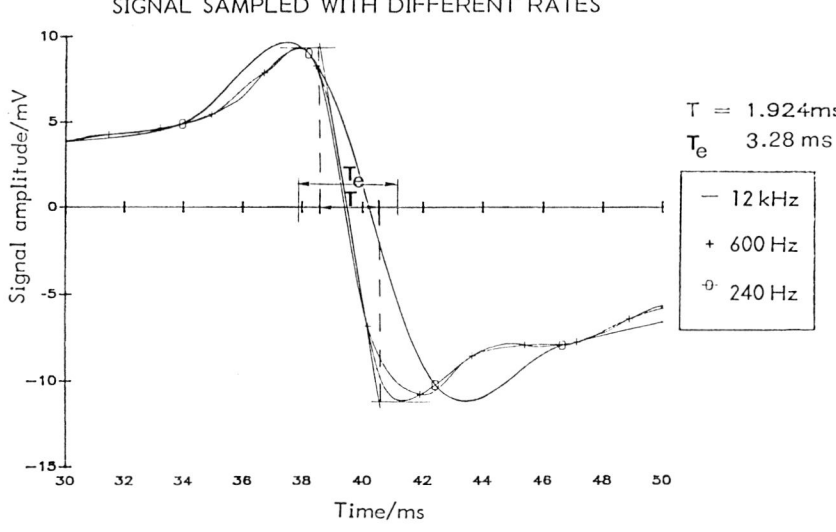

Figure 11. Signal distortion by insufficient sampling rate. The first curve was gained with a sampling rate of 12 kHz, the second sampled at 600 Hz already deviates slightly from the original, and the curve sampled at 240 Hz inadequately represents the intrinsic deflection as the amplitude is reduced and the decay time is remarkably increased.

electrodes regardless of area, shape, material, and surface structure perform nearly equally well [2,4]. Statements in the literature that special lead designs should have higher signal amplitudes reveal the investigators' mismatch between lead impedance and amplifier input.

REFERENCES

1. Kahn W, Greatbatch W. Physiologic electrodes. In: Ray CD, editor. Medical Engineering. Chicago: Year Book Medical, 1974:1073–82.
2. Irnich W. Intracardiac electrograms and sensing test signals: Electrophysiological, physical, and technical considerations. PACE 1985;8:870–88.
3. Arai Y, Yamazoe M, Toeda T et al. Optimal pacemaker sensing with respect to amplitude and slew rate of intracardiac electrograms: theoretical analysis by computer simulation. PACE 1984;7:778–83.
4. Kleinert M, Elmqvist H, Strandberg H. Spectral properties of atrial and ventricular signals. PACE 1979;2:11–9.
5. Irnich W. Einführung in die Bioelektronik. Stuttgart: Georg Thieme, 1975:125.

6. Bornzin G, Stokes K. The electrode-biointerface: Sensing. In: Barold SS, editor. Modern cardiac pacing. Mount Kisco: Futura, 1985:79–95.
7. Myers GH, Kresh YM, Parsonnet V. Characteristics of intracardiac electrograms. PACE 1978;1:90–103.
8. Parsonnet V, Myers GH, Kresh YM. Characteristics of intracardiac electrograms II. PACE 1980;3:406–17.

20. Unipolar versus bipolar leads

IVO KERSSCHOT

INTRODUCTION

A unipolar lead is a single conductor lead with an electrode located at the tip. A bipolar lead has two separate and isolated conductors within a single-lead; the distal electrode is located at the tip of the lead and the other one is usually about 2 cm more proximal. Several types of bipolar lead exist: those with two parallel conductors, the currently used coaxial leads, and the single coil type [1], allowing for small lead diameters comparable to the currently available unipolar leads.

Since both pacing and sensing are electrical phenomena, current flows from one pole to the other; in bipolar pacing these phenomena occur at the two different poles located at the tip of the lead; on the other hand, unipolar systems use the single pole at the tip of the lead, the electrical loop being closed by the pacemaker can and the body tissues. Some modern pacemakers, if connected to a bipolar lead, are suitable for both unipolar and bipolar pacing and/or sensing according to telemetric programming, allowing for maximal flexibility after implantation.

Both unipolar and bipolar pacing systems have been used since the first decade of cardiac pacing [2,3]. While bipolar leads are generally applied for temporary pacing, most leads used in implanted pacing systems are still unipolar; this can be explained by the smaller diameter and greater flexibility of unipolar leads, allowing for easier introduction and intracavitary positioning of the lead. On the other hand, bipolar leads are expected to approximate the mechanical properties of their unipolar counterparts in the next future.

DIFFERENCES IN ELECTRICAL OUTPUT

A unipolar pacing system consists of a large electrical loop between the pacemaker can in the pectoralis regio and the electrode located at the tip of the lead near the right ventricular apex. The resulting stimulus can easily be picked up by the amplifier of an electrocardiographic (ECG) recorder, resulting in clearly visible spikes on the surface ECG coincident with each pacing output. On the contrary, bipolar pacing results in very small stimulus artefacts which are hardly visible on the ECG due to the proximity of both electrodes. This can complicate the interpretation of complex ECG tracings and analysis of the waveform of the pacing pulse during pacemaker follow-up. On the other hand, modern telemetric facilities can largely compensate for this loss of information.

Both atrial and ventricular thresholds are comparable between unipolar and bipolar lead systems [4–7]. The impedance of bipolar leads is consistently higher due to the smaller surface of the anode, permitting less battery current drainage and possibly longer pacemaker longevity.

Due to the proximity of the anode (pacemaker can) to the pectoralis muscle in unipolar systems, current leakage during stimulation can result in inappropriate muscle twitching. If this phenomenon occurs in a bipolar lead system, degradation of the outer insulation should be suspected.

DIFFERENCES IN SENSING BEHAVIOR

Electrogram sensing

Several studies compared intracardiac electrograms in unipolar and bipolar systems, demonstrating that bipolar leads have comparable [8–11] or even better [4] amplitudes and slew rates. Furthermore, a much better signal-to-noise ratio (e.g. QRS signal in the atrial lead) clearly favors bipolar sensing. The feature of polarity programming in combination with bipolar leads allows for maximal flexibility in dealing with sensing problems after implantation.

Sensing of extracardiac signals

Electromagnetic interference (EMI) can induce currents in the pacing lead by the antenna effect, influencing the sensing circuit of the pacemaker and resulting in inappropriate pacemaker behavior [12]. Due to the much smaller antenna, bipolar pacing systems seem to be much less sensitive to EMI [13].

Skeletal muscle oversensing. Contraction of the ipsilateral pectoralis muscle can influence the sensing circuit of an unipolar pacing system due to the proximity of the anode to the muscle. This can result in inappropriate pacemaker inhibition in VVI systems; the atrial channel seems much more susceptible than the ventricular channel due to the higher sensitivity settings, resulting in premature ventricular triggering and, eventually, the induction of pacemaker-mediated tachycardias. If pectoralis muscle interference is ob-

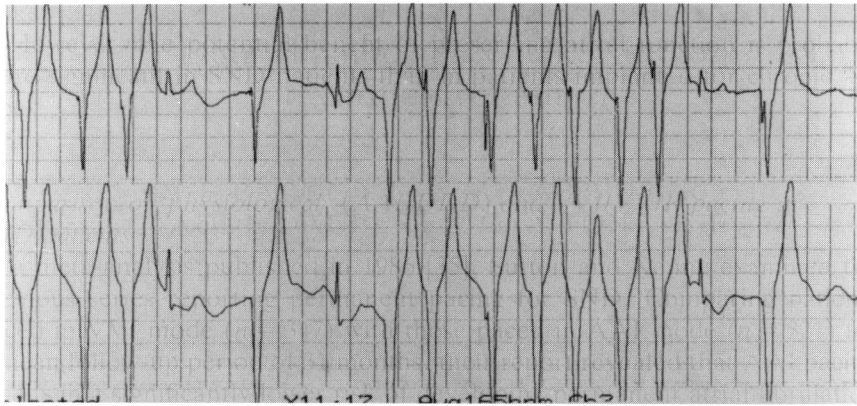

Figure 1. Two-channel Holter recording during normal daily activity in a patient with a bipolar ventricular pacing system; the pacemaker was programmed to the VVT mode because of recurrent syncope. Premature ventricular stimulation is evident from the tracing, suggesting pectoralis muscle oversensing, which could easily be confirmed with provocative maneuvers. At reoperation, a very low lead impedance was found which is typical for insulation failure. One division equals 200 ms.

served in a bipolar system, lead insulation degradation must be suspected (Figure 1).

Crosstalk is defined as the inappropriate interference between the two channels in a dual chamber pacemaker; most commonly, crosstalk refers to the inhibition of the ventricular output by the atrial stimulus and afterdepolarizations. Unipolar pacing systems are more vulnerable to this dangerous phenomenon because of their larger stimulus artefact. Besides lowering the atrial output pulse, duration, and ventricular sensitivity, the problem can be overcome by increasing the ventricular blanking period or switching to safety or committed pacing.

Mechanical differences

Owing to their thickness and construction, coaxial bipolar leads are stiffer than their unipolar counterparts. The difference in size and flexibility can interfere with the introduction and manipulation of the lead during implantation; furthermore, the stiffness of the distal tip of the bipolar leads has been suggested as a contributing factor in the possibly higher incidence of myocardial perforation with bipolar leads [14]. Several authors have reported on the problem of polyurethane degradation in pacemaker leads [15–18] leading to insulation defects. Several mechanisms have been proposed, including crush injury (clamping of the lead between the clavicle and the first rib), metal ion oxidation, environmental stress cracking, and wear [16,19]. Some reports suggest that bipolar leads are more prone to insulation failure [15,20], resulting in sensing problems, higher stimulation thresholds, and premature battery depletion. In order to overcome these problems, much effort has been put into researching new bipolar leads with better mechanical properties [1].

CONCLUSIONS

Bipolar leads are undoubtedly superior as regards sensing characteristics due to their better signal-to-noise ratio; the incidence of EMI and skeletal muscle oversensing and pectoralis muscle stimulation is extremely low. On the other hand, the currently available coaxial bipolar leads have some mechanical disadvantages, including a possibly higher incidence of insulation failure. Small and flexible bipolar leads with excellent long-term performance still remain one of the challenges in cardiac pacing for the future.

REFERENCES

1. Adler SC, Foster AJ, Sanders RS, Wuu E. Thin bipolar leads: a solution to problems with coaxial bipolar designs. PACE 1992;15:1986–90.
2. Furman S, Schwedel JB. An intracardiac pacemaker for Stokes–Adams seizures. N Engl J Med 1959;261:943–8.
3. Chardack WM. A myocardial electrode for long-term pacemaking. Ann N Y Acad Sci 1964;111:893–907.
4. Kay GN, Epstein AE, Plumb VJ. Comparison of unipolar and bipolar active fixation atrial pacing leads. PACE 1988;11:544–9.
5. Mond H, Strathmore N, Hunt P et al. Bipolar and unipolar permanent pacing leads – which is superior? (abstract). PACE 1989;12:678.
6. Anderson N, Mathivanar R, Skalsky M, Tunstell A, Ng M, Harman D. Active fixation leads: long-term threshold reduction using a drug-infused ceramic collar. PACE 1991;14:1767–71.
7. Soldati E, Bongiorni MG, De Simone L et al. Acute bipolar and unipolar sensing and pacing parameters. A within-patient study. In: Antonioli GE, Aubert AE, Ector H, editors. Pacemaker Leads. Amsterdam: Elsevier, 1991: 413–8.
8. DeCaprio V, Hurzeler P, Furman S. A comparison of unipolar and bipolar electrograms for cardiac pacemaker sensing. Circulation 1977;56:750–5.
9. Breivik K, Ohm O-J, Engedal H. Long-term comparison of unipolar and bipolar pacing and sensing, using a new multiprogrammable pacemaker system. PACE 1983;6:592–600.
10. Binner L, Richter P, Wieshammer S et al. Bipolar versus unipolar mode in dual chamber pacing. Comparison of myopotential interference, acute and long-term pacing and sensing thresholds. PACE 1987;10:646.
11. Klementowicz P, Andrews C, Furman S. Superior bipolar sensing: a prospective study. J Am Coll Cardiol 1987;9:31A.
12. Marco D, Eisinger G, Hayes DL. Testing of work environments for electromagnetic interference. PACE 1992;15:2016–27.
13. Toivonen L, Valjus J, Hongisto M, Metso R. The influence of elevated 50 Hz electric and

magnetic fields on implanted cardiac pacemakers: the role of the lead configuration and programming of the sensitivity. PACE 1991;14:2114–22.
14. Cameron J, Mond H, Ciddor G, Harper K, McKie J. Stiffness of the distal tip of bipolar pacing leads. PACE 1990;13:1915–20.
15. Furman S, Benedek ZM. The implantable lead registry. Survival of implantable pacemaker leads. PACE 1990;13:1910–4.
16. Hayes DL, Graham KJ, Irwin M et al. A multicenter experience with a bipolar tined polyurethane ventricular lead. PACE 1992;15:1033–9.
17. Mugica J, Daubert JC, Lazarus B, Henry L, Duconge R, Lespinasse P. Is polyurethane lead insulation still controversial? PACE 1992;15:1967–70.
18. Woscoboinik JR, Maloney JD, Helguera ME et al. Pacing lead survival: performance of different models. PACE 1992;15:1991–5.
19. Phillips R, Frey M, Martin RO. Long-term performance of polyurethane pacing leads: mechanisms of design-related failures. PACE 1986;9:1166–72.
20. Raymond RD, Nanian KB. Insulation failure with bipolar polyurethane pacing leads. PACE 1984;7:378–80.

21. Single lead VDD pacing: an update

GIOVANNI ENRICO ANTONIOLI, LUCIA ANSANI,
ROBERTO AUDOGLIO, GABRIELE GUARDIGLI,
GIANFRANCO PERCOCO & TIZIANO TOSELLI

INTRODUCTION

A widespread use of P-synchronous pacing became possible in the mid to late 1970s, although that system was available from the early 1960s as VAT mode [1]; at that time, in fact, this mode of pacing required two leads, one to sense atrial depolarization and the other to pace the ventricle, but the insertion of two leads through a single vein was very difficult because of the limited lead technology. The development of a system able to assure a reliable AV synchrony via a single AV lead would have been the ideal solution to the problems of implant, simplifying the venous approach and representing a suitable treatment for patients with complete AV block (CHB) and normal sinoatrial function (SAF) who do not require atrial pacing.

Different theoretical and experimental solutions were proposed in the mid-1970s [2–7], some of those similar to the "P-sensing ventricle stimulating lead" we presented in 1979 in Montreal [8,9]; nevertheless, only this last lead passed through the prototype phase and underwent a true process of development.

EXPERIMENTAL OBSERVATIONS AND FIRST CLINICAL APPLICATIONS

The single AV lead for P-synchronous pacing was conceived in the mid-1970s when we observed that unipolar electrodes 'floating' in the mid-to-high right atrium were able to detect atrial electrograms (EGMs) consistently similar to those recorded in the right appendage, except for amplitude. In particular, the atrial deflection was larger and sharper than the far-field ventricular component, showing interesting characteristics which could be potentially useful for a dedicated sensing circuit (Table 1).

The first experiences of temporary and permanent VAT/VDT pacing by properly designed single AV leads and pulse generators were made between the late 1970s and the early 1980s [8–11]. However, those early experiences

Table 1. Atrial electrogram characteristics detected by 25 unipolar tip electrodes floating in the mid-to-high atrium directly connected to the high impedance ECG recorder. Average values and ranges of amplitude in mV, major intrinsic deflection duration t in ms, dv/dt, and frequency content.[a]

	Amplitude (mV)		t	dv/dt		Frequency
	Min	Max	(ms)	Min	Max	content (Hz)
Mean	1.11	2.16	7.64	0.15	0.29	72.42
SD	±0.67	±1.07	±2.43	±0.09	±0.15	±24.25
Minimum	0.50	0.90	4.00	0.05	0.12	41.66
Maximum	3.00	4.80	13.00	0.43	0.69	125.00

[a] Calculated with the simplified formula Hz = 1:2t. Amplitude = 80% of peak-to-peak amplitude of the atrial signal; SD = standard deviation; Min = minimum observed value; Max = maximum observed value.

were conducted with unipolar floating atrial electrodes which may detect interfering signal, such as electromagnetic interferences (EMI), myopotentials, and far-field ventricular signal. To solve those problems, different atrial bipolar configurations were developed in the 1980s (Figure 1).

First the orthogonal configuration was developed, more or less contemporarily to a short longitudinal dipole (5 mm) [12–14]. In the late 1980s, a wide longitudinal dipole (30 mm) and a short diagonal dipole (DAB, 7 mm) were introduced into clinical use [15,16]. All the bipolar systems (regardless of their configuration) provided a better discriminating capability than the un-

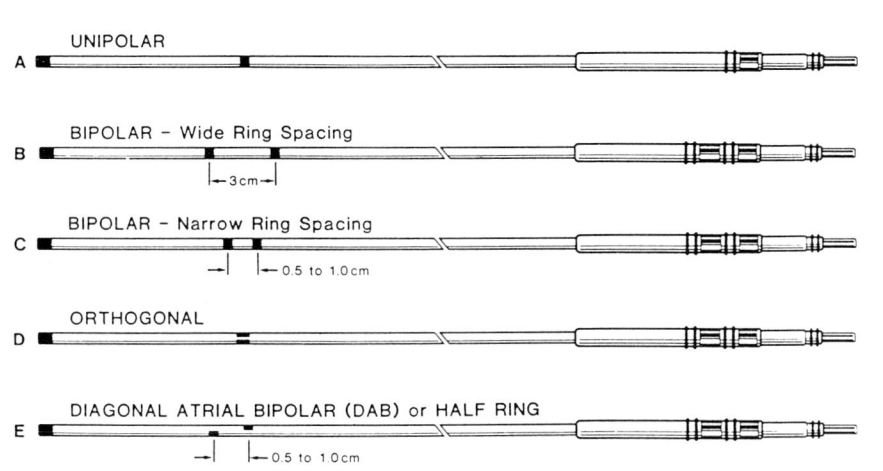

Figure 1. Five configurations of atrial sensing electrodes mounted on a ventricular pacing catheter. All but two (A and D) are in use.

ipolar system, detecting atrial depolarization of greater amplitude and dV/dt characteristics.

We prefer a floating short atrial dipole spacing, because it can be placed close to the atrial wall, allowing more effective sensing of the atrial depolarization. This concept is based on earlier observations recently confirmed in an investigational study we conducted with a temporary experimental quadripolar lead introduced into the right atrium in 34 patients during electrophysiologic study [17,18].

As shown in Figure 2, the 1-cm spacing provides sharper atrial signals and better A/V ratios compared with the 3-cm spacing. Figure 3 graphically shows the mean signal amplitudes and A/V ratios (A = A wave EGM, V = ventricular far-field EGM) as measured from different dipole spacings. The most outstanding feature of these data is that the ventricular signal is the highest with the 3-cm dipole compared with all the other interelectrode spacings at all locations. The highest P wave levels are derived from the A-B (1 cm) electrode pair in the high atrial location and the A-C (2 cm) pair in the high medium atrial location. The P-wave levels from the A-D (3 cm) electrode pair exceed those from the B-C (1 cm), B-D (2 cm), and C-D (1 cm) electrode pairs. The A/V ratios are the best in all 1-cm-spaced electrodes except for the atrial floor location, where it is similar to the 3-cm spacing ratio.

Extrapolating these data, one can postulate that at the atrial floor both electrodes would most likely be held to the greatest distance from the atrial wall by the transit of a hypothetical permanent catheter through the tricuspid valve. Also, comparing the A-C (2 cm) pair to the B-C (1 cm) pair, the data suggest that the A electrode is most likely positioned closer to the atrial wall than the B electrode, thus influencing the result. The A-C (2 cm) pair also provides a greater signal than the B-D (2 cm) pair, probably for the same reason, i.e., the A electrode is probably closer to the active tissue. The likelihood of a closer orientation of these respective A electrodes relative to the atrial wall on a hypothetical permanent catheter is credible given the more central location of the tricuspid valve compared with the lead entry site into the atrium, just below the superior vena cava, the location of electrode A. For this reason alone, modest spacing of the dipole is desirable, since both active electrodes can be placed closer to the active tissue, allowing the first derivative processing to occur with an effective high-magnitude signal sensed on both electrodes and thereby eliciting an enhanced resultant intrinsic deflection. Further, restricting the electrode pair to the mid-to-high atrium aids in the ventricular far-field rejection process due to the greater distance of the electrodes from the ventricular myocardium, another feature obvious from the data. Also, the Fast Fourier analysis of the atrial EGM shows that the best frequency range for sensing is provided by a short dipole floating in the mid-to-high right atrium.

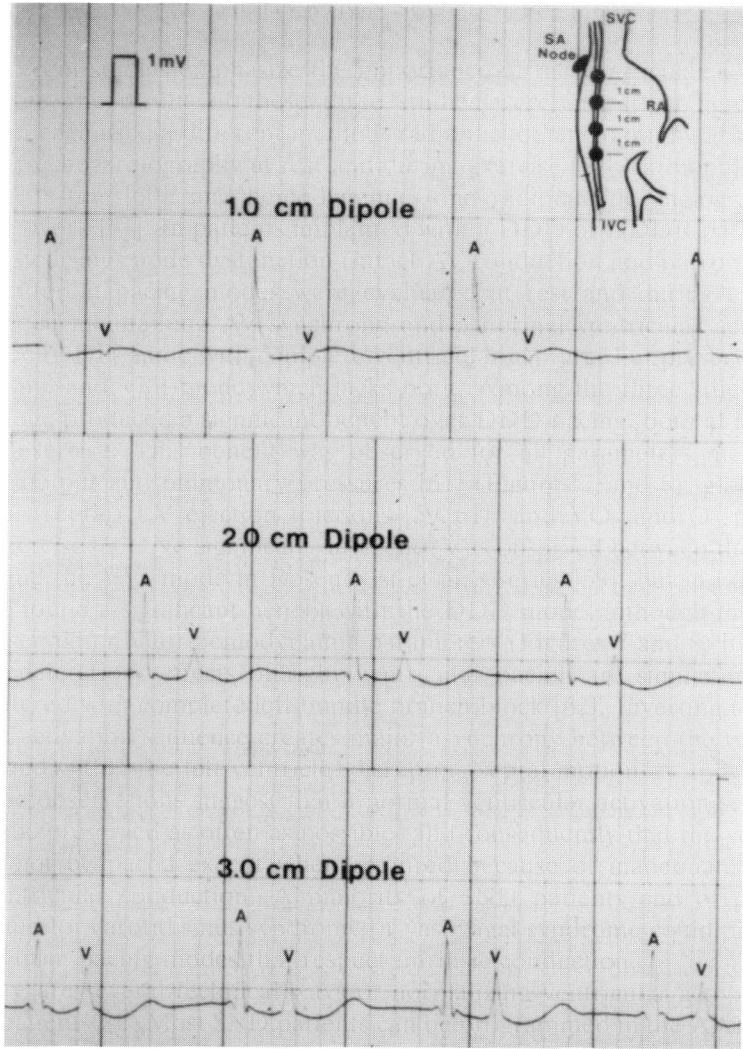

Figure 2. Examples of acute electrograms recorded from narrowly and widely spaced electrodes. The 1-cm dipole corresponds to the A-B pair; the 2-cm dipole, to the A-C pair; the 3-cm dipole, to the A-D pair.

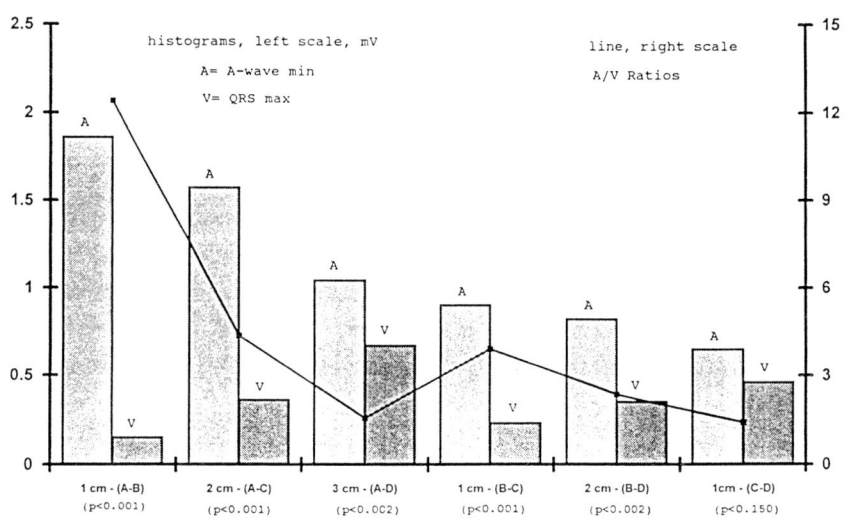

Figure 3. Mean signal amplitudes recorded by the different dipoles of an experimental multipolar catheter in the right atrium in 34 patients. Histograms represent the A wave minimum value compared with the QRS wave maximum value detected by the differently spaced dipoles. The continuous line indicates the A/V ratios. The reported *p* values refer to the comparison between atrial and ventricular signal amplitudes.

EXTENSIVE CLINICAL EXPERIENCE

A series of extensive clinical studies has been conducted in Europe and the USA with the single lead systems. The most important series are the following:

- the CPI Ultra II system, which uses the unipolar configuration of the atrial electrode and includes 250 cases in Italy, 98 of which represent our personal contribution to the series [19];
- the Medico Phymos system, which uses the wide longitudinal dipole and includes 1002 cases in Europe [20];
- the Lem Biomedica Twinal 30 system, which uses the short DAB dipole and includes 514 cases in Italy [21];
- the CCS-MAESTRO SAVVI 305/A-Track system, which is exactly the same system in the USA using the short DAB dipole manufactured in Italy by LEM-Biomedica [22–25];
- the 'newborn' experience conducted in the USA with the Intermedics VDDR system, which is still continuing [26].

The results of the two Italian extensive clinical studies cited, in which we participated as coordinating centre, are highly significant to address the reliability of the single AV lead VDD pacing. The first one was conducted with the CPI Ultra II system. Ninety-eight patients were followed-up on average 36 months after the implant (range 16–63 months). Of those patients, 16 died of pacing-unrelated reasons; 10 were lost to follow-up, but their VDD units were working correctly at the last check-up; 72 are still being followed. Five of these 72 patients had their pacing mode converted to VVI because of a complete loss of sensing (2 patients at 1 and 3 years after implantation) and chronic atrial fibrillation (3 patients, at 24, 30, and 33 months after implantation). Of the 72 patients, 67 (93%) are still paced in VDD mode; the telemetric evaluations of the atrial EGM show a constantly high quality signal.

The second study concerns the LEM Biomedica Twinal 30 system and includes 514 patients followed-up on average for 15.6 months (range 1–42 months). Twenty patients died of pacing-unrelated causes; one patient was lost to the follow-up, but his unit was working perfectly at the last check-up. Of the 493 patients still in follow-up 461 (93.5%) are paced in VDD mode; 27 units (5.48%) were converted to VVI mode because of a complete loss of atrial sensing (15 patients, 3.04%), chronic atrial fibrillation (11 patients, 2.23%), and development of a marked sinus bradycardia (1 patient); 5 patients underwent system revision for an inconstant detection of the atrial signal. If present, the loss of atrial sensing was related to a displacement of the atrial dipole, without displacement of the ventricular tip. Paroxysmal atrial fibrillation occurred in 4 patients and resolved spontaneously or with drug therapy. Sustained pacemaker-mediated tachycardia (PMT) was reported in 37 patients, but in all cases it was solved by the reprogramming of one or more parameters such as sensitivity, band-pass filter, and refractory period [27].

The results of these two studies indicate without any doubt the reliability of the single AV lead VDD pacing systems. However, our more than 10-year experience with these systems leads us to believe that their successful functioning strictly depends on the attention paid to the following points: (1) patient selection; (2) implant procedures; (3) pacemaker programming.

Patient selection. The ideal candidates for the single AV lead VDD pacing are those with CHB and uncompromised SAF, and possibly those with a mild sinus node dysfunction. The lack of sinus and atrial pathology or related symptoms is the first mandatory requirement to adopt this pacing mode. Atrial size and SAF must be carefully evaluated in order to exclude potential arrhythmologic risk. Supraventricular tachycardia, sinus bradycardia, sinus arrest, and occasional atrial flutter or fibrillation episodes exclude SAF integrity. A satisfactory chronotropic function with respect to the patient's age should also be assessed. Exercise tests and Holter monitoring yield important information about the variations of the sinus rates in daily life.

Implant procedures. The following conditions affect the floating atrial EGM quality: (1) spacing between dipoles; (2) distance from the myocardial wall (attenuation, biological filtering, i.e. blossoming of the extracellular field); (3) interference pattern (relative distances of adjacent myocardium,

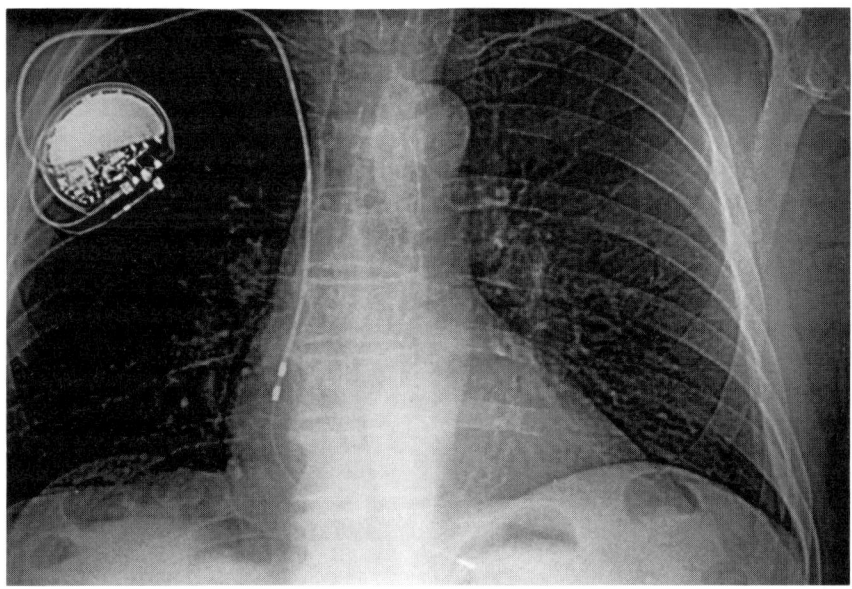

Figure 4. Example of X-radiograph in frontal view showing an implanted single lead VDD system (Lem Biomedica Twinal 30) with correct positioning of the atrial dipole in the mid-to-high right atrium and the ventricular tip anchored at the right ventricle apex.

boundary effects, aging of cardiac muscle and development of interfiber collagen); (4) electrode size (field potential averaging, source and load impedance imbalance). Furthermore, the floating condition induces by itself morphology and amplitude variations of the signal, mainly during deep breathing, coughing, postural changes, etc.

After the fixation of the ventricular tip in the selected position, the lead should be manoeuvred in order to place the dipole as close as possible to the mid-to-high atrial wall, as shown in Figure 4. A floating atrial signal no lower than 0.5 mV should be constantly detected during all the above-mentioned situations. A good quality atrial EGM is extremely important to obtain a reliable synchronization during all daily activities and movements.

Since the atrial electrode floats in the bloodstream, anatomical changes do not affect the detected signal. Chronic measurements at reintervention or by telemetry did not show significant variations of the atrial EGMs. Consequently, a loss of atrial sensing cannot be attributed to a chronic signal attenuation.

Pacemaker programming. The single AV lead VDD system programming is similar to that for a DDD system. These units should feature algorithms and protection mechanisms against premature ventricular contractions and retrograde conduction, in order to avoid sustained PMTs. The wider the

Table 2. Primary characteristics of AV single leads for VDD pacing available today.

Manufacturer	Model	Atrial configuration	Ventricular configuration	Atrial dipole spacing (mm)	Atrial elect. surface (mm^2)	AV distance (cm)	Body size (fr.)
In clinical use:							
Cardiac Control Systems, Inc. Palm Coast, FL	A-track 333	D.A.B.	Unipolar	5.0	8.6	13.5 (16.5)	6.6
Lem Biomedica SRL Florence, Italy	Synkel PLU 113	D.A.B.	Unipolar	7.0	6.0	13.5 (11.5–15.5)	6.5
Medico Italia SRL Rubano, Italy	Phymos 830S lead	Ring.-bip.	Unipolar	30.0	15.9	14.5 (12.5–17.5)	11.0
Under clinical evaluation:							
ELA Medical, SA Montrouge, France	Various models	Ring.-bip.	Unipolar Bipolar	15.0–30.0	n.a.	Various	n.a.
Intermedics, Inc. Angleton, TX	UniPass 425-04/06	D.A.B.	Unipolar	5.0	8.6	13.5 and 16.5	6.6
Lem Biomedica SRL Florence, Italy	Synkel PLU 113 GEA	Ring.-bip.	Unipolar	5.0	25.0	13.0	6.6
Medtronic, Inc. Minneapolis, MN	CapSure VDR 5032	Ring.-bip.	Bipolar	8.6	12.5	13.5	8.5
Siemens, AG Solna, Sweden	1324C–1326C 1328C	Ring.-bip.	Bipolar	12.0	32.0	9.6–11.6–13.6	7.7
Vitatron, BV Dieren, The Netherlands	IMP 15Q	Ring.-bip.	Bipolar	8.6	12.5	13.5 (11.5)	8.0

Table 3. Primary characteristics of implantable cardiac pulse generators specifically designed for single lead VDD pacing.

Manufacturer	Model	Pacing modes	Atrial sensing (mV)	Atrial bandwidth (Hz)	Rate responsivity algorithm	Rate adaptive AV delay	Intracardiac EGM
In clinical use:							
Cardiac Control Systems, Inc. Palm Coast, FL	Maestro Savvi 305	VDD, VVI VVT, VOO	0.1–5.0 13 steps	Low: 20–110 High: 40–200	None	No	Yes
Cardiac Control Systems, Inc. Palm Coast, FL	Maestro Savvi 333	VDD, VVI VVT, VOO	0.1–5.6 16 steps	Low: 21–100 High: 39–170	None	No	Yes
LEM Biomedica SRL Florence, Italy	Twinal 30S	VDD, VDT VVI, VVT, VOO	0.1–5.6 16 steps	Low: 21–100 High: 39–170	None	No	Yes
Medico Italia SRL Rubano, Italy	Phymos ADV	VDD, VVI, VOO	0.1–0.2 2 steps	80–140	None	Yes (1 step)	Markers
Under clinical evaluation:							
ELA Medical, SA Montrouge, France	Chorus 6234 VDD single lead	VDD, VVI VVT, VOO	0.4–4.0 14 steps	n.a.	None	Yes	Yes
Intermedics, Inc. Angleton, TX	Unity 292-07	VDD, VVI VVT, VOO, OOO	0.1–1.6 11 steps	n.a.	Activity (VDD–VVI)	Yes	Yes
Medtronic, Inc. Minneapolis, MN	Thera VDR	VDD, VVI, VVT VOO, ODO, OSO	0.25–4.0 9 steps	n.a.	Activity (VVI–VOO)	Yes	Yes
Siemens, AG Solna, Sweden	Avilog P64	VDD, VVI VVT, VOO, OOO	0.1–5.0 15 steps	n.a.	Activity (all modes)	Yes	Yes
Siemens, AG Solna, Sweden	Addvent 2060 LR	VDD, VVI VVT, VOO, OOO	0.1–5.0 15 steps	n.a.	Activity (all modes)	Yes	Yes
Vitatron, BV Dieren, The Netherlands	Saphir 600 VDDR	VDD, VVI VVT, VOO, OOO	0.1–7.5 26 steps	26–160	Activity + QT (all modes)	Yes	Markers

programmability range of the pacemaker used, the rarer are the adaptation problems faced during implantation and follow-up. The atrial sensitivity should be at least one step lower than the minimum signal detected during implantation. The AV delay must be programmed according to the hemodynamically most effective value found during the exercise test. The post ventricular atrial refractory period (PVARP) should be extended enough to overcome any possible retrograde P wave. If algorithms to prevent PMT are not available, the PVARP extension can limit the sinus tracking rate during exercise.

CONCLUSION

The single AV lead VDD pacing mode has attained sufficient flexibility and reliability to be used extensively and to be included in the ACC/AHA guidelines for pacemaker implantation [28]. As a consequence of the popularity gained by the system, most manufacturers have recently developed new single AV leads and dedicated pacemakers for VDD pacing which are now undergoing clinical evaluation. The most important characteristics of all the old and new systems are summarized in Tables 2 and 3. It is worthwhile to remember that the system performance depends absolutely on the combination of high quality technology with optimum knowledge of the implanting surgeons of the indications and limits of the system and the strategies for its full use.

REFERENCES

1. Nathan DA, Samet P, Center S et al. Long-term correction of complete heart block. Clinical and physiologic studies of a new type of implantable synchronous pacer. Progr Cardiovasc Dis 1964;6:538–65.
2. Chamberlain DA, Wollons DJ, White HM et al. Synchronous A-V pacing with a single pervenous electrodes (abstract). Br Heart J 1973;35:559.
3. Babotai I, Turina M. New atrio-ventricular electrode. In: Meere C, editor. Cardiac Pacing. Pace Symp, Montreal, 1979; Chap 29-1.
4. Cameron JR, Crisholm AW, Harrison AV et al. A single catheter for all modes of pacing. In: Feruglio GA, editor. Cardiac Pacing (Europacing Florence 1981). Padova: Piccin, 1982:1091–2.
5. Sowton E, Crick J, Wainwright RJ. The crown of thorns. A single pass electrode for physiological pacing. In: Feruglio GA, editor. Cardiac Pacing (Europacing Florence 1981). Padova: Piccin, 1982;1089–90.
6. Audoglio R, Aquilina M, Moracchini PV et al. New single endocardial lead for VDD pacing with variable interelectrode length. Concepts and clinical experience. Cardiostim '84, RBM Revue Européenne Technologie Biomedicale 1984;6:259.
7. Curry PVL, Raper DA. Single lead for permanent physiological cardiac pacing. Lancet 1978;2:757–9.
8. Antonioli GE, Grassi G, Baggioni GF et al. A simple P-sensing ventricle stimulating lead

driving a VAT generator. In: Meere C, editor. Cardiac Pacing. PaceSymp, Montreal, 1979: Chap 34-9.
9. Antonioli GE, Grassi G, Baggioni GF et al. A simple new method for atrial triggered pacemaker. G Ital Cardiol 1980;10:679–89.
10. Antonioli GE, Grassi G, Marzaloni M et al. A new implantable VDT pacemaker using a single, double-electrode catheter. In: Feruglio GA, editor. Cardiac Pacing (Europacing Florence 1981). Padova: Piccin, 1982:1093–9.
11. Antonioli GE. Single pass lead: what is the future? In: Perez-Gomez F, editor. Cardiac Pacing: Electrophysiology, Tachyarrhythmias. Madrid: Editorial Grouz, 1985:986–92.
12. Goldreyer BN, Olive AL, Leslie J et al. A new orthogonal lead for P-synchronous pacing. PACE 1981;4:638–44.
13. Aubert AE, Ector H, Denys BG et al. Sensing characteristics of unipolar and bipolar orthogonal floating atrial electrodes: morphology and spectral analysis. PACE 1986,9:343–59.
14. Antonioli GE, Sermasi S, Marzaloni M et al. A comparison study of intra-atrial electrograms from different types of floating atrial electrodes. Cardiostimolazione 1984;2:25–9.
15. Curzio G, Aquilina M, Morgagni W et al. A-wave endocavitary sensing by means of floating electrodes: three different approaches. In: Perez-Gomez F, editor. Cardiac Pacing: Electrophysiology, Tachyarrhythmias. Madrid: Editorial Grouz, 1985:865–73.
16. Brownlee RR. Toward optimizing the detection of atrial depolarization with floating bipolar electrodes. PACE 1989;12:431–42.
17. Antonioli GE, Brownlee RR, Audoglio R. Science, theory and clinical considerations related to sensing atrial depolarization in single-lead VDD pacing. In: Antonioli GE, Aubert AE, Ector H, editors. Pacemaker Leads 1991. Amsterdam: Elsevier, 1991:115–33.
18. Barbieri D, Ansani L, Guardigli G et al. High-resolution and frequency content analysis of floating endo-atrial signals at different dipole lengths. In: Antonioli GE, Aubert AE, Ector H, editors. Pacemaker Leads 1991. Amsterdam: Elsevier, 1991:135.
19. Antonioli GE, Ansani L, Barbieri D et al. Single-lead VDD pacing. In: Barold SS, Mugica J, editors. New Perspective in Cardiac Pacing 3. Mount Kisco, NY: Futura, 1993: 359–82.
20. Crick JCP. European multicenter prospective follow-up study of 1002 implants of a single lead VDD pacing systems. PACE 1991;14:1742–4.
21. Antonioli GE, Ansani L, Barbieri D et al. Italian multicenter study on a single lead VDD pacing system using a narrow atrial dipole spacing. PACE 1992;15:1890–3.
22. Varriale P, Pilla AG, Tekriwal M. Single-lead VDD pacing system. PACE 1990;13:757–66.
23. Longo E, Catrini V. Experience and implantation techniques with a new single-pass lead VDD pacing system. PACE 1990;13:927–36.
24. Furman S, Gross J, Andrews C. Single lead VDD pacing. In: Antonioli GE, Aubert AE, Ector H, editors. Pacemaker Leads 1991. Amsterdam: Elsevier, 1991:183–97.
25. Gross JN, Andrews C, Ben-Zurn UM et al. VDD pacing: chronic efficacy, incidence of atrial fibrillation and evolution of sinoatrial dysfunction (abstract). PACE 1993;16:881.
26. Lau CP, Tai YT, Leung SK et al. Improved aerobic capacity with single lead atrial synchronous pacing with a rate adaptive sensor (abstract). JACC 1993;21:383A.
27. Sermasi S, Marconi M. VDD single pass lead pacing: Sustained pacemaker mediated tachycardias unrelated to retrograde activation. PACE 1992;15:1903–7.
28. Dreifus LS, Fisch C, Griffin JC et al. Guidelines for implantation of cardiac pacemaker and antiarrhythmia devices. ACC/AHA Task Force Report. Circulation 1991;84:455–67.

22. Substantial improvement of screw-in electrodes

PETRAS STIRBYS

INTRODUCTION

The goal of developing an ideal electrode design still exists. Attempts are being made to reduce an incidence rate of electrode-related complications. Numerous requirements for implantable electrodes constrain the construction tempo of new models. There is the possibility of derangement of the settled balance between many clinical and engineering characteristics of applied electrodes. It is known that such peculiarities as the electrode's surface area, composition material, geometric form, and fixing elements are in close interrelationship. The mechanical fixation capabilities and the electric performance of electrode are nearly equally important. Finally, the precondition of all modifications of approved electrodes is that their characteristics of easy insertion and removal as necessary must be retained. Screw-in electrodes are likely to be the most preferable ones. They already have clear biomedical advantages and overwhelmingly positive clinical results and could be improved further. This report presents a new approach to electrode design and is based on theoretical and practical considerations. Accurate shaping of the fixation elements has resulted in numerous new and original patterns.

CLINICAL BACKGROUND

Retractable or fixed screw helices were introduced in the mid-1970s as a solution to the high incidence of lead displacements seen at that time [1]. These leads are also isodiametric, which should contribute to the ease of insertion and may improve their chronic removability if so required [1, 2].

Unfortunately, we still face the problem of electrode displacement. The complication rate for atrial leads varies between 4.5% and 18% [1, 3–8]. In 1985–1987 the implanting of atrial leads was a major problem for some surgeons, resulting in a disappointingly high incidence of complications, especially dislocations [6, 7]. As to the reliability of atrial screw-in leads,

Markewitz et al. [2] have declared that the complication rate (loss of sensing and capture) might be far below 10% and with well-trained surgeons, below 5%.

In early 1986, screw-in leads were characterized as 'modern electrodes'. At that time, these leads appeared to be highly effective. Therefore, they were preferred by some users [9]. The screw fixation mechanism offers advantages over a nonscrew (passive fixation) mechanism, including a reduced incidence of lead dislodgement and the ability to place the lead tip in different atrial positions (including interatrial septum) to ensure optimal sensing [1, 2, 10, 11]. However, some apparent disadvantages, e.g. atrial wall perforation by the screw or poor handling, leading to the screw being stuck to the venous wall, are simply a matter of surgical experience [2].

In 1989 in the USA [12], active fixation leads, such as corkscrew types, were used most frequently in the atrium (62% of cases). Early electrode problems such as dislodgement and perforation were encountered seldom, but in the ventricle were more common with passive than with active fixation electrodes; late electrode problems were also uncommon, but in the ventricle occurred more frequently with passive fixation electrodes [12]. Nevertheless, the statement of Brownlee and Hirst [13] certainly must be kept in mind: 'The complication rate of atrial leads is higher than ventricular leads and must be taken into consideration when selecting the pacing mode for a particular patient, but that in the majority the advantages of physiological pacing justify the additional problems.'

With the introduction of dual chamber pacing, atrial electrode displacement was a constant source of pacemaker malfunction and, unfortunately, delayed the general introduction of physiological dual chamber pacing for several years [14]. Recently, Shandling et al. [15] pointed out that a spring-loaded retracting mechanism may cause more endocardial trauma than other active fixation leads. However, these leads are now gaining in popularity in institutions implanting dual or single chamber pacemakers during 'same-day' surgery [1]. Atrially placed screw-in leads continue to compare favourably with nonscrew leads over time [10].

Depending on the manufacturer, the helical screw-in mechanism has a different length, and therefore the depth of its penetration may vary as follows: 2.1 mm (Accufix, Telectronics), 1.5–1.6 mm (DY, YR, Biotronic), 0.9 mm (FH, Biotronic). A corkscrew-type spiral has two and a half turns, whereas double screw-in elements (sickle-shaped anchoring hooks) have only a half-turn. Although double screw-in electrodes demonstrate reliable intracardiac stability, the incidence rate of displacement is on average 0.67% [16]. A special provocative dislodgement test has revealed a superior fixation quality of double screw-in electrodes over other types [16].

Sintered platinum or carbon-coated atrial screw-in leads have a proven long-term reliability with satisfying long-term results concerning pacing and sensing threshold [2, 17–19].

In general, this shows that the current environment is undoubtedly favourable for electrodes of the screw-in class. That is why the conceptual development of such a type of electrode is being pursued. This article contains our previous approach to the fundamental principles of constructing electrodes with active fixation [3] and is supplemented with several innovative solutions. The concept elaborated starts from its embryonic stage with a subsequent evolution and incorporation of widely approved still unknown as patterns as well. In appearance, the fundamental theory of electrode improvement is based on the purely mechanistic electrode-tissue interaction. However, the theory covers both the electrode's improved mechanical (fixation) properties and electric performance. Also, another important feature forms the focus for our theory: an electrode of a new design must be subjected to extraction when necessary.

A STEPWISE PRINCIPLE OF EVOLUTION OF A PIN-LIKE ELECTRODE RESULTING IN NEW ALLOWABLE PATTERNS

Every innovation claims to be the ideal version. In order to design an ideal or even an acceptable appliance, device, or technology, the old rule of developing from simple towards complex may still be used. Another driving force leading to a new venture or discovery is the establishment of the so-called golden mean of a pattern. These two criteria have served as a foundation for tentative studies.

It is known that the electrode's resistivity to spontaneous defixation increases in proportion to the degree of shaping of its piercing part (or parts). From the mechanical point of view, every given pattern of a penetrating part that pierces easily may also be easily removed (dislodged) and vice versa. In other words, the force required to insert the piercing part into the endocardium (juxtaendocardium or myocardium) is proportionally related to the force needed for extracting it.

Our starting position is represented by two extreme patterns (Figure 1). The first one is represented by a primitive (straight sharp pin) piercing element without tines which is easily pierced and removed (Figure 1A). The two versions (Figures 1B, C) of the other pattern – unilateral and bilateral (arrow-like) anchor – are equivalent from the functional point of view, i.e. they are relatively easily to insert but not to remove. The latter pattern possesses a superior fixational quality that unfortunately is inapplicable in clinical practice, because its removal requires vigorous and drastic efforts. Thus, the ideal electrode might be ranked between the two patterns. While searching for the 'golden mean', two approaches are possible: (1) gradual shaping of the straight sharp pin or (2) gradual simplification of the anchor-like piercing element. Let us consider the first one.

A straight sharp pin has no tines, and therefore, it is not feasible to fix it in the heart wall. A dislodgement rate close to 100% may be anticipated. That is why this primitive fixing element has no practical value other than

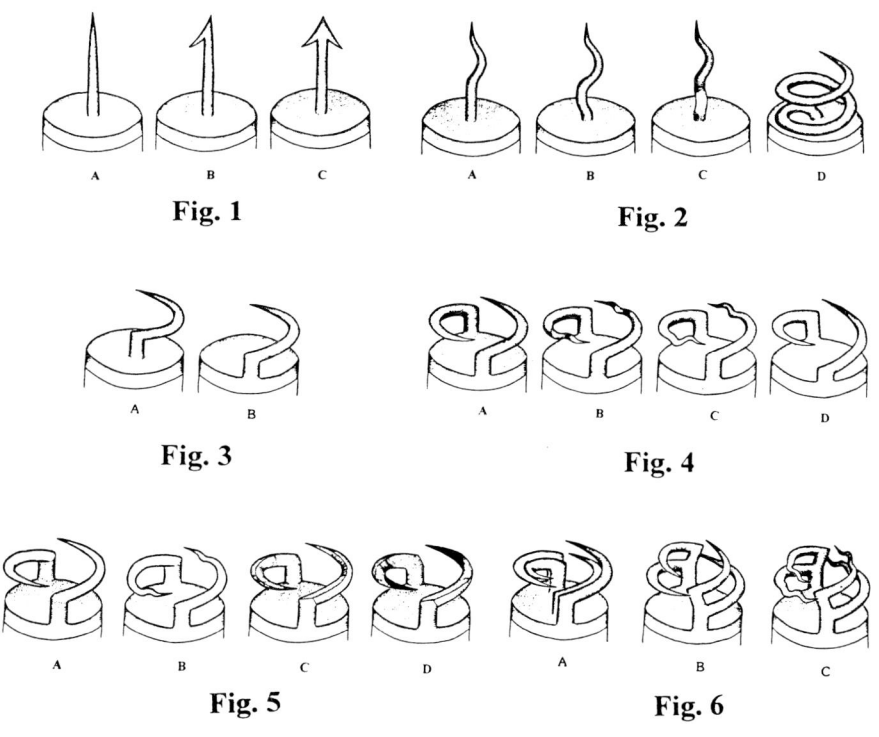

Figures 1–6. Schematic representation of electrode design evolution (see details in text).

serving as a basic pattern (primordial) for its further remodelling. Figure 2 represents sharp pin patterns with an axial bending(s): unilateral curvature (A), bilaterally 'curled' on the same plane (B), bilaterally curved on different perpendicular planes (C), and spiral-like cork-screw type (D) being widely produced by many manufacturers (Medtronic, Biotronic, etc). Subsequent angular bending gives us two unusual patterns with a centric (Figure 3A) and excentric (Figure 3B) localization of the hooks. Every hook has a round form in cross-section. They may be inserted into the superficial juxtaendocardium or subadjacent myocardium. However, remote fixation and removal of the electrode are impossible. To promote a remote control and reliable fixation, two symmetrical, excentric hooks are needed (Figure 4A). Reciprocity of the two hooks promotes their quick penetration and fixation. This electrode is called the 'double screw-in' and has been in use since 1978 [20] with excellent clinical results [16]. However, a zero rate of electrode displacement has yet to be achieved. Probably, the fixation capabilities of the electrode could be improved by combining angular and axial bendings: curling in the horizontal (Figure 4B) and vertical (Figure 4C) planes. Two asymmetric, half-turn hooks with a different length of hook support (Figure 4D) might be useful since each hook will pierce the tissues at different angles. Therefore, self-loosening is hindered and stability enhanced.

Another generation of electrodes is represented by a double screw-in electrode with sharp-edged, sickle-like hooks (Figure 5A). These hooks maximize the concentration of the current density, thereby resulting in the efficient and economic function of pacemaker batteries, ensuring and extending pacemaker longevity. A slight twist of these double screw-in hooks (Figure 5B) improves their fixation capabilities [21]. A similar electric performance could be demonstrated for an electrode containing triangular double screw-in hooks (Figure 5C). An electrode with triangular, spiral-like, twisted hooks (Figure 5D) is even more effective.

Mechanical fixation capabilities might be nearly doubled by building into the design two double screw-in hooks on separate hook supports (Figure 6A) or by arranging two pairs of hooks on two single hook supports (Figure 6B). The latter one has been patented [22]. Another model (Figure 6C) possesses an extreme steadfastness; this type of electrode is presumably unremovable following fibrous encapsulation.

The biocompatibility and electric performance of the electrodes presented can be enhanced by covering the tip and its hooks with carbon-vitreous particles or black platinum. Currently, some new patterns are being patented. New designs involve hook straightening during the extraction of the lead.

REFERENCES

1. Ormerod D, Walgren S, Heil R. Design and evaluation of a threshold, porous tip lead with a mannitol coated screw-in tip ('sweet tip'). PACE 1988;11:1784–90.
2. Markewitz A, Wenke K, Weinhold C. Reliability of atrial screw-in leads. PACE 1988;11:1777–83.
3. Stirbys P. Theoretical approach to fundamental principles in construction of electrodes with active fixation. In: Ergeb exp Med 52. Berlin: Verlag Gesundheit, 1990:257–60.
4. Dodinot B, Medeiros F, Golvao S. Tined or screw in atrial leads. PACE 1985;8:A-81.
5. Molajo AO, Bowes RJ, Fananapazir L et al. Comparison of vitreous carbon and elgiloy transvenous ventricular pacing leads. PACE 1985;8:261–65.
6. Dodinot B, Medeiros F, Golvao S et al. Tined or screw in atrial leads. In Aubert AE, Ector H, editors. Pacemaker Leads. Amsterdam: Elsevier, 1985:75.
7. Hill PE. Complications of permanent transvenous cardiac pacing: a 14 year review of all transvenous pacemakers inserted at one community hospital. PACE 1987;10:567.
8. Lemke B, Dryander S, Grosskurth D et al. Longterm results of actively fixed pacemaker leads in atrial and ventricular position. Abstracts of 2nd international symposium on pacing leads, Ferrara 1991:35.
9. Parsonnet V, Bernstein A. Pacing in perspective: concepts and controversies. Circulation 1986;73, 6:1087–93.
10. Shandling AH, Castellanet MJ, Thomas LA et al. The influence of endocardial electrode fixation status on acute and chronic atrial stimulation threshold and atrial endocardial electrogram amplitude. PACE 1990;13:1116–22.

11. Stirbys P. Permanent interatrial septal pacing: feasibility and advantages. PACE 1986;9:209–11.
12. Bernstein A, Parsonnet V. Survey of cardiac pacing in the United States in 1989. Am J Cardiol 1992;69:331–8.
13. Brownlee W, Hirst R. Six years experience with atrial leads. PACE 1986;9:1239–42.
14. Dreifus LS. In search of atrial sensing and capture. PACE 1988;11:381–3.
15. Shandling A, Nolasco V, Floro J et al. Comparative implantation characteristics of spring-loaded retracting active fixation atrial electrodes (abstract). PACE 1991;14:740.
16. Stirbys P, Skucas J, Andziukevicius G. A method for estimating endocardial electrode stability. PACE 1990;13:1860–3.
17. Markewitz A, Meiser B, Weinhold C. Which tip tops in atrial screw-in leads: sintered platinum vs. carbon? PACE 1991;14:740.
18. Markewitz A, Meiser B, Weinhold C. Removal of infected pacemaker leads. Abstracts of 2nd International symposium on pacing leads. Ferrara 1991:40.
19. Pioger G, Girodo S, Ripart A. Vitreous carbon screw-in leads: clinical results. Abstracts of 2nd international symposium on pacing leads, Ferrara 1991:78.
20. Bredikis J, Stirbys P et al. Double screw-in electrode. Patent no. 663410; priority registered in January 6, 1978.
21. Stirbys P. Implantable double screw-in electrode. Patent no. 4680696/30-14(0370790); priority registered in March 15, 1989.
22. Stirbys P. Implantable endocardial electrode. Patent no. 1621231; priority registered in March 15, 1989.

23. Physiological cardiac pacing: an individual objective

J. CLAUDE DAUBERT, PHILIPPE MABO, DANIEL GRAS, CHRISTOPHE LECLERCQ & THIERRY LELIÈVRE

INTRODUCTION

A physiological pacemaker is one which preserves or best restores the three fundamental elements which determine cardiac performance in chronically paced patients, i.e. chronotropic function, atrial function by optimal AV synchronization, and finally, normal ventricular activation sequence. The goal of a physiological pacemaker must, of course, encompass optimal cycle by cycle instantaneous cardiac performance, but also long-term preservation of the heart's fundamental function, including both mechanical (atrial, valvular, and ventricular) and electrical (prevention of arrhythmia) stability. There is a wide range of highly individualized technical solutions which make it possible to meet this goal. Pacing modes vary from extremely sophisticated systems to the simplest units, for example, an ordinary VVI pacemaker programmed for patients with normal baseline ECG and chronotropic function.

CHRONOTROPIC FUNCTION

Normal cardiac response to exercise: a predominant role for heart rate adaptation

During physical exercise, the heart adapts to metabolic demand by increasing both stroke volume and heart rate. The stroke volume adapts by increased contractility, as seen by the reduced endsystolic volume, and also by improved ventricular filling, the ventricle then being able to cope with the increased venous inflow. Improved filling is itself the consequence of accelerated endsystolic relaxation, increased diastolic compliance, and more efficient atrial systole [1]. The atrial contribution to stroke volume amounts to about 20% in the normal resting subject and increases to 30% on average during submaximal exercise. This holds true, however, only for one cardiac cycle.

Thus, compared with the average 200% increase in cardiac output resulting from increased contractility alone [2] and the 200–300% increase resulting from normal chronotropic function, the physiological role of atrial systole in the cardiac function adaptation to exercise is actually quite limited.

Increased heart rate is the preferential adaptation mechanism and the first to come into play. This is particularly so for low and moderate exercise levels and in subjects with little or no prior physical training [3]. At load-constant exercise levels, the heart rate rises immediately, before any increase in stroke volume. These two factors then follow a parallel course up to the point where the stroke volume stops increasing, and the increased cardiac output can only result from a supplementary rise in heart rate [4]. This physiological situation illustrates the importance of preserving the heart's chronotropic function as closely as possible to normal and, in the case of chronotropic incompetence, of restoring normal function.

Chronotropic function in pacemaker patients

Chronotropic incompetence (CI) may be defined as the ineffective adaptation of the heart rate to metabolic demand, especially during exercise. CI is frequently seen in candidates for permanent cardiac pacing. The incidence, however, varies greatly from one series to another, depending on the authors' diagnostic criteria. Actually, there is no generally accepted statistical definition of CI [5]. In clinical practice, it is less important to know whether the heart rate for a given exercise level or at peak exercise is below a particular percentage of the predicted normal heart rate than to know whether this insufficient acceleration causes functional symptoms or not and whether there is a real limitation of exercise capacity. Thus, a functional definition would be more useful than a purely statistical definition. Taking into consideration all indications, the incidence of CI can include 58% of pacemaker patients [6]. However, the incidence varies widely, depending on the indication for pacing and according to whether the CI is ventricular, atrial or both.

Ventricular chronotropic incompetence
High-degree AV block. CI is almost always present in patients with high-degree AV block because the ventricular escape rhythm is unable to accelerate fast enough to meet the demands of exercise. The intra- or subhisian rate-dependent AV blocks are typical examples. These blocks are not seen at rest (1:1 AV conduction) but appear suddenly during exercise when the sinus rate overruns a critical threshold and provokes an abrupt fall in heart rate and subsequent severe hemodynamic dysfunction [7]. There are, however, several exceptions. In young subjects, certain AV blocks located in the AV node can partially, or even totally, regress during exercise so that the heart rate adaptation becomes nearly normal. Such a situation is most often seen in trained athletes [8]. In other patients, the AV block persists during

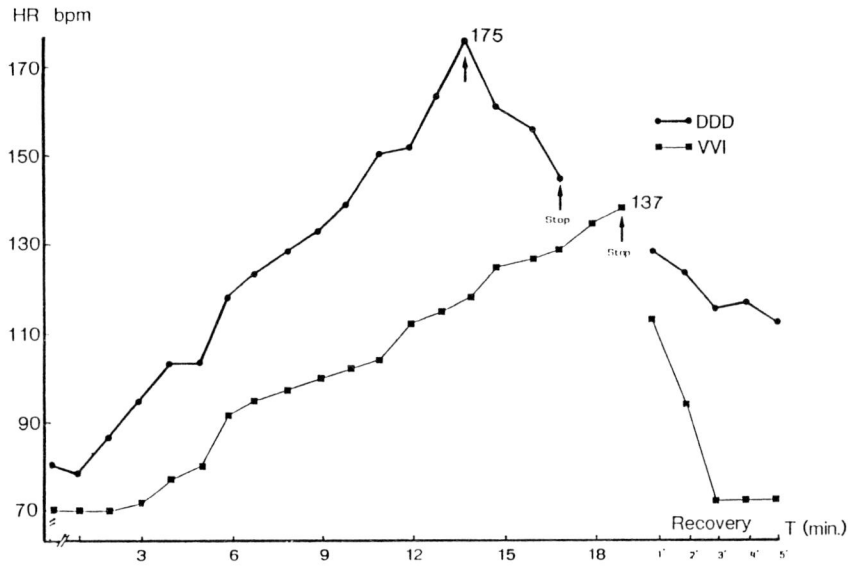

Figure 1. Exercise capacity of a chronically paced patient for congenital complete AV block. Comparison of the VVI mode (fixed pacing rate = 70 bpm) and of the DDD mode (upper rate limit = 175 bpm) during standardized exercise testing on cycloergometer (30 watts/3-min steps starting from 30 W workload until exhaustion). In the DDD mode, the spontaneous sinus rate reaches the upper rate limit (URL) after 14 min of exercise, triggering the Wenckebach association and inducing rate slowing. The test was stopped by exhaustion at 17 min. In the VVI mode, the intrinsic ventricular rate progressively accelerates from the 3rd min of exercise to the 19th min up to a maximum of 137 bpm, resulting in a complementary gain (versus DDD) of 2 min in exercise duration and of 30 watts in sustained workload.

exercise, but the intrinsic ventricular rate increases sufficiently to provide exercise adaptation equal to or even better than that produced by an apparently 'physiological' pacing system (Figure 1). As a general rule, ventricular CI becomes all the more frequent and all the more severe as the patient becomes older and as the AV block is located more distally in the His-Purkinje system.

Pacemaker patients with chronic atrial fibrillation. A majority of the patients with chronic atrial fibrillation requiring permanent ventricular pacing for bradycardia support at rest have an abnormal chronotropic response to exercise. In the series from Corbelli et al. [9], the heart rate adapted normally in only 21% of patients. Three different types of abnormal chronotropic response were observed: inappropriate tachycardia throughout the exercise; permanent inappropriate bradycardia during exercise; or an alternation of both with, in most cases, inappropriate tachycardia in the early stages of exercise followed by inappropriate bradycardia during the late stages of exercise. Finally, 58% of patients showed abnormally depressed heart rates during part or all of the exercise duration, and could potentially benefit from a rate adaptative pacing system.

Atrial chronotropic incompetence
Sinus node disease. (SND) is the most frequent cause of atrial chronotropic incompetence (ACI). In six studies defining ACI as a peak exercise heart rate <120 bpm, the average incidence was 40% [10]. Such statistical definitions, however, do not account for patient age and do not necessarily imply a significant limitation of exercise capacity. This is particularly true for elderly patients with limited physical activity. In order to determine the real needs for a corrective rate adaptive pacing system, it would be best to consider only those patients with symptomatic ACI. Using this basic criteria, Kallryd et al. [11] found that the need for rate-responsiveness was 25% of SND patients at the time of first implant. Nevertheless, the incidence and the severity of ACI increase with time [6, 12]. This fact would justify wider indications for sensor-driven pacemakers (AAIR or DDDR mode) at initial implant, even if the rate-responsiveness is not immediately needed. The pacemaker could be programmed later if symptomatic ACI developed.

Chronic AV block. Sinoatrial disease has been reported to occur in 20–30% of patients with complete AV block [13, 14], but even in the absence of overt SND, ACI is not uncommon. Evidence may be found when investigating patients chronically paced in the VDD/DDD mode. In a personal series of 50 consecutive patients (unpublished data), atrial chronotropic competence was evaluated during a cycloergometer exercise test conducted with 10 W/l-min steps from a starting load of 30 W until exhaustion. The pacemaker's total atrial refractory period (AV delay + postventricular atrial refractory period) was reprogrammed in such a way as to raise the upper pacing rate above the individual (PMHR). CI, defined by a peak HR < 75% PMHR, was found in 15 of 50 patients (30%). In this subgroup, 9 (60%) showed no sign of sinus dysfunction at the preoperative electrophysiologic study. Higher incidences of ACI of up to 46% [6] have been noted in other series. Based on these observations, in one-third or more of the patients this is probably of no clinical importance, but in an unknown proportion, the best pacing mode would probably be DDDR rather than DDD.

Heart transplant patients. CI or at least a certain form of it is almost always present in denervated hearts. Compared with matched normal controls, transplant patients with an orthotopic heart or a heart-lung graft have a significantly faster resting heart rate, but a significantly lower heart rate during exercise at comparable oxygen uptake (VO_2) [15]. The capacity of heart transplant patients to accelerate their heart rate during exercise is thus reduced significantly, or even totally annulled. In most cases, this lack of heart rate adaptation is well tolerated except when it is associated with severe resting bradycardia resulting from significant postoperative SND. In prospective studies, SND has been found to occur relatively frequently, up to 44% [16], but it is often minor and temporary. In a few patients, approximately 7–10% of the total heart transplant population, SND is more severe and may persist long enough to justify implanting a permanent pacemaker. CI is always severe and symptomatic in these patients, who need a rate-variable pacing mode. However, the resting heart rate and chronotropic response to exercise may progressively improve or even normalize with time, even in these cases [17].

Apparently idiopathic ACI. Occasionally, ACI appears to be independent of any detectable abnormality in cardiac automaticity or conduction [5]. Cardioneuropathies with autonomic nervous system dysfunction have been hypothesized. When symptomatic, these apparently idiopathic ACIs may justify the implantation of a rate-responsive pacemaker (AAIR or DDDR). However, before correcting the CI in these patients, 'silent myocardial ischemia' must be exluded. Early work in this field [18, 19] suggested that CI could be a marker of myocardial ischemia, even without any chest pain or, significant ST-T changes during exercise. These studies revealed that CI was three times more frequent in coronary artery disease patients than in those free of coronary insufficiency. Moreover, the prognostic significance seems to be important. Ellestad and Wan [18] reported a five-year mortality of 20% and a total incidence of cardiac events (unstable angina, myocardial infarction, and sudden death) of 60% in the group with ACI and no ST segment depression during exercise, while the respective rates in the group of patients without ACI was extremely low (5% for all cardiac events).

How can the normal chronotropic response be restored in chronically paced patients?

There are two different pacing methods for adapting heart rate and restoring a normal, or nearly normal, chronotropic response to exercise in CI patients.

P wave synchronous pacing
In the late sixties, *P wave synchronous pacing* (VAT mode) was introduced to treat chronic AV block in patients with normal sinus node function. Twenty-five years later, sinus activity (when normal both at rest and during exercise) is still the best sensor for adapting the pacing rate. Sinus activity is the only physiological sensor that perfectly reflects metabolic demand. When optimally programmed, VDD (with the possibility of a single-pass lead) and DDD units are the only pacemakers capable of restoring a truly physiological chronotropic response. Conversely, inadequate programming may result in persistent or even aggravated CI. In VDD/DDD pacing, exercise tolerance depends above all on the highest HR at which 1:1 AV synchrony can be sustained. Theoretically, the highest possible upper rate limit should be programmed not only to guarantee normal AV synchrony up to high sinus rates, but also to avoid an undesirable triggering of the algorithms for

Table 1. Hemodynamic consequences of triggering ventricular protection algorithms during exercise in DDD pacing.

	1:1	W	2:1	F	Variance
VR (bpm)	138 ± 12	95 ± 12	72 ± 6	86 ± 11	0.0001
AR (bpm)	138 ± 12	148 ± 13	146 ± 14	144 ± 21	0.0025
Systolic AP (mmHg)	226 ± 12	205 ± 29	206 ± 25	210 ± 34	ns
Diastolic AP (mmHg)	92 ± 10	70 ± 17	63 ± 10	68 ± 10	0.0001
Mean AP (mmHg)	144 ± 14	121 ± 23	116 ± 16	121 ± 18	0.0001
Rate presure product	3126 ± 371	2098 ± 445	1502 ± 217	1793 ± 246	0.0001
AV reassociation (s)		35 ± 20	85 ± 35	97 ± 24	0.001

Atrial rate (AR, bpm), ventricular rate (VR, bpm) and atrial pressure (systolic, diastolic, and mean AP; mmHg) were continuously monitored during four consecutive exercise tests at a constant workload corresponding to the maximum sustained during a previous training test. 1:1 AV association, Wenckebach (W), 2:1 block and fallback (F) were tested in random order. AR was the lowest with 1:1. Time to 1:1 AV reassociation during recovery was shorter with W than with F and 2:1. 1:1 provided the highest VR, diastolic and mean AP, and rate pressure product. Finally, the worst mode was 2:1, and W was less deleterious.

ventricular protection, especially 2:1 block and Wenckebach association. Recent studies have clearly shown that these algorithms are hemodynamically deleterious (Table 1) [20]. However, the maximal pacing rate must remain compatible with the physiological and pathological status of the individual patient, taking into account age, physical activity, presence of ischemic heart disease or congestive heart failure, and especially potential risk for atrial tachyarrhythmias. In VDD/DDD pacing, the maximal pacing rate cannot exceed the 2:1 point corresponding to the total atrial refractory period (TARP). Programming a long TARP dramatically decreases the upper pacing rate and potentially the patient's exercise capacity. So to achieve an optimal exercise adaptation, TARP must be programmed to the shortest acceptable value, by acting either on postventricular atrial refractory period (PVARP), or on AV delay, or on both. PVARP can be adapted by programming short fixed values or by using an automatic rate-responsive algorithm. Such a programming produces an increased risk for pacemaker-mediated tachycardias (PMTs), especially during exercise [21], and can only be used with devices equipped with reliable algorithms for the detection and automatic reduction of PMTs [22]. Consequently, AV delay rate modulation algorithms appear to be the most convenient way to shorten TARP and to raise the maximal pacing rate in order to maintain 1:1 AV synchrony in all daily activities. This can be done either abruptly from one cycle to the next one by the 'AV delay hysteresis' or progressively by tracking the spontaneously increasing atrial rate with an automatic rate-adaptative AV delay. These two algorithms can be combined in perfect synergy to achieve optimal adaptation [23].

Dual atrium pacing. P wave sensing may also be used for driving atrial pacing. This technique was initially proposed to restore the normal chrono-

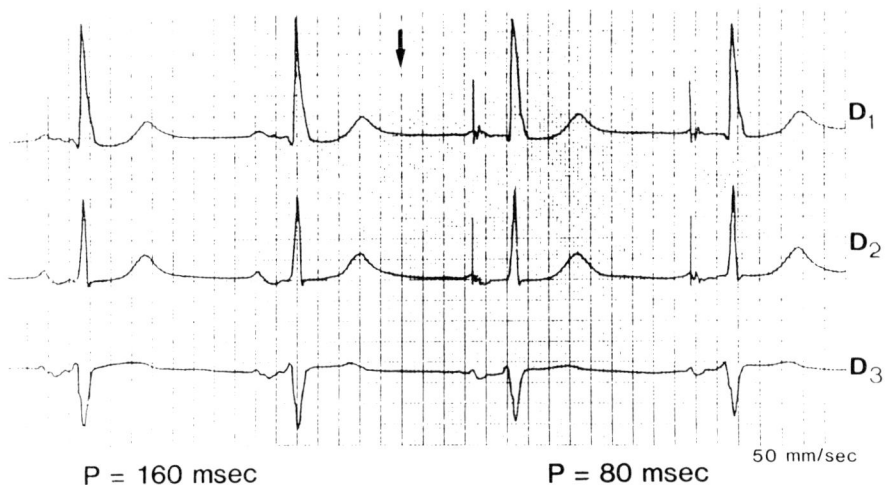

Figure 2. Dual atrium pacing in high-degree interatrial conduction block. P wave synchronous left atrial pacing (arrow) normalizes P wave duration and corrects interatrial asynchrony.

tropic response in heart transplant patients requiring permanent pacing for severe SND + ACI. In this indication, the recipient's sinus activity (this implies that the recipient's atrium is of good quality) is sensed to trigger pacing in the donor's atrium via another screw-in lead. The pacing system may be a conventional DDD pacemaker, eventually programmed in a DAT mode [24], or better a SSI pacemaker programmed in AAT mode with bipolar sensing and pacing configuration [25].

Dual atrium pacing may also be used to treat major interatrial conduction blocks. The pacing system is very similar, using a right atrial lead to pick-up the P wave and a coronary sinus lead to pace the left atrium [26]. This allows not only permanent atrial resynchronization (Figure 2), but also a significant improvement in chronotropic capacity by clearly reducing the optimal programmable value of AV delay and so the TARP (at least when the system is used in a pseudo-triple chamber configuration with permanent ventricular pacing: see below).

Sensor-driven pacing
Over the last few years, technological advances have provided us with multiple sensors to adapt the pacing rate either in the atrium (AAIR mode) or in the ventricle (VVIR mode) or both (DDDR mode). These different sensors detect signals which are more or less physiological and more or less closely related to metabolic demand. The most physiological sensors detect internal changes consequent upon exercise such as the QT interval, respiratory changes (minute ventilation and respiratory rate), central venous tem-

perature, mixed venous O_2 saturation, venous blood pH, hemodynamic parameters (stroke volume, dp/dt, preejection time, right ventricular ejection time, right atrial pressure), etc. Others are less physiological because they detect external changes resulting from exercise, such as body movement and acceleration forces. We cannot, of course, give a detailed description here of the advantages and disadvantages of each of these different systems which are either currently available or under investigation nor discuss their use alone or in combination. But, for example, by combining two or more sensors (QT + activity or minute ventilation + activity) one could expect to 'smooth out' certain inconveniences, one sensor compensating for the other. Precise descriptions of these different systems can be found in reference volumes [27]. In any case, however, none of these systems is perfect, and none can recreate the same quality of chronotropic function as the normal sinus response. These systems are nevertheless major technical advances which very significantly improve exercise tolerance in CI patients who have no sinus atrial activity or an abnormal sinus node response to exercise. In all situations, the sensor programming must be highly individualized in order to obtain the rate-responsiveness most adapted to the individual needs of each patient. We must avoid the useless discussion about a choice between a hypokinetic sensor which does not react in daily life activities and inversely a hyperkinetic sensor which would induce an inappropriate heart rate acceleration for minimal exercise levels or even without exercise. Optimal programming is usually best evaluated by standardized programs of daily life activities (walking, climbing stairs) whose effects on the heart rate can be evaluated by ECG Holter monitoring or by interrogating event counters and rate histograms of the pacemaker, rather than by conventional treadmill exercise testing.

ATRIAL FUNCTION AND AV SYNCHRONY

The atrial single chamber pacing modes (indicated in SND patients with intact AV conduction) and the dual chamber pacing modes (AV block and SND plus abnormal AV conduction) make it possible to preserve or to restore a fully efficient atrial function, whenever it is technically feasible and physiologically useful, i.e. when the atrium's electrophysiologic (acceptable electrical stability, pacing thresholds, and A wave amplitude) and mechanical characteristics are suitable for permanent pacing. An extensive use of atrial pacing is encouraged by the considerable reduction in the rate of failure during the past few years, due to advances in lead technology (screw-in leads which can be implanted at any site in the right atrium, steroid eluting leads allowing efficient pacing even in very diseased atria, new coronary sinus leads to pace and sense the left atrium when the right atrium cannot be used, etc.).

The physiological importance of atrial function

The atria have many physiologically important roles [28, 29]. They serve as a primer pump, completing ventricular filling, lowering filling pressures to the optimal minimum, and assuring presystolic closure of the AV valves. All these functions result from the atrial systole, but also from the release of atrial natriuretic peptides. Consequently, the atria are directly or indirectly involved in regulation systems controlling all the determinants of cardiac function: preload and ventricular filling, inotropism, endsystolic relaxation, afterload, and even myocardial O_2 consumption.

However, the hemodynamic importance of preserving an optimal atrial function varies greatly from one patient to another, depending on several physiological and pathological factors, especially age (the atrial contribution to stroke volume increases progressively with age), the anatomic and functional status of the atrium, LV systolic function (there is an inverse relationship between atrial contribution and LV ejection fraction) [30], LV relaxation and compliance (the transport function of the atrium is significantly increased when endsystolic relaxation and diastolic compliance are altered by physiological ageing or pathological processes, such as hypertrophy, ischemia, or fibrosis), and the quality of AV synchrony, of course.

In conclusion, the atrial contribution may be considered as relatively minor in normal hearts, particularly in young people. It becomes much more important in diseased hearts, especially in hypertrophic cardiomyopathies (primary or secondary), chronic ischemic heart diseases, and chronic LV dysfunctions of other causes, at least within certain limits [28, 29]. However, recent reports [31, 32], suggest that preserving the maximal atrial contribution via an optimized AV synchrony should be of interest even in the endstage of idiopathic dilated cardiomyopathy. The authors reported significant short- and long-term functional improvement after the implantation of a DDD pacemaker with a short (100 ms) programmed AV delay.

The benefit of preserving atrial function in permanent cardiac pacing

Although there has been no randomized study either in SND patients or in chronic AV block patient published, comparing the long-term outcome of two identical groups, one paced in a 'physiological' (DDD/AAI) mode, the other in the VVI/VVIR mode, enough presumptive evidence has been accumulated to suggest strongly that atrial function and optimal AV delay must be preserved whenever possible in permanent cardiac pacing.

Limits and adverse effects of VVI/VVIR pacing

Indirect evidence supports the analysis of the limits and adverse effects of the ventricular single chamber pacing modes. They result principally from the loss of normal AV synchrony. Excepting patients with chronic atrial arrhythmia, ventricular pacing produces either complete AV dissociation or 1:1 VA conduction. *Complete AV dissociation* is usually observed in patients implanted for high-degree AV block. The hemodynamic consequences are often moderate, with a mean decrease of 10-15% in cardiac output and an average increase of 20-30% in pulmonary pressures [33]. This relatively good tolerance may be explained by the changing relations between atrial and ventricular contractions from one cycle to another, with alternating normal or nearly normal AV synchrony and complete disynchrony. *1:1 VA conduction* is relatively rare in patients implanted for chronic AV block, but much more frequent in SND patients. The hemodynamic consequences are more severe, with a decrease of 20-50% in cardiac output, a major increase in pulmonary pressures, and in some patients, severe arterial hypotension [33]. These deleterious effects can be explained by the occurrence of the atrial systole against closed AV valves with a total loss of contribution to stroke volume and by major atrial stretching, resulting in the activation of atrial reflexes and an acute production of atrial natriuretic peptides.

Associated with the alteration in the ventricular activation sequence (see below), the loss of normal AV synchrony (and thus of atrial contribution) is a major determinant of the long-term adverse effects frequently observed in ventricularly paced patients [33]: '*pacemaker syndrome*' is an unclearly defined entity that includes all unpleasant symptoms and deleterious hemodynamic effects which appear or are significantly aggravated after pacemaker implantation. Depending on the diagnostic criteria used, its incidence varies from 5 to 83% of the VVI/VVIR patients. It is generally accepted that about 20% of patients are affected by mild to moderate symptoms and could thus benefit from pacemaker upgrading. All indications considered, permanent ventricular pacing induces or aggravates symptoms of *congestive heart failure* (CHF) in 15-20% of patients. The mechanisms of hemodynamic deterioration with ventricular pacing are complex. In addition to those previously mentioned, the development of atrial tachyarrhythmias and of valvular regurgitations and a progressive alteration in LV systolic and diastolic function probably play an important role. *Valve malfunction*, and especially tricuspid regurgitations, has an estimated incidence of 10% in ventricularly paced patients, significantly higher than in those paced physiologically. *Atrial tachyarrhythmias and thromboembolic events*: whatever the indication for pacing, the long-term incidence of chronic atrial fibrillation is 4 to 5 times higher in VVI-paced patients than in those implanted with a DDD pacemaker. This probably results in an increasing risk for thromboembolic events. *Patient survival*: the study of large cohorts of chronically paced patients shows a significant decrease in survival in those implanted with a VVI/VVIR pacemaker [34].

However, the potential benefit of preserving atrial function is probably more significant in SND patients than in patients implanted for chronic AV block.

Comparison of 'physiological' (AAI/DDD) and VVI/VVIR pacing in SND patients

In a meta-analysis published in 1986 [35], Sutton and Kenny examined the previous series reporting permanent pacing for SND. Comparing patients paced in VVI mode ($n = 347$) with those paced in AAI mode ($n = 321$) for a mean follow-up period of 31 months, their report revealed that AAI pacing results in a significantly lower risk of developing permanent atrial fibrillation (3.9% vs. 22.3%; $p < 0.001$) and a lower risk of thromboembolic events (1.6% vs. 12.3%; $p < 0.001$).

Method errors plague many comparative series, but the reports by Rosenquist et al. [36] are the most reliable. They compared the pacing experience of two Swedish hospitals with different pacing strategies. In one, all SND patients were paced in AAI mode ($n = 89$), and in the other, all SND patients were paced in VVI mode ($n = 79$). At inclusion, the two groups were correctly matched for age, sex, associated heart disease, and NYHA class. At the end of the follow-up (4 years), there was a significant reduction in the incidence of congestive heart failure, permanent atrial fibrillation, and overall mortality in the AAI group. The decrease in incidence of thromboembolic events which was significant at 2 years (4.5% vs. 13%; $p < 0.01$) was no longer found at 4 years (12% vs. 15%; NS).

More recently, Santini et al. [37] published the results of a retrospective study in a large population of SND patients ($n = 339$) either paced in AAI ($n = 135$), DDD ($n = 79$), or VVI ($n = 125$) mode. These authors unfortunately gave little information on the characteristics of the patients in each of the three groups. They only indicated that the prevalence of patients aged over 70 years was identical in the AAI (54.8%) and the VVI (55.5%) groups. With a mean follow-up of 5 years, the incidence of permanent atrial fibrillation, the overall mortality, and the cardiac mortality were significantly lower in the AAI group. Mortality due to stroke was only lower in patients aged over 70 years. For each of the parameters studied, the incidence of events tended to be higher in the DDD group than in the AAI group, but the difference was only significant for permanent atrial fibrillation (13% vs. 4%; $p < 0.02$). Finally, a significant reduction in global mortality was observed in those two studies and in another one from Alpert et al. [38].

We can conclude from these different studies that compared with VVI mode, pacing modes which maintain atrial activity and normal AV synchrony can significantly lower the risk of permanent atrial fibrillation, overall and cardiovascular mortality, and probably the risk of thromboembolic events and congestive heart failure in SND patients.

Comparison of DDD and VVIR pacing in patients with chronic AV block
During the last few years, many studies [39, 44] have investigated the acute and short-term effects of VVIR compared with DDD pacing in patients implanted for complete heart block. In acute studies, no significant differences were observed for exercise tolerance (time of exercise, maximal sustained workload, VO_2 and VCO_2), hemodynamics (cardiac output, coronary sinus blood flow, MVO_2), and sympathetic activity (plasma epinephrine and norepinephrine). The only difference concerned atrial natriuretic peptide release, which was significantly higher with VVIR pacing in the two studies in which it was evaluated [40–43].

Double-blind crossover comparisons with 4 [41], 6 [40], or 12 [44] weeks in each pacing mode provide partially conflicting results. However, in the two studies with the longest follow-up, the sum of symptom scores (symptoms of general well-being) was significantly lower in the DDD mode. The only study that investigated cognitive functioning [44] also showed a significant improvement with DDD pacing. Thus, the maintenance of AV synchrony seems to add further symptomatic relief and to provide a better quality of life compared with rate increase alone.

In the same way, we can probably expect a long-term benefit from dual chamber pacing, similar to that observed in SND patients [29]. Two studies have shown a significant reduction in mortality with DDD pacing compared with VVI/VVIR, but only in patients with congestive heart failure at the time of implant [45, 46].

The importance of AV synchrony optimization

Whatever the indication for pacing, a fully efficient atrial function can only be expected when AV synchrony is optimized individually.

DDD/DDDR pacing: the optimal AV delay
Experience in DDD/DDDR pacing has demonstrated the importance of the opinion expressed by Wish et al. [47] in 1989: 'The benefit of dual-chamber pacing has been generally underestimated by lack of an appropriately programmed AV delay.'

In DDD/DDDR pacing in which the ventricle is paced permanently, the cardiac performance is mainly dependent on the quality of the atrial contribution and thus on programming the optimal AV delay, individually adapted both at rest and during exercise. An optimal AV delay means that at every cardiac cycle, the programmed electrical AV interval produces exactly the delay required for the left atrial systole to make its maximum contribution to stroke volume. Unfortunately, there is no correlation between the electrical interval applied at the pacing sites (usually in the right heart) and the optimal mechanical delay which concerns the left heart. This lack of correlation results from the important interindividual differences in electrical and electromechanical intervals both in the atria (electromechanical delay within the right atrium, interatrial conduction time, electromechanical delay within the left atrium) and in the ventricles (especially the interventricular conduction time).

This explains the wide variablility in optimal individual delays, not only for the basic AV delay measured at rest in sequential AV pacing but also for the difference in AV delay between a paced atrial cycle and a sensed atrial cycle. This dictates which value should be programmed for the AV delay hysteresis.

In everyday clinical practice, it is easy to determine these different optimal AV delays with Doppler echocardiography [48]. In healthy individuals at rest, the optimal basic AV delay generally lies between 150 and 200 ms. Nevertheless, its value may vary greatly from one patient to another as a function of several physiologic and pathologic factors including age (the optimal AV delay is shorter in young people), the quality of left ventricular function, etc. Likewise, individual values of the AV delay hysteresis vary between 42 and 83 ms (mean = 70 ± 12 ms) according to Rey et al. [49], 35 and 260 ms (mean = 90 ± ms) according to Wish [50] who included patients with very long interatrial conduction times, and between 16 and 90 ms (mean = 70 ± 24 ms) according to Ritter et al. [20].

This individual optimization of AV delay is not only needed at rest but also during exercise. In DDD pacing, the dynamic nature of the optimal AV delay should come as close as possible to the physiological adaptation of the PR interval to heart rate (HR) in the normal individual. It is well-known that the PR interval shortens progressively as the HR increases. Precise electrophysiological studies have shown an almost perfect linear relationship between PR and HR during exercise [51].

Most of the modern DDD pacemakers have an algorithm of automatic rate-adaptative AV delay. Some of them may perfectly mimic physiology by adapting the sensed AV delay to HR cycle by cycle, with a true linear shortening. In two studies using similar protocols, one based on measurements of hemodynamic performance [52] and the other on a cardiopulmonary evaluation [53], the hemodynamic benefit of such algorithms during exercise was clearly demonstrated in patients paced permanently for complete AV block.

The hemodynamic benefit acquired by cycle to cycle optimization of the left atrial contribution is not the only important reason for individually programming an adapted basic AV delay and the algorithms of AV delay hysteresis and rate-adaptative AV delay. Another important reason is to optimize the upper rate response of DDD and DDDR pacemakers and consequently the patient's exercise tolerance (see above).

How to solve the problem of very long interatrial conduction times? Al-

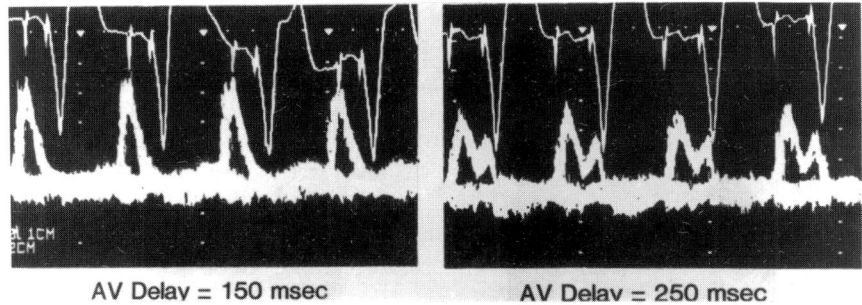

Figure 3. Doppler-echocardiographic demonstration of the deleterious consequences of advanced interatrial block in patients paced in DDD mode. No A wave can be seen on the transmitral flow when the AV delay is programmed at the 'usual' value of 150 ms. It is necessary to prolong the AV delay to 250 ms to recover a correctly synchronized A wave.

though rare in the general population [54], the prevalence of interatrial blocks is relatively high in pacemaker patients and has been estimated (personal data) at 12% of patients implanted for high-degree AV block and 35% of patients implanted for sinoatrial disease. Even in these latter patients, high-degree interatrial block is often associated with AV conduction disorders requiring, in the case of permanent pacing, a dual chamber mode. If a 'classical' 150–200 ms AV delay is programmed in these patients, the greatly extended interatrial conduction time (mean = 145 ± 32 ms in our series) results in a very delayed left atrial systole. The atrial kick occurs during ventricular contraction when the mitral valve is closed. Thus, the hemodynamic efficacy of the atrial systole is completely lost (Figure 3). The only solution to restoring an effective atrial systole is to program a very long AV delay of 250–300 ms. This has two major inconveniences. First, the interatrial asynchrony remains untouched, with the resulting risk of recurrent atrial tachyarrhythmias and especially of atypical atrial flutter [54]. Second, the pacemaker must have a very long TARP, which substantially lowers its URL and reduces the patient's capacity for exercise adaptation. In order to solve this two-fold problem, we have proposed resynchronizing the electrical and mechanical activity of the two atria by pacing them simultaneously [26]. The system uses two atrial leads, one placed in the usual position in the right atrium and the other into the coronary sinus to pace and sense the left atrium at its inferior wall. A 'triple chamber pacemaker' paces the two atria simultaneously, in synchrony with the ventricular pulse delivery. The effectiveness of this system in preventing atrial tachyarrhythmias [26] and in optimizing cardiac performance [55] has been demonstrated with regularly programmed values for AV delay and a significantly shorter TARP. The hemodynamic benefit is illustrated in Figure 4 and in Table 2. For a mean optimal AV delay of 175 ms, dual atrial pacing increased cardiac output by

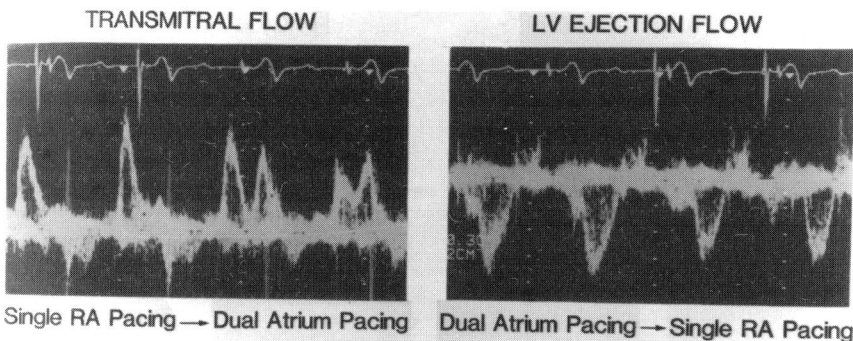

Figure 4. Mechanical benefit of permanent atrial resynchronization in patients with advanced interatrial block paced in DDD mode. Doppler-echo study of the transmitral flow and of the LV ejection flow. For a fixed AV delay of 150 ms, switching from a single right atrium pacing mode to a simultaneous dual atrium pacing mode produces the recovering of a well synchronized A wave and increases significantly V_{max} and the time velocity integral of the ejection flow.

Table 2. Hemodynamic benefits of simultaneous dual atrium pacing in patients with advanced interatrial block, paced in DDD mode.

Cardiac output (l/mn)				Optional AV delay (ms)		
Patient no.	Uni	Dual	Δ	Dual	Uni	Δ
1	5.7	6.5	+14%	150	250	100
2	4.6	5.9	+28%	200	?	?
3	5.1	6.8	+33%	150	200	50
4	4.9	6	+23%	150	250	100
5	4.3	5	+16%	250	?	?
6	6.6	8.1	+23%	150	250	100
M ± SD	5.2 ± 0.8	6.4 ± 1	23 ± 6%	175 ± 30		
Pulmonary capillary wedge pressure (mm Hg)						
1	14	12	−14%	200	?	?
2	22.5	15	−33%	200	?	?
3	15	7.5	−50%	125	250	125
4	12	8.5	−30%	100	200	100
5	20	18	−10%	250	?	?
6	12	9	−25%	150	250	100
M ± SD	16 ± 3	12 ± 3	27 ± 13%	171 ± 45		

Comparison of a single right atrium pacing mode (Uni) and a simultaneous dual atrium pacing mode (Dual) at identical pacing rates in six patients. Δ = difference (%) between Dual and Uni; ? = non determinable.

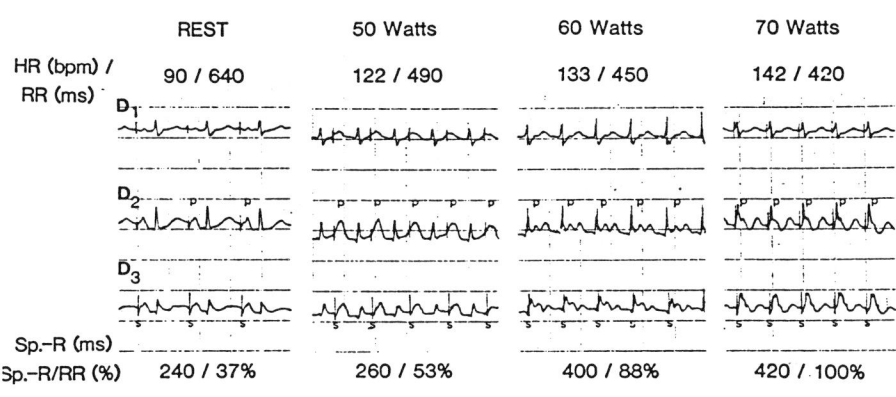

Figure 5. AAIR pacemaker syndrome. Due to a paradoxical and major increase in the atrial stimulus-R wave interval during exercise, the P waves produced come within the R wave of the preceding cycle.

23 ± 6% and decreased pulmonary capillary wedge pressure by 27 ± 13% in comparison with single right atrial DDD pacing. Indeed, to reach a similar degree of performance with the DDD mode, the AV delay has to be lengthened by 100 ms (mean).

Optimal AV synchrony and AAI/AAIR pacing
Single chamber atrial pacing (AAI-AAIR) is the most appropriate therapy for symptomatic SND patients because it is the only mode capable of preserving both atrial function and the normal ventricular activation sequence. However, these objectives can only be achieved in the case of narrow QRS and strictly normal AV conduction both at rest and during exercise. If the latter condition is not met, major AV dysynchrony may result. A typical example is the lack of adaptation to heart rate, or even a paradoxical prolongation, of the spike-R interval during exercise. This situation may produce P waves coming either immediately after or even within the preceding R wave, thus nullifying the atrial contribution (Figure 5) and sometimes resulting in severe exercise-related functional symptoms [56]. In a personal series [57], this abnormal behavior was observed in 30% of the AAIR-paced patients, although there was no apparent conduction defect at the pre-implant electrophysiologic study. We found that the principal determinants of this nonadaptation phenomenon were the existence of a bradytachy syndrome (in comparison with isolated SND) and the need for cardiodepressor drugs.

Although it has no direct relation to AAI pacing, *spontaneously very long*

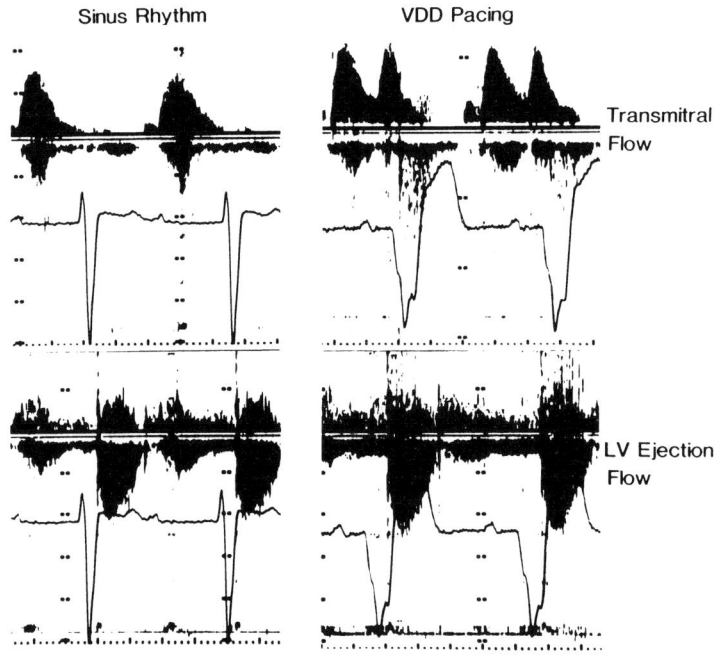

Figure 6. Adverse hemodynamic effects of very long PR intervals: Doppler-echocardiographic demonstration. No A wave is seen on transmitral flow in sinus rhythm. Temporary DDD pacing with a 150 ms AV delay produces recovery of a well synchronized A wave and significantly increases the V_{max} and time velocity integral of the LV ejection flow.

PR intervals persisting on exercise represents a very similar situation. It has been recently demonstrated that permanent DDD pacing with optimized AV delay provides a significant functional and hemodynamic benefit by restoring an effective left atrial function despite the necessary ventricular capture (Figure 6) [58].

These two examples clearly illustrate a frequent dilemma when choosing the optimal pacing mode in the individual patient. What is most important when the PR interval is long or moderately prolonged? Is it to optimize AV synchrony which would usually mean ventricular pacing and thus an altered activation sequence? Or is it to maintain a normal ventricular activation sequence at the price of an altered AV synchrony and reduced atrial contribution? The only answer to this dilemma lies in an evaluation of each patient's own hemodynamic and exercise behavior, both in the AAI mode and in the DDD mode with complete ventricular capture, using noninvasive techniques.

THE IMPORTANCE OF PRESERVING A NORMAL VENTRICULAR ACTIVATION SEQUENCE

Three recent studies emphasize the importance of the ventricular activation sequence. The results of these three studies were in perfect agreement, although each used a different method: radionuclide angiography at rest and Doppler-echocardiography at rest and during exercise [59], cardiopulmonary exercise testing [60], and hemodynamics and radionuclide angiography in our own work [61]. In patients implanted with a DDD or DDDR pacemaker for isolated sinus node dysfunction (intact AV conduction and narrow QRS), three different pacing modes were evaluated at rest and during exercise: AAI mode maintaining AV synchrony and a normal ventricular activation sequence; DDD mode with complete ventricular capture, but preserving AV synchrony, and VVI mode which lacks both. Among the three studies, the AAI mode produced a significant benefit over DDD pacing, both at rest and during exercise. This benefit was observed for all parameters measured: cardiac output and pulmonary pressures [61] (Figures 7 and 8), global and regional (septal) LV ejection fractions [59, 61], and VO_2 and O_2 pulse at peak exercise [60]. No significant difference was observed between the DDD mode and the VVI mode in Rosenqvist et al.'s series [59], but in our study [61] we found a significant benefit with the DDD mode, although the effect was observed only for hemodynamic parameters (Figures 7 and 8) [61].

The deleterious effects of right ventricular pacing are similar to those encountered with complete left bundle branch block [62]. Inverting the ventricular activation sequence creates major asynchrony between the two ventricles and within the left ventricle, disrupting septal motion.

These observations suggest that a normal ventricular activation sequence should be preserved as often as possible, and consequently that the ventricle should not be paced except when required because of inadequate AV or intraventricular conduction. A majority of SND patients and of patients implanted for carotid sinus syndrome or vasovagal syndrome could probably benefit from pacing modes that respect intrinsic conduction.

There are several technical ways of normalizing ventricular activation in paced patients: (a) Most SND patients can be programmed in the AAI mode; the risk of secondary AV block should not be exaggerated, especially since most of them are suprahisian blocks which develop progressively. The pacemaker can always be reprogrammed later to the DDD mode. (b) Programming in the DDD or DDI mode with a basic AV delay longer than the spontaneous PR or A stimulus-R interval, but this solution has the major inconvenience of increasing TARP and of limiting URL. (c) The use of an automatic algorithm which maintains the AAI mode as long as AV conduction is normal and switches to the DDD mode when the PR interval critically lengthens or when a nonconducted P wave occurs (ELA Medical Chorus II DDD pacemaker).

Another direction for the future would be to pace the distal His bundle

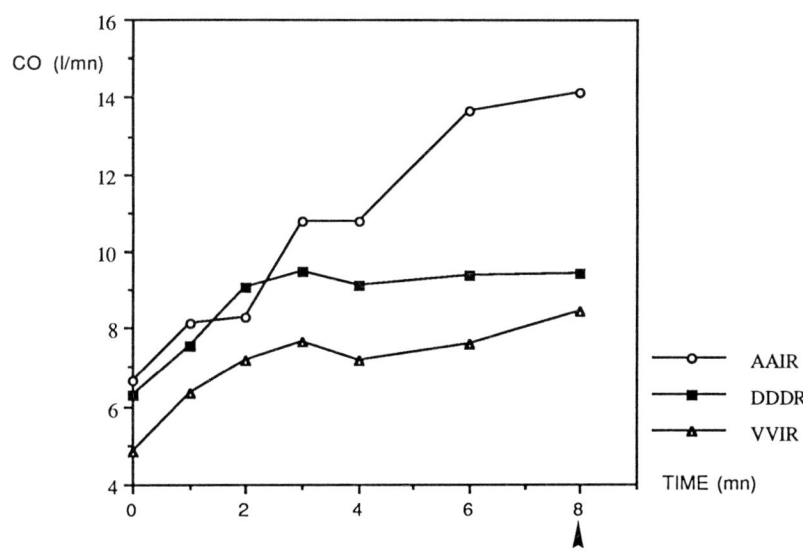

Figure 7. Hemodynamic importance of preserving a normal sequence of ventricular activation. Comparison of three pacing modes (AAI, VVI, and DDD) at identical pacing rates during exercise, in a patient chronically implanted for sinus node disease with intact AV conduction and narrow QRS. Cardiac output (CO) is significantly higher in the AAI mode than in the DDD and VVI modes at each exercise level and especially at peak exercise (arrowhead).

by implanting a screw-in lead in the upper portion of the interventricular septum [63].

The particular problem of hypertrophic obstructive cardiomyopathy (HOCM)
HOCM is the only exception to this rule. It has been demonstrated since the early 1960s that RV apical pacing with complete ventricular capture (CVR) can reduce or even abolish the left ventricular outflow tract (LVOT) gradient [64]. This effect was attributed to the inversion in the septal activation sequence, causing the septum to move away from the LV free wall during systole, resulting in an increase in LVOT dimensions and hence in a reduction in LVOT blood velocities. A decrease in hyperkinesia was also postulated.

However, a maximal hemodynamic benefit can only be expected if a fully efficient left atrial systole is preserved. This implies using DDD pacemakers with an optimally programmed AV delay that is in practice the longest compatible with CVR. In some patients with short PR intervals in sinus rhythm, a prolonged AV conduction time may be required, using pharmacological or physical (radiofrequency ablation) support [65]. All published stud-

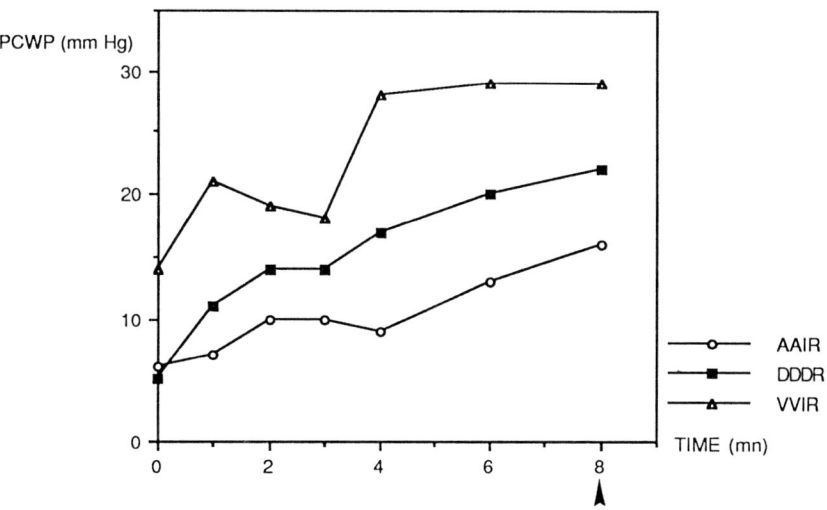

Figure 8. Hemodynamic importance of preserving a normal sequence of ventricular activation. Comparison of three pacing modes (AAI, VVI, and DDD) at identical pacing rates during exercise, in a patient chronically implanted for sinus node disease with intact AV conduction and narrow QRS. Pulmonary capillary wedge pressure (PCWP) is significantly lower in the AAI mode than in the DDD and VVI modes at each exercise level, and especially at peak exercise (arrowhead).

ies in chronically implanted patients [65–68] indicate a highly significant short- and long-term improvement in functional status (especially dyspnea and chest pain) and in exercise tolerance. The LVOT gradient is reduced by an average of 60–80%. Thus, DDD pacing may be considered an effective alternative to surgery in most patients with HOCM with drug-refractory symptoms. This is the first example of cardiac pacing used as a primary treatment of an organic heart disease independently of any conduction defect.

CONCLUSION

Today, pacemaker technology offers the means of providing each individual patient with optimal pacing adapted to his or her particular needs. In many cases, the patient can benefit from truly physiologic pacing capable of restoring normal or nearly normal heart function in all the different situations of everyday life. But this goal can only be reached after a highly rigorous preimplantation evaluation of the patient's needs, careful selection of the pacing system which will perfectly adapt to the patient's needs, and optimal programming of the different pacing parameters and algorithms. In the near future, we shall undoubtedly see intelligent pacemakers capable of automatic mode adaptation to the patient's changing needs. Cardiac pacing will then have become truly physiological.

REFERENCES

1. Higginbotham MB, Morris KG, Williams RS et al. Regulation of stroke volume during submaximal and maximal upright exercise in normal man. Circulation Res 1986;58:281–91.
2. Kruse I, Arnman K, Conradson TBJ et al. A comparison of the acute and long term hemodynamic effects of ventricular inhibited and atrial synchronous ventricular inhibited pacing. Circulation 1982;65:846–55.
3. Hammond HK, Froelicher VF. Normal and abnormal heart rate responses to exercise. Prog Cardiovasc Dis 1985;27:271–96.
4. Loeppky JA, Greene ER, Hoekenger DE et al. Beat-by-beat stroke volume assessment by pulsed Doppler in upright and supine exercise. J Appl Physiol 1981;50:1173–82.
5. Daubert C, Mabo P, Pouillot C, Lelong B. Atrial chronotropic incompetence: implications for DDDR pacing. In: Barold S, Mugica J, editors. New Perspectives in Cardiac Pacing, 2, NY: Mount Kisco, Futura 1991:251–71.
6. Gwinn N, Lemen R, Kratz J et al. Chronotropic incompetence: a common and progressive finding in pacemaker patients. Am Heart J 1992;123:1216–9.
7. Paillard F, Mabo P, Ben Slimane A et al. Les blocs auriculo-ventriculaires démasqués à l'épreuve d'effort. Ann Cardiol Angéiol 1990;39:55–60.
8. Levy S, Danis C, Broustet JP et al. Blocs auriculo-ventriculaires idiopathiques du sujet jeune: intérêt de l'épreuve d'effort et l'épreuve à l'atropine pour la localisation du trouble conductif. Arch Mal Coeur 1982;75:11–9.
9. Corbelli R, Masterson M, Wilkoff BL. Chronotropic response to exercise in patients with atrial fibrillation. PACE 1990;13:179–87.
10. Rosenqvist M. Atrial pacing for sick sinus syndrome. Clin Cardiol 1990;13:43–7.
11. Kallryd A, Kruse I, Ryden L. Atrial inhibited pacing in the sick sinus node syndrome: clinical value and the demand for rate responsiveness. PACE 1989;12:954–61.
12. Vardas PE, Fitzpatrick A, Ingram A et al. Natural history of sinus node chronotropy in paced patients. PACE 1991;14:155–68.
13. Daubert C, Mabo P, Druelles P, Ritter P, Paillard F. Dysfonction sinusale et anomalies de la conduction auriculo-ventriculaire. Stimucoeur 1988;16:206–10.
14. Fromer M, Kappenberger L, Steinbrunn W. Binodal disease: diseased sinus node and atrioventricular block. Z Cardiol 1983;72:4l0–3.
15. Banner NR, Lloyd MH, Hamilton RD et al. Cardiopulmonary response to dynamic exercise after heart and combined heart-lung transplantation. Br Heart J 1989;61:215–23.
16. Heinz G, Hirsch M, Buxbaum P et al. Sinus node dysfunction after orthotopic cardiac transplantation: postoperative incidence and long-term implications. PACE 1992;15:731–7.
17. Di Biase A, Ise TM, Schnittger I et al. Frequency and mechanism of bradycardia in transplant recipients and need for pacemaker. Am J Cardiol 1991;67:1385–9.
18. Ellestad MHJ, Wan MKC. Predictive implications of stress testing. Follow-up of 2700 subjects after maximum treadmill stress testing. Circulation 1975;51:363–9.
19. Wiens RD, Lafla P, Marder CM et al. Chronotropic incompetence in clinical exercise testing. Am J Cardiol 1984;54:74–8.
20. Ritter P, Mabo P, Varin C et al. Effects of 1:1, Wenckebach, 2:1 AV associations and Fallback on arterial pressure and cycle to cycle arterial pressure variability during exercise in DDD pacing (abstract). PACE 1990;14:682.
21. Cazeau S, Daubert C, Mabo P et al. Dynamic electrophysiology of ventriculoatrial conduction: implications for DDD and DDDR pacing. PACE 1990;13:1646–55.

22. Limousin M, Bonnet JL. A new algorithm to solve endless loop tachycardia in DDD pacing: a multicenter study of 91 patients. PACE 1990:13;867-74.
23. Daubert C, Ritter P, Mabo P, Varin C, Leclercq C. AV delay optimization in DDD and DDDR pacing. In: Barold S, Mugica J, editors. New Perspectives in Cardiac Pacing, 3, Mount Kisco, NY: Futura, 1993:259-87.
24. Markewitz A, Kemkes B, Reble E et al. Particularities of dual chamber pacemaker therapy in patients after orthotopic heart transplantation. PACE 1987;10:326-32.
25. Kacet S, Molin F, Lacroix D et al. Bipolar atrial triggered pacing to restore normal chronotropic responsiveness in an orthotopic cardiac transplant patient. PACE 1991;14:1444-7.
26. Daubert C, Berder V, Mabo P et al. Arrhythmia prevention by permanent atrial resynchronization in advanced interatrial blocks (abstract). Circulation 1990;82:181.
27. Chu-Pak Lau. Rate adaptative cardiac pacing: single and dual chamber. Mount Kisco, NY: Futura, 1993.
28. Channer KS, Jones JV. Atrial systole: its role in normal and diseased hearts. Clin Sci 1988;75:1-4.
29. Daubert C, Ritter P, Mabo P, Druelles P. Hemodynamic response to cardiac pacing in DDD mode. In: Barold S, Mugica J, editors. New Perspectives in Cardiac Pacing, 1. Mount Kisco, NY: Futura, 1988:27-44.
30. Hamby RI, Noble WJ, Murphy DH et al. Atrial transport function in coronary artery disease: relation to the left ventricular function. J Am Coll Cardiol 1983;1:1011-7.
31. Hochleitner M, Hörtnagl H, Ng CK, Hörtnagl H, Gschnitzer H, Zechman W. Usefulness of physiologic dual-chamber pacing in drug resistant idiopathic dilated cardiomyopathy. Am J Cardiol 1990;66:198-202.
32. Hochleitner M, Hörtnagl H, Hörtnagl H, Fridrich L, Gschnitzer F. Long-term efficacy of physiologic dual-chamber pacing in the treatment of end-stage idiopathic dilated cardiomyopathy. Am J Cardiol 1992;70:1230-5.
33. Daubert C, Mabo P, Leclercq C, Gras D. Limits and adverse effects of VVI and VVIR pacing. In: Santini M, Pistolese M, Alliegro A, editors. Progress in Clinical Pacing, 1992, Mount Kisco, NY: Futura, 1993:141-66.
34. Hesselson AB, Parsonnet V, Bernstein AD, Bonavita GJ. Deleterious effects of long-term single chamber ventricular pacing in patients with sick sinus syndrome: the hidden benefits of dual-chamber pacing. J Am Coll Cardiol 1992;19:1543-9.
35. Sutton R, Kenny RA. The natural history of sick sinus syndrome. PACE 1986;9:1110-3.
36. Rosenqvist M, Brandt J, Schüller H. Long-term pacing in sinus node disease: effects of stimulation mode on cardiovascular morbidity and mortality. Am Heart J 1988;118:16-22.
37. Santini M, Alexidou G, Ansalone G et al. Relation of prognosis in sick sinus syndrome to age, condution defects and modes of permanent cardiac pacing. Am J Cardiol 1990;65:729-35.
38. Alpert MA, Curtiss JJ, Sanfelippo JF et al. Comparative survival following permanent ventricular pacing and dual-chamber pacing for patients with chronic symptomatic sinus node dysfunction with and without congestive heart failure. Am Heart J 1987;113:958-65.
39. Rossi P, Rognoni G, Ochetta E et al. Respiration-dependent ventricular pacing compared with fixed ventricular and atrio-ventricular synchronous pacing: aerobic and hemodynamic variables. J Am Coll Cardiol 1985;6:646-52.
40. Menozzi C, Brignole M, Moracchini PV et al. Intrapatient comparison between chronic VVIR and DDD pacing in patients affected by high degree AV block without heart failure. PACE 1990;13:1816-22.
41. Oldroyd KG, Rae AP, Carter R, Wingate C, Cobbe SM. Doubleblind crossover comparison of the effects of dual-chamber pacing (DDD) and ventricular rate adaptative (VVIR) pacing on neuroendocrine variables, exercise performance, and symptoms in complete heart block. Br Heart J 1991;65:188-93.
42. Linde-Edelstam C, Hjemdahl P, Pehrsson SK, Astrom H, Nordlander R. Is DDD pacing

superior to VVIR? A study on cardiac sympathetic nerve activity and myocardial oxygen consumption at rest and during exercise. PACE 1992;15:425-34.
43. Blanc JJ, Mansourati J, Ritter P et al. Atrial natriuretic factor release during exercise in patients successively paced in DDD and rate matched ventricular pacing. PACE 1992;15:397-402.
44. Linde-Edelstam C, Nordlander R, Unden AL, Orth-Gomer K, Ryden L. Quality of life in patients treated with atrioventricular synchronous pacing compared to rate modulated ventricular pacing: a long-term, double-blind, crossover study. PACE 1992;15:1467-76.
45. Alpert MA, Curtis JJ, Sanfelippo JF et al. Comparative survival after permanent ventricular and dual-chamber pacing for patients with high degree atrioventricular block with and without pre-existent congestive heart failure. J Am Coll Cardiol 1986;7:925-32.
46. Linde-Edelstam C, Gullbert G, Nordlander R, Pehrsson K, Ryden L. Effects of atrial synchronous pacing on survival in patients with high degree AV block and congestive heart failure (abstract). J Am Coll Cardiol 1991;17:289A.
47. Wish M, Fletcher RD, Cohn A. Hemodynamics of AV synchrony and rate. J Electrophysiol 1989;3:170-5.
48. Lascault G, Bigonzi F, Frank R et al. Non-invasive study of dual chamber pacing by pulsed Doppler. Prediction of the hemodynamic response by echocardiographic measurements. Eur Heart J 1989;10:525-31.
49. Rey JL, Slama MA, Triboulloy C et al. Etude par écho-Döppler des variations hémodynamiques entre modes double-stimulation et détection de l'oreillette chez des patients porteurs d'un stimulateur double-chambre. Arch Mal Coeur 1990;83:961-6.
50. Wish M, Fletcher RD, Gotdiener JS et al. Importance of left atrial timing in the programming of dual chamber pacemaker. Am J Cardiol 1987;60:566-71.
51. Daubert C, Ritter P, Mabo P et al. Physiological relationship between AV interval and heart rate in healthy subjects: applications to dual chamber pacing. PACE 1986;9:1032-9.
52. Mabo P, Ritter P, Varin C, et al. Intérêts d'un algorithme d'adaptation automatique du délai AV à la fréquence atriale instantanée en stimulation cardiaque DDD. Arch Mal Coeur 1992;85:1443-8.
53. Ritter P, Vai F, Bonnet JL et al. Rate adaptative atrioventricular delay improves cardiopulmonary performances in patients implanted with a dual chamber pacemaker for complete heart block. Eur J CPE 1991;1:31-8.
54. Bayes de Lunà A, Cladellas M, Oter R et al. Interatrial conduction block with retrograde activation of the left atrium and paroxysmal supraventricular tachyarrhythmias. Eur Heart J 1988;9:1112-8.
55. Daubert C, Mabo P, Berder V et al. Simultaneous dual atrium pacing in high degree interatrial blocks: hemodynamic results (abstract). Circulation 1991;84:453.
56. Den Dulk K, Lindemans FW, Brugada P et al. Pacemaker syndrome with AAI rate variable pacing: importance of atrioventricular conduction properties, medication and pacemaker programmability. PACE 1988;11:1226-33.
57. Mabo P, Pouillot C, Kermarrec A et al. Lack of physiological adaptation of the atrioventricular interval to heart rate in patients chronically paced in the AAIR mode. PACE 1991;14:2133-42.
58. Mabo P, Cazeau S, Forrer A et al. Isolated long PR interval as only indication of permanent DDD pacing (abstract). J Am Coll Cardiol 1992;19:66.
59. Rosenqvist M, Isaaz K, Botvinick EH et al. Relative importance of activation sequence compared to atrioventricular synchrony in left ventricular function. Am J Cardiol 1991;67:148-56.
60. Harper GR, Pina IL, Kutalek SP. Intrinsic conduction maximizes cardiopulmonary performance in patients with dual chamber pacemakers. PACE 1991;14:1787-91.
61. Leclercq C, Mabo P, Le Helloco A et al. Hemodynamic interest of preserving a normal sequence of ventricular activation in permanent cardiac pacing (abstract). J Am Coll Cardiol 1992,19:150.

62. Grines C, Bashore T, Boudoulas H, et al. Functional abnormalities in isolated left bundle branch block: the effects of interventricular asynchrony. Circulation 1989,79:845–53.
63. Karpawich PP, Justice CD, Chang CH, Gause CY, Kuhns LR. Septal ventricular pacing in the immature canine heart: a new perspective. Am Heart J 1991;121:827–33.
64. Bourdarias JP, Lockhart A, Ourbak P, Ferrane J, Scebat L, Lenègre J. Hémodynamique des myocardiopathies obstructives. Arch Mal Coeur 1964;57:737–8.
65. Gras D, Guillo P, Mabo P et al. Permanent DDD pacing with complete ventricular capture as an alternative to surgery in hypertrophic obstructive cardiomyopathy (abstract). Circulation 1992;86:272.
66. McDonald K, McWilliams E, O'Keefe B, Maurer B. Functional assessment of patients treated with permanent dual chamber pacing as a primary treatment for hypertrophic cardiomyopathy. Eur Heart J 1988;9:893–8.
67. Fananapazir L, Cannon RO, Tripodi D, Panza JA. Impact of dual-chamber permanent pacing in patients with obstructive hypertrophic cardiomyopathy with symptoms refractory to verapamil and β-adrenergic blocker therapy. Circulation 1992;85:2149–61.
68. Jeanrenaud X, Goy JJ, Kappenberger L. Effects of dual-chamber pacing in hypertrophic obstructive cardiomyopathy. Lancet 1992;339:1318–23.

24. Pacemaker syndrome during atrial-based pacing

S. SERGE BAROLD

INTRODUCTION

Ausubel and Furman defined the pacemaker syndrome as a clinical complex of "signs and symptoms related to the adverse hemodynamic and electrophysiologic consequences of ventricular pacing" [1] in the presence of a normally functioning implanted ventricular pacemaker. Recent studies have indicated that the incidence of the pacemaker syndrome (including subtle manifestations) is considerably higher than previously believed as most patients with dual chamber pulse generators prefer the DDD (VDD) to the VVI mode, with only a small number showing no preference. Schüller and Brand [2] recently suggested that the pacemaker syndrome be redefined more broadly as follows: "The pacemaker syndrome refers to symptoms and signs present in the pacemaker patient which are caused by inadequate timing of atrial and ventricular contractions". This new definition is more appropriate because the introduction of pacing modes more physiologic than the VVI or VVIR modes has not entirely eliminated the pacemaker syndrome, which can also occur under certain circumstances with atrial-based pacing in the presence of "inadequate timing of atrial and ventricular contractions" (Table 1). During VVI(R) pacing, the pacemaker syndrome is more commonly related to retrograde ventriculoatrial (VA) conduction than the random timing of atrial and ventricular activity. Similarly during atrial-based pacing, the continual occurrence of an atrial event after a ventricular event engenders the pacemaker syndrome more commonly than AV dissociation.

PACEMAKER SYNDROME WITH DUAL CHAMBER PACING

Obviously, some malfunction of dual chamber pacing such as loss of effectual atrial pacing due to a high threshold can cause the pacemaker syndrome by producing VVI pacing with retrograde VA conduction [2]. However, under certain circumstances, a DDD or DDDR pacemaker can cause the pace-

Table 1. Causes of pacemaker syndrome during atrial-based pacing.

1. Single chamber rate-adaptive pacing
   AAIR on exercise
2. Dual chamber pacing
   (i) DDI, DDD, DDIR, DDDR: Marked delay of left atrial activation at rest and/or exercise.
   (ii) VDD, DDD, DDDR: Sinus tachycardia with long programmed AV interval on exercise.
   (iii) VDD, VDDR: Sinus bradycardia at rest slower than programmed lower rate.
   (iv) VDDR: Atrial chronotropic incompetence on exercise with conversion to the VVIR mode when sinus rate is slower than sensor-driven rate.
   (v) DDI, DDIR: At rest and/or during exercise.
   (vi) DDI, DDD, DDIR, DDDR: Repetitive nonreentrant ventriculoatrial synchrony at rest and/or during exercise.
3. Automatic mode switching from dual chamber to single chamber ventricular pacing
   (i) Reset from the DDD (DDDR) to the VVI (VOO) mode consequent to activation of the elective replacement indicator or sensing electromagnetic interference at rest.
   (ii) Mode switching from DDDR (DDD) to VVIR (VVI) as a protective mechanism against unphysiologic supraventricular tachyarrhythmias, at rest and/or during exercise.

maker syndrome during normal function of a pacing system thought to be appropriately programmed [3]. Pacemaker syndrome can occur if the AV delay is programmed either too long or too short [4].

In patients with AV block equipped with a DDD or VDD pacemaker with a long and fixed AV interval (e.g., 250 ms), vigorous exercise can place the sensed P wave too close to the previous paced ventricular beat (but still beyond the relatively short postventricular atrial refractory period, PVARP). This situation can produce unfavorable hemodynamic consequences or the pacemaker syndrome on exercise [5].

Delayed left atrial systole

Although it is difficult to predict the optimal AV delay for any given patient [6–12], it is reasonable after implantation to program the AV interval in most patients at 200 ms after atrial pacing and 150 ms after atrial sensing. Clinical follow-up will then determine the need for noninvasive hemodynamic studies to optimize the AV interval. As a rule, the AV interval initiated by atrial pacing (i.e., DVI cycle) should be about 50 ms longer than the AV interval initiated by atrial sensing (i.e., VDD cycle) to provide similar mechanical AV relationships on the left side of the heart [7,8,13,14]. In the individual patient, the determination of the stroke volume by Doppler-echocardiography at various AV intervals (after atrial pacing and sensing) is the only way to determine precisely the AV delay providing optimal hemodynamic benefit [8].

A DDD pacemaker senses and paces on the right side of the heart. Yet the timing relationships of atrial and ventricular mechanical activity on the left side of the heart determine the hemodynamic performance. In the presence of severe atrial disease, the propagation of electrical activity from the right atrium to the left atrium can be markedly delayed because of (1) increased latency (delay from onset of pacemaker stimulus to the beginning of an identifiable atrial depolarization; probably a rare phenomenon) [15] and (2) delayed interatrial conduction. With delayed left atrial activation, the programmed AV delay may no longer provide an adequate time for effective mechanical left atrial systole before mechanical left ventricular systole and in extreme cases left atrial systole begins after the onset of ventricular systole [13,16,17]. Several groups have measured the interatrial conduction time (IACT) from the onset of the atrial stimulus of DDD or AAI pacemakers to the onset [13,18] or the peak deflection [19] of the "left" P wave recorded by an esophageal lead. A wide range of IACT can be recorded in patients with implanted pacemakers as shown by the following studies: Wish et al. [13] ($n = 16$) IACT = 70 ± 380 ms (mean 144 ± 82), Chirife et al. [18] ($n = 16$) IACT = 35–130 ms (mean 73), and Stierle et al. [19] ($n = 27$) IACT = 36.6–210 ms (mean 116 ± 32.1). Wish et al. [13] reported three patients with a programmed AV delay of 150 ms in whom the IACT was longer than the AV interval, i.e., left atrial depolarization followed ventricular activation. Such a situation produces the equivalent of ventriculoatrial pacing. Wish et al. [13] found that the IACT of all patients whose optimal programmed AV delay was 150 ms was significantly less (90 ± 14 ms) than that of patients whose optimal delay was 200 and 250 ms (148 ± 56 ms) ($p < 0.05$).

With significant interatrial conduction delay and/or latency, programming an AV delay of 150–200 ms during DDD (DDDR) pacing may not provide the hemodynamic benefit of AV synchrony and cause the pacemaker syndrome because delayed left atrial systole occurs when the mitral valve has already closed. Such inappropriate matching of left atrial and left ventricular systole could conceivably occur early after device implantation or much later without a change in the programmed AV delay due to progression of atrial disease and/or a drug-induced atrial conduction delay. M-mode and Doppler-echocardiography are invaluable in making the diagnosis by demonstrating the position of the mitral A wave and the Doppler A wave of transmitral flow in relation to the ventricular stimulus and onset of left ventricular systole.

Some DDDR pacemakers can shorten the AV interval (atrial paced/ventricular paced) on exercise automatically according to the sensor input. However, when exercise produces little or no associated improvement in interatrial conduction and/or latency, an adequate AV interval (atrial paced/ventricular paced) at rest could paradoxically become inappropriate on exercise (because of rate-adaptive shortening), thereby creating an exercise-induced pacemaker syndrome if left atrial systole begins after the onset of left ventricular systole [20].

Rarely with a very long IACT, considerable shortening of the AV delay (e.g. 25 ms) may allow optimal left atrial activation [13]. The atrial stimulus causes delayed atrial activation well beyond the paced QRS complex that terminates the AV interval: atrial activation is so displaced that its close proximity to the succeeding paced ventricular beat may provide a better AV relationship. This paradoxical effect is similar to a very prolonged first-degree AV block in which the P wave before a QRS gives rise to the succeeding delayed QRS complex and not the one that immediately follows it.

The restoration of AV synchrony in patients with substantial interatrial conduction block may require programming an exceedingly long AV interval that a dual-chamber device may not be able to provide. A very long AV interval, as pointed out by Daubert et al. [21], has two major disadvantages: (1) interatrial asynchrony is unaffected and predisposes to atrial arrhythmias, and (2) the need for a long PVARP with significant lowering or limitation of the upper rate and exercise response.

The electrophysiologic and hemodynamic consequences of high-degree interatrial conduction block can also be corrected with permanent resynchronization of the two atria, a concept introduced by Daubert et al. [21–25]. The system uses two atrial leads, one in the right atrial appendage and the other in the coronary sinus (to pace and sense the left atrium) connected via a Y connector to (1) an SSI pacemaker ("dual atrial pacemaker") programmed to the AAT mode with bipolar pacing and sensing configuration, an arrangement suitable only in patients with intact AV conduction, and (2) the atrial port of a DDDR pacemaker ("triple chamber pacemaker") to produce dual atrial and AV sequential pacing. In this way, the triple pacemaker paces the two atria simultaneously and then delivers its ventricular stimulus to produce a more appropriate AV interval. In patients with substantial interatrial conduction delay, atrial resynchronization by triple-chamber pacing increases the cardiac output and lowers the wedge pressure compared with the identical rate of pacing with a standard dual-chamber pulse generator [21,24]. Resynchronization can also prevent atrial tachyarrhythmias in patients with advanced interatrial block. Daubert et al. [25] recently reported that atrial resynchronization remained effective in 17 of 19 patients with interatrial conduction block during a follow-up period of 21 ± 12 months. The work of Daubert et al. [21–25] will probably renew interest in atrial pacing from the coronary sinus. Indeed, conventional dual-chamber pacing with left atrial pacing via the coronary sinus rather than triple pacing may be sufficient in some patients with high-degree interatrial block to achieve atrial resynchronization and optimize mechanical AV synchrony.

VDD Mode

The VDD mode functions like the DDD mode without an atrial output. In the absence of sensed atrial activity, the VDD mode will continue to pace effectively in the VVI mode at the programmed lower rate. Thus, when the sinus rate drops below the lower rate, VVI pacing may cause the pacemaker syndrome, particularly in young and active patients who have sinus bradycardia at rest [26,27]. VDD-induced pacemaker syndrome was virtually eliminated when dedicated VDD devices were replaced by DDD pulse generators, but it may reappear because recent favorable experience with single lead VDD pacing will probably lead to a renaissance of dedicated VDD devices [27–29]. The recently introduced single lead VDDR mode of pacing carries the risk of inducing the pacemaker syndrome both at rest and upon exercise [30]. Patients with VDDR systems should be carefully evaluated for the development of atrial chronotropic incompetence that would favor the conversion of the VDD mode to the VVIR mode on exercise.

DDI and DDIR Modes

In dual chamber pulse generators with ventricular-based lower rate timing (lower rate interval controlled by ventricular events, constant atrial escape interval), the DDI mode is equivalent to the DDD mode with the upper rate (interval) equal to the lower rate (interval) [31,32]. In the DDI mode (ventricular based), the pacemaker avoids competitive atrial pacing by sensing atrial activity (which therefore inhibits release of the atrial stimulus at the completion of the atrial escape interval). Unlike the ventricular response of traditional DDD and VDD modes, the paced ventricular rate in the DDI mode cannot exceed the programmed lower ventricular rate (the functional equivalent of no atrial tracking). Similarly, in the DDIR mode the ventricular pacing rate can never exceed the sensor-driven rate. For this reason, the DDI and DDIR modes have achieved a modest success for the treatment of patients with alternating bradycardia and supraventricular tachyarrhythmias, mostly in patients with atrial chronotropic incompetence [33,34].

In the DDD mode, sensing of retrograde P waves beyond the PVARP causes endless loop tachycardia (pacemaker-mediated tachycardia). In the DDI mode, a slower but hemodynamically significant pacemaker endless loop can occur (without tachycardia as in the DDD mode) at the programmed fixed ventricular pacing rate, an arrangement capable of causing the pacemaker syndrome similar to the VVI mode with retrograde VA conduction [35] (Figure 1).

In the DDI mode, AV synchrony is maintained in only two situations: (1) when the programmed lower rate exceeds the spontaneous atrial rate so that both channels pace sequentially and (2) in patients with sick sinus syndrome and *relatively normal AV conduction* if the spontaneous atrial rate exceeds the programmed lower rate (P-P interval < lower rate interval). The conducted QRS inhibits the pulse generator, and there will be no advantage over DDD pacing, particularly in the presence of atrial tachyarrhythmias that conduct to the ventricle. In contrast, AV synchrony does not occur in the DDI mode in patients with AV block when the sinus rate exceeds the pro-

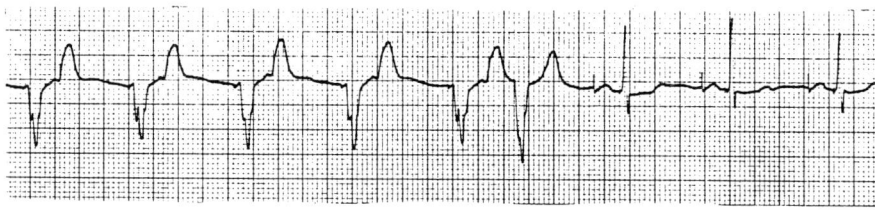

Figure 1. DDI mode with endless loop response. Lower rate = 70/min, postventricular atrial refractory period (PVARP) = 200 ms. On the left, each ventricular paced beat is followed by a retrograde P wave sensed by the pulse generator beyond its PVARP. A ventricular extrasystole associated with VA conduction block (because of prematurity) allows return of AV synchrony. Sensing of retrograde P waves can be eliminated by programming a longer PVARP. (Reproduced with permission from [55]).

grammed lower rate (Figure 2, upper strip). In the latter case, the P waves sensed by the atrial channel gradually march through the pacing cycles, moving closer and closer to the preceding paced ventricular beat, thereby producing constantly changing AV intervals, mostly unphysiologic in duration. In this situation, the pacemaker functions like the VVI mode (with AV dissociation) except when a P wave falling in the PVARP is unsensed, whereupon which the pulse generator delivers an atrial stimulus at the termination of the atrial escape interval provided the sinus (or atrial) rate is not excessively fast. Thus, with a normal sinus mechanism and AV block, the DDI mode presents no real hemodynamic advantage over VVI pacing. The relatively long period of AV dissociation favored by a relatively short PVARP (release of atrial stimuli are inhibited by the sensed P waves) may not be tolerated in some patients, creating a pacemaker syndrome at rest (even in the absence of retrograde VA conduction). In this respect, Sulke et al. [36] demonstrated (in patients with implanted pacemakers, allowing comparison of the DDD, DDI, and VVI modes in the same individual) that in the DDI mode "mode switching" from the DDI mode (with AV sequential pacing) to the functional VVI mode with mild exertion associated with an increase in atrial rate was not acceptable to most patients. The perceived general well-being was similar when the DDI mode was compared to the VVI mode. A comparable situation associated with the pacemaker syndrome can occur in the DDIR mode upon exercise in patients with complete AV block when the sinus rate exceeds the sensor-driven interval, and the pacemaker functions essentially like the VVIR mode (Figure 2, lower strip).

Patients with AV block (spontaneous or induced by ablation), a normal sinus mechanism, and intractable paroxysmal supraventricular tachyarrhythmias fare better with retained AV synchrony by using appropriately programmed DDD or DDDR devices designed with a protective algorithm

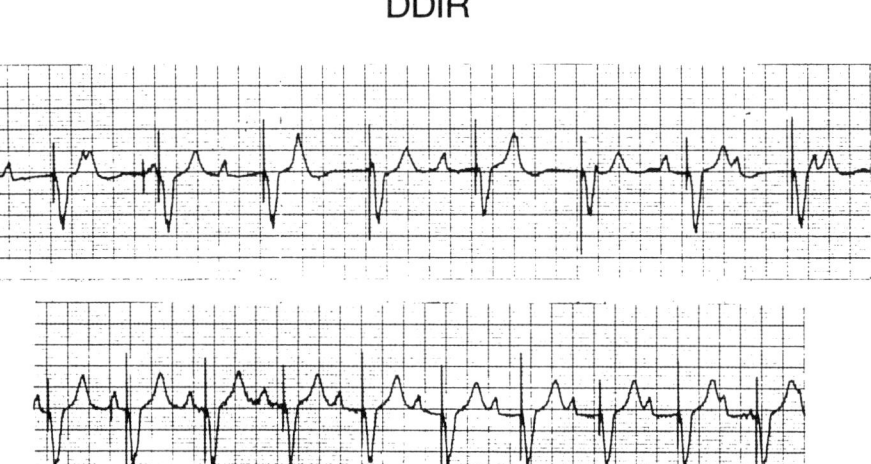

Figure 2. ECG of a patient who developed the pacemaker syndrome with the DDIR pacing mode. A dual chamber pulse generator was implanted after His bundle ablation for intractable paroxysmal atrial fibrillation. (top) The DDIR mode at rest functions at the programmed lower rate of 60/min, slower than the prevailing sinus rate. Note that sinus P waves march through the cardiac cycle, producing AV dissociation. The P wave following the first ventricular paced beat falls in the 300 ms postventricular atrial refractory period (PVARP) and is unsensed, thereby allowing the release of an atrial stimulus at the end of the atrial escape interval initiated by the first ventricular paced complex. (bottom) On exercise, when the sinus rate slightly exceeds the sensor-driven rate, sinus P waves march through the cardiac cycle producing AV dissociation. The pulse generator does not sense the P wave following the first ventricular paced beat because it falls in the PVARP. This allows release of an atrial stimulus at the termination of the sensor-driven atrial escape interval initiated by the first ventricular paced beat. (Reproduced with permission from [55]).

for the recognition of supraventricular tachyarrhythmias and prevention of rapid ventricular paced rates (e.g., fallback or automatic mode switching to a slower ventricular rate whenever the atrial rate exceeds a given rate, usually the programmed upper rate) [37]. This approach prevents the pacemaker syndrome caused by almost continual AV dissociation related to the DDI and DDIR modes.

Repetitive nonreentrant ventriculoatrial synchrony

Repetitive retrograde VA conduction in patients with dual chamber pacemakers can cause two forms of VA synchrony [38]. (1) Endless loop tachycardia (pacemaker-mediated tachycardia) or repetitive reentrant VA synchrony

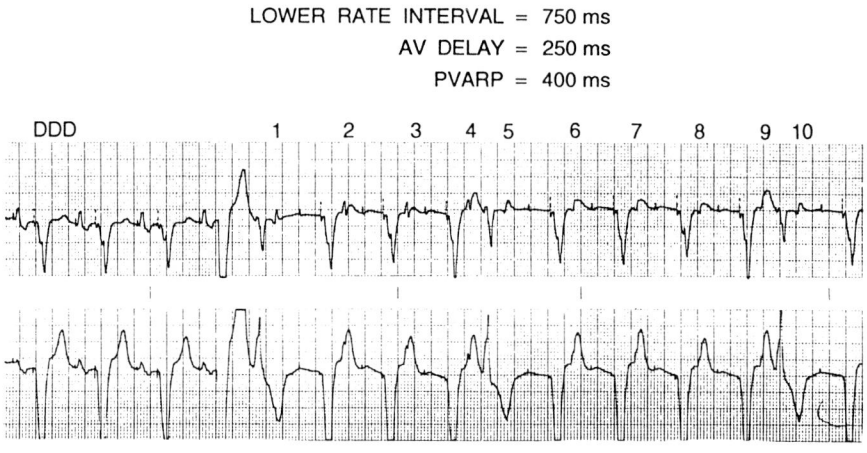

Figure 3. Initiation of repetitive nonreentrant VA synchrony (AV desynchronization arrhythmia) by a ventricular extrasystole during DDD pacing (parameters shown above the electrocardiogram). The numbers indicate retrograde P waves. The 4th and 5th complexes are ventricular extrasystoles (VE). The second initiates retrograde VA conduction (1). The succeeding atrial stimulus is ineffectual because it falls within the myocardial atrial refractory period related to retrograde P wave no. 1. The accompanying ventricular paced beat perpetuates VA conduction (2), thereby starting repetitive nonreentrant VA synchrony. VEs with retrograde VA conduction (5 and 10) during the arrhythmia do not disturb the basic mechanism. Two electrocardiographic leads were recorded simultaneously. (Reproduced with permission from [38]).

occurs when the pacemaker senses retrograde P waves. Traditionally, endless loop tachycardia is not classified as a cause of pacemaker syndrome, but according to the definition by Schüller and Brandt [2], the situation really represents a form of it. (2) VA synchrony can also occur without endless loop tachycardia when a paced ventricular beat engenders an *unsensed* retrograde P wave falling within the PVARP of a DDI, DDD, or DDDR pacemaker. Under certain circumstances this form of VA synchrony may become self-perpetuating because the pacemaker continually delivers an *ineffectual* atrial stimulus during the atrial myocardial refractory period generated by the preceding retrograde atrial depolarization (Figure 3). By definition, the amplitude of the atrial stimulus must exceed the atrial pacing threshold tested during atrial pacing with a normal relationship of atrial and ventricular events. Originally I called this form of VA synchrony "AV desynchronization arrhythmia", but I now prefer the term repetitive nonreentrant VA synchrony or VA synchrony nonreentrant arrhythmia [38–40]. Schüller and Brandt have called this situation "pseudo-atrial exit block".

A long AV interval and/or a relatively fast lower rate (or sensor-driven rate with DDDR or DDIR pacing) favor the development of repetitive

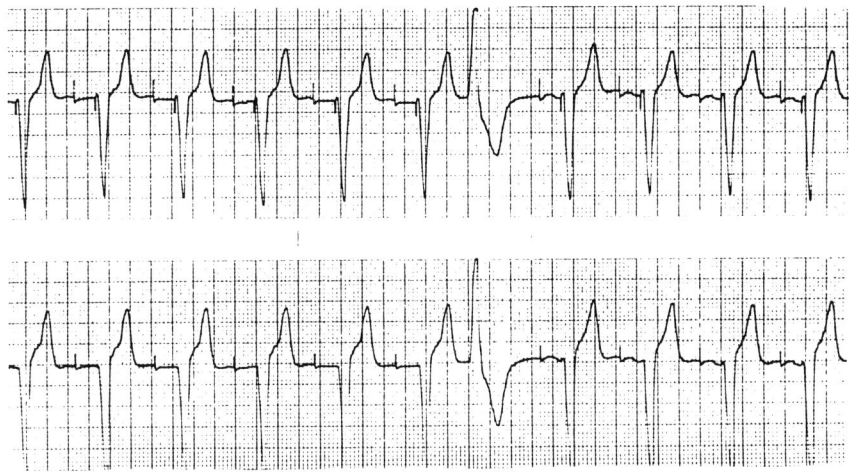

Figure 4. Sustained repetitive nonreentrant VA synchrony terminated by ventricular extrasystole associated with block of retrograde VA conduction which therefore allows the succeeding stimulus to cause atrial capture.

nonreentrant VA synchrony, usually in the setting of relatively long retrograde VA conduction with retrograde P waves in the PVARP. A retrograde P wave beyond the PVARP but unsensed because of a low amplitude or low sensitivity of the atrial channel can also initiate a hemodynamic situation similar to repetitive nonreentrant VA synchrony. Rarely AV synchrony (with atrial capture) and VA synchrony (retrograde P waves) coexist in the same cardiac cycle whenever a relatively long AV interval (e.g., 250 ms) favors retrograde VA conduction. Both endless loop tachycardia and repetitive nonreentrant VA synchrony depend on retrograde VA conduction and are physiologically similar [38]. Both share similar initiating and terminating mechanisms (Figures 3, 4), and under certain circumstances one arrhythmia may convert spontaneously to the other [38]. Repetitive nonreentrant VA synchrony is not uncommonly unsustained (as discussed later), but its termination is often unrelated to a spontaneous change of retrograde VA conduction (conduction block or improved conduction, thereby allowing the subsequent atrial stimulus to fall beyond the atrial myocardial refractory period with resultant atrial capture).

Once repetitive nonreentrant VA synchrony is initiated, three scenarios are possible. (1) The atrial stimulus continually falls in the absolute atrial myocardial refractory period and is always ineffectual even if the atrial output of the pacemaker is increased to its maximal value. (2) The atrial stimulus falls within the relative refractory period of the atrial myocardium so that the threshold for atrial pacing is increased. After the induction of repetitive nonreentrant VA synchrony, the higher atrial pacing threshold seems to decrease gradually and then stabilize (all other parameters remaining unchanged) over a period of less than 1 min to a value greater than the one tested during atrial pacing with a normal relationship of atrial and ventricular events. Recent observations on the effect of atrial pressure or dimension on the atrial pacing threshold do not provide a good explanation for this threshold behavior [41,42]. In terms of the pacing threshold, one of two situations can then occur: (a) spontaneous return of atrial capture without any change of the pacemaker parameters when the atrial pacing threshold attains a value equal to the atrial output of the pacemaket [46] or (b) repetitive nonreentrant VA synchrony persists until atrial capture is promoted by an increase in the atrial output of the pacemaker.

When sustained, repetitive nonreentrant VA synchrony can cause unfavorable hemodynamics similar to the pacemaker syndrome during the normal function of a DDD or DDI (DDDR, DDIR) pulse generator [43]. Because the duration of the atrial escape (pacemaker VA) interval can be easily controlled, repetitive nonreentrant VA synchrony should not be an important problem with conventional DDD or DDI pulse generators. However, DDDR or DDIR pulse generators could induce repetitive nonreentrant VA synchrony upon exercise when the sensor-driven increase in pacing rate shortens the atrial escape (pacemaker VA) interval. Conceivably, during exercise a ventricular extrasystole could precipitate repetitive nonreentrant VA synchrony with the perpetuation of retrograde VA conduction, thereby negating the potential beneficial effect of AV synchrony by producing a VVIR-like pacemaker syndrome (Figure 5).

A pacemaker can be easily designed with an algorithm to terminate repetitive nonreentrant VA synchrony by automatic prolongation of the atrial escape interval for one cycle whenever the pacemaker detects a predetermined number of P waves within the PVARP. In this respect, the automatic mode switching function of the Telectronics Meta DDDR pacemaker from the DDDR to the VVIR mode upon the detection of supraventricular tachycardia (by omission of the succeeding atrial stimulus whenever the pacemaker detects a P wave within the PVARP) could be adapted to terminate repetitive nonreentrant VA synchrony automatically [37] (Figure 6). Repetitive nonreentrant VA synchrony that starts with a ventricular extrasystole and associated retrograde VA conduction can be prevented by lengthening the atrial escape interval after a ventricular extrasystole, a feature already available in the Siemens-Pacesetter Synchrony DDDR pulse generators (Figure 7) [44].

PACEMAKER SYNDROME WITH AAIR PACING

When patients are carefully selected for AAIR pacing in the absence of drug therapy, the PR interval should shorten or at least remain constant during

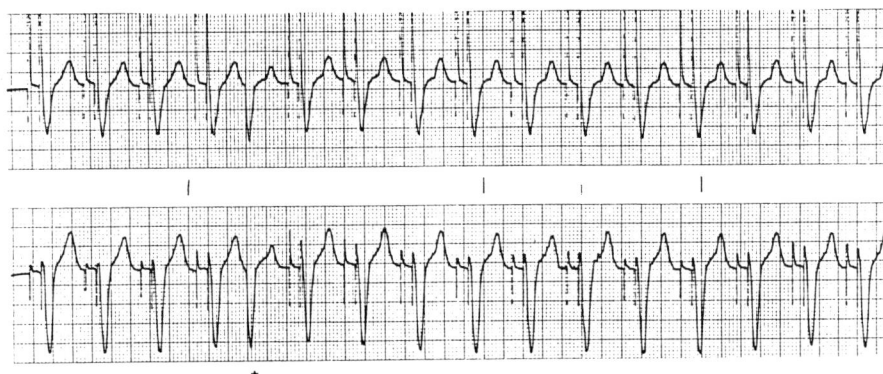

Figure 5. AV desynchronization arrhythmia initiated by ventricular extrasystole (star) during rapid AV sequential pacing by a DDD pulse generator programmed as follows: lower rate interval = 560 ms, AV delay = 100 ms. The ventricular extrasystole causes retrograde ventriculoatrial conduction so that the succeeding atrial stimulus falls in the atrial myocardial refractory period generated by retrograde atrial depolarization. The following ventricular paced beat leads to retrograde VA conduction with initiation of repetitive non-reentrant VA synchrony. The latter in this example occurs with a short AV interval because of the rapid pacing rate. A similar situation could occur during DDDR pacing. (Reproduced with permission from [40]).

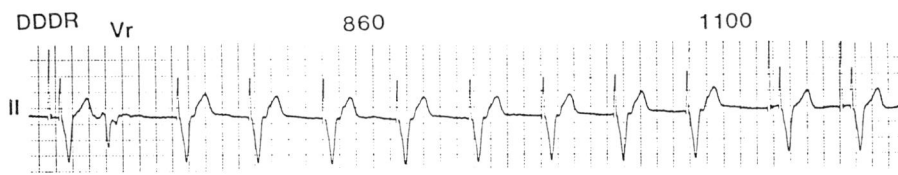

Figure 6. Behavior of Telectronics Meta DDDR pacemaker showing an eight-beat sequence with the terminal 240 ms extension of the atrial escape interval. The second beat (Vr) is a ventricular extrasystole with retrograde VA conduction. Each paced ventricular beat is associated with retrograde VA conduction. The pacemaker senses atrial depolarization within the postventricular atrial refractory period (PVARP) (beyond the initial 100 ms absolute refractory period). After the eighth beat, the atrial escape interval extends from 880 to 1120 ms (for one cycle only) that allows atrial pacing to break the retrograde VA sequence. In this way, a similar algorithm with sensing of a predetermined number of retrograde P waves (in the PVARP) during repetitive nonreentrant VA synchrony could terminate the arrhythmia automatically simply by lengthening the atrial escape interval. (Reproduced with permission from [37]).

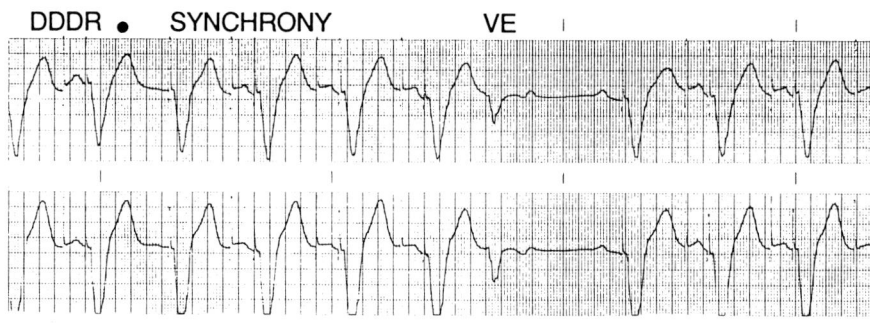

Figure 7. Response of the Pacesetter-Siemens Synchrony I DDDR pacemaker to a sensed ventricular extrasystole (VE). Two ECG leads were recorded simultaneously. The solid black circle marks sensing of a P wave beyond the postventricular atrial refractory period. The VE disengages the atrial escape interval from the sensor drive for one cycle so that the atrial escape interval lengthens to 830 ms. If the VE had caused retrograde VA conduction, the initiation of repetitive nonreentrant VA synchrony would have been prevented by the long atrial escape interval. (Reproduced with permission from [44]).

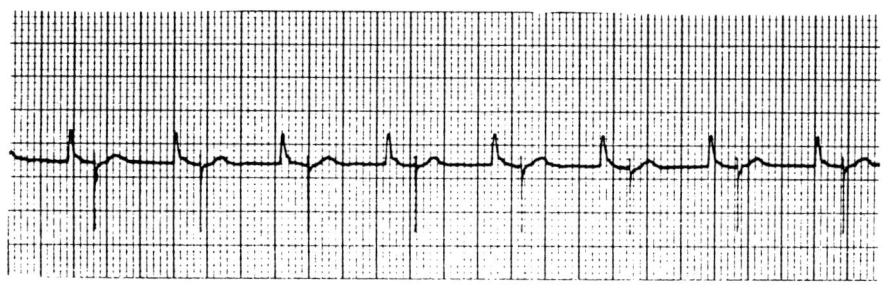

Figure 8. Electrocardiogram of a patient on beta-blocker therapy and with a DDDR pulse generator implanted for sick sinus syndrome. When the device was programmed to the AAIR mode, mild exercise caused a substantial increase of the PR interval with an unfavorable hemodynamic response consistent with the AAIR pacemaker syndrome.

exercise as the heart rate increases [45–49]. During atrial pacing, a marked delay between the pacemaker stimulus and the onset of ventricular systole can produce atrial systole against closed AV valves, a situation hemodynamically identical to VVI or VVIR pacing with retrograde VA conduction (Figure 8). This form of pacemaker syndrome is highly unlikely with the pacing rates ordinarily used in the AAI mode, but can occur in the AAIR mode when the atrial pacing rate increases [46,50,51].

Mabo et al. [46] studied the effect of exercise in 17 patients with AAIR pacemakers. The spike-R interval shortened in 6 patients, remained unchanged in 6 (2 were taking drugs), and was paradoxically prolonged in 5 patients. Three of the 5 patients in the last group were asymptomatic, but 2 complained of severe symptoms during exercise, absent before pacemaker implantation, i.e., they developed the AAIR pacemaker syndrome. Four of the 5 patients that exhibited paradoxical prolongation of the PR interval were taking drugs (beta-blockers). Possible causes of the lack of PR interval shortening in the study of Mabo et al. [46] included (1) associated organic heart disease, (2) heart transplant recipient (denervated heart), (3) drugs such as beta-blockers and Class I antiarrhythmic agents, (4) characteristics of the activity sensor. A fast activity sensor response in the AAIR mode with a sudden increase in the atrial rate disproportionate to the degree of exercise can lengthen the PR interval before the expected catecholamine surge has the opportunity to improve or shorten AV conduction. Thus, the AAIR mode poses the risk of "overstimulation" with fast pacing rates above the requirement at low-level exercise with resultant undesirable paradoxical prolongation of the PR interval. This behavior tends to correct itself as the sympathetic tone progressively increases during exercise. In this respect, elderly people do not need rates of 120–130 bpm. In most patients, a pacing rate of 90 bpm during normal walking is quite satisfactory, and an AAIR device should be programmed accordingly.

Drugs that impair AV conduction should be used cautiously in patients with AAIR pacemakers because paradoxical prolongation of the AV interval on exercise usually occurs in patients taking drugs that depress AV conduction [45,48,51]. As a rule, if the clinical situation suggests the patient will require antiarrhythmic or beta-blocker therapy at the time of pacemaker implantation, a dual chamber pacemaker should be used.

PACEMAKER SYNDROME DUE TO AUTOMATIC SWITCHING OF THE PACING MODE

Pacemaker reset from the DDDR or DDD mode to the VVI or VOO mode consequent to activation of the elective replacement indicator or as a response to interference can cause the pacemaker syndrome or even the development of congestive heart failure in susceptible patients [52]. The pacemaker syndrome can also occur at rest or upon exercise in patients with pulse generators capable of automatic switching of the pacing mode from dual chamber to VVI or VVIR as a protective mechanism against unphysiologic rapid ventricular pacing triggered by supraventricular tachyarrhythmias (Figure 9). Theoretically, during physical exertion if sinus tachycardia exceeds the programmed upper rate of a DDD pacemaker, conversion to the VVI or VVIR mode (fallback or automatic mode switching) leads to a loss of AV synchrony and a decrease in the ventricular pacing rate at a time when it is most needed. This problem may be minimized or eliminated by

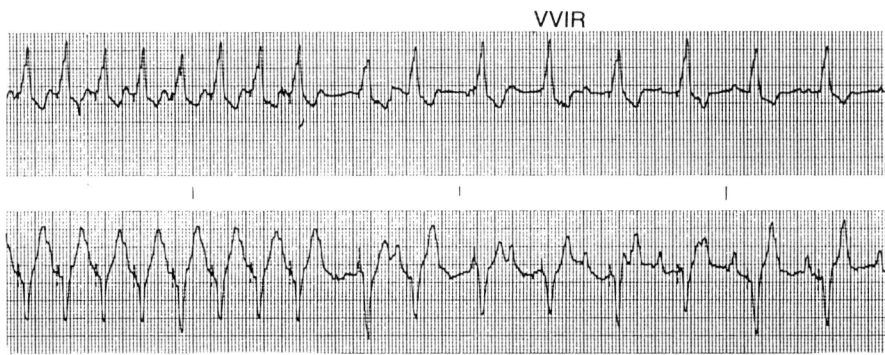

Figure 9. Response of Telectronics Meta DDDR pacemaker (minute ventilation sensor) to exercise. The programmed parameters are shown above the electrocardiogram. Two electrocardiographic leads were recorded simultaneously. When the sinus rate exceeds the programmed upper rate of the pacemaker (145/min), the pacemaker switches automatically from 1:1 AV synchrony to VVIR pacing at a considerably slower rate, a situation that can produce the pacemaker syndrome. The marked slowing of the pacing rate upon conversion to the VVIR mode can be prevented by increasing the programmed upper rate and/or adjusting the sensor response to exercise. (Reproduced with permission from [55]).

appropriate programming of the pulse generator with an upper rate above the patient's sinus node response on exercise, but below the atrial rate observed during supraventricular tachycardia.

CONCLUSION

Although atrial-based pacemakers can prevent the traditional pacemaker syndrome that occurs with single lead ventricular pacing, they can also produce it at rest and/or during exercise whenever inappropriate programming and/or selection of the pacing mode result in "inadequate timing of atrial and ventricular contractions" (Table 1) [20,53]. The pacemaker syndrome with atrial-based pacing, as with single lead ventricular pacing, is an eminently treatable complication. The pacemaker syndrome is preventable and should not occur when the appropriate device is implanted, provided it is properly programmed and functioning correctly [54].

REFERENCES

1. Ausubel K, Furman S. The pacemaker syndrome. Ann Intern Med 1985;103:402.
2. Schüller H, Brandt J. The pacemaker syndrome: Old and new causes. Clin Cardiol 1991;14:336.
3. Torresani J, Ebagosti A, Allard-Latour G et al. Pacemaker syndrome with DDD pacing. PACE 1984;7:1148.
4. Travill CM, Sutton R. Pacemaker syndrome: An iatrogenic condition. Br Heart J 1992;68:163.
5. Stierle U, Potratz J, Taubert G et al. Schrittmachersyndrom bei AV-synchronisierter Stimulation des Herzens. Dtsch Med Wochenschr 1991;116:1907.
6. Iwase M, Sotobata I, Yokota M et al. Evaluation of pulsed Doppler echocardiography of the atrial contribution to left ventricular filling in patients with DDD pacemakers. Am J Cardiol 1986;58:104.
7. Janosik DL, Pearson AC, Buckingham TA et al. The hemodynamic benefit of differential atrioventricular delay intervals for sensed and paced atrial events during physiologic pacing. J Am Coll Cardiol 1989;14:499.
8. Pearson AC, Janosik DL, Redd RM et al. Hemodynamic benefit of atrioventricular synchrony: Prediction from baseline Doppler echocardiographic variables. J Am Coll Cardiol 1989;13:1613.
9. Ronaszeki A, Ector H, Denef B et al. Effect of short atrioventricular delay on cardiac output. PACE 1990;13:1728.
10. Haskell RJ, French WJ. Optimum AV interval in dual chamber pacemakers. PACE 1986;9:670.
11. Lascault G, Bigonzi F, Abergel E et al. Non-invasive study of dual chamber pacing by pulsed Doppler. Prediction of the haemodynamic response by echocardiographic measurements. Eur Heart J 1989;10:525.
12. Rockey R, Quinones MA, Zoghbi WA et al. Influence on left atrial systolic emptying on left ventricular early filling dynamics by Doppler in patients with sequential atrioventricular pacemakers. Am J Cardiol 1988;62:968.
13. Wish M, Fletcher RD, Gottdiener JS et al. Importance of left atrial timing in the programming of dual-chamber pacemakers. Am J Cardiol 1987;60:566.
14. Alt EU, Von Bibra H, Blömer H. Different beneficial AV intervals with DDD pacing after sensed and paced atrial events. J Electrophysiol 1987;1:250.
15. Grant SCD, Bennett DH. Atrial latency in a dual chambered pacing system causing inappropriate sequence of cardiac chamber activation. PACE 1992;15:116.
16. Wish M, Gottdiener JS, Cohen AI et al. M-mode echocardiograms for determination of optimal left atrial timing in patients with dual chamber pacemakers. J Am Coll Cardiol 1988;11:317.
17. Wish M, Fletcher RD, Cohen A. Hemodynamics of AV synchrony and rate. J Electrophysiol 1989;3:170.
18. Chirife R, Ortega DF, Salazer AI. Nonphysiologic left heart AV intervals as a result of DDD and AAI "physiological" pacing. PACE 1991;14:1752.
19. Stierle U. Schmücker G, Potratz J et al. Interatrial conduction in AV-sequential pacing (abstract). Eur Heart J 1991;12(Suppl):304.
20. Sutton R. The atrioventricular interval—What considerations influence its programming? Eur J Cardiac Pacing Electophysiol 1992;2:169.
21. Daubert C, Ritter P, Mabo P et al. AV delay optimization in DDD and DDDR pacing. In: Barold SS, Mugica J, editors. New perspectives in cardiac pacing, 3. Mount Kisco, NY: Futura, 1993:259.
22. Daubert C, Berder V, DePlace C et al. Hemodynamic benefits of permanent atrial resynchronization in patients with advanced interatrial blocks paced in the DDD mode. PACE 1991;14:650.

23. Daubert C, Berder V, Mabo P et al. Arrhythmia prevention by permanent atrial resynchronization in advanced interatrial blocks. Circulation 1990;82(Suppl III):181.
24. Daubert C, Mabo P, Berder V et al. Simultaneous dual atrial pacing in high degree interatrial block: Hemodynamic results. Circulation 1991;84:II-453.
25. Daubert C, Mabo P, Berder V et al. Permanent dual atrium pacing in major interatrial conduction blocks: A four years experience. PACE 1993;16 (Part II):885.
26. Levine PA, Seltzer JP, Pirzada FA. The "pacemaker syndrome" in a properly functioning physiologic pacing system. PACE 1983;6:279.
27. Antonioli CE, Ansani L, Barbieri D et al. Italian multicenter study on a single lead VDD pacing system using a narrow atrial dipole spacing. PACE 1992;15:1890.
28. Crick JCP. European multicenter prospective follow-up study of 1002 implants of a single lead VDD pacing system. PACE 1991;14:1742.
29. Sutton R. The second coming of VDD. Eur J Cardiac Pacing Electrophysiol 1992;4:225.
30. Lau CP, Tai YT, Leung SK et al. Improved aerobic capacity with single lead atrial synchronous pacing with a rate adaptive sensor. J Am Coll Cardiol 1993;21:383A.
31. Barold SS. The DDI mode of cardiac pacing. PACE 1987;9:480.
32. Barold SS, Falkoff MD, Ong LS et al. All dual chamber pacemakers function in the DDD mode. Am Heart J 1988;115:1353.
33. Sutton R, Ingram A, Kenny RA et al. Clinical experience of DDI pacing. In: Belhassen S, Feldman S, Cooperman Y, editors. Cardiac Pacing and Electrophysiology. Proceedings of the VIIIth World Symposium on Cardiac Pacing and Electrophysiology, Jerusalem. R&L Creative Communications. 1987:161.
34. Vanerio G, Maloney JD, Pinski SL et al. DDIR versus VVIR pacing in patients with paroxysmal atrial tachyarrhythmias. PACE 1991;14:1630.
35. Cunningham TM. Pacemaker syndrome due to retrograde conduction in a DDI pacemaker. Am Heart J 1988;115:478.
36. Sulke N, Dritsas A, Bostock J et al. "Subclinical" pacemaker syndrome: A randomized study of symptom free patients with ventricular demand (VVI) pacemakers upgraded to dual chamber devices. Br Heart J 1992;67:57.
37. Barold SS, Mond HG. Optimal antibradycardia pacing in patients with paroxysmal supraventricular tachyarrhythmias: Role of fallback and automatic mode switching mechanisms. In: Barold SS, Mugica J, editors. New Perspectives in Cardiac Pacing, 3. Mount Kisco, NY: Futura 1993:483.
38. Barold SS. Repetitive reentrant and non-reentrant ventriculoatrial synchrony in dual chamber pacing. Clin Cardiol 1991;14:754.
39. Barold SS, Falkoff MD, Ong LS et al. AV desynchronization arrhythmia during DDD pacing. In: Belhassen B, Feldman S, Cooperman Y, editors. Cardiac Pacing and Electrophsiology. Proceedings of the VIIIth World Symposium on Cardiac Pacing and Electrophysiology, Jerusalem. R&L Creative enterprises, 1987:177.
40. Barold SS. Repetitive non-reentrant ventriculoatrial synchrony in dual chamber pacing. In: Santini M, Pistolese M, Alliegro A, editors. Progress in Clinical Pacing. Amsterdam: Excerpta Medica, 1990:451.
41. Calkins H, El-Atassi R, Kalbfleisch S et al. Effects of an acute increase in atrial pressure on atrial refractoriness in humans. PACE 1992;15:1674.
42. Katsumoto K, Nijbori T, Watanabe Y. Rate-dependent threshold changes during atrial pacing. Clinical and experimental studies. PACE 1990;13:1009.
43. Chien WW, Foster E, Phillips B et al. Pacemaker syndrome in a patient with DDD pacemaker for long QT syndrome. PACE 1991;14:1209.
44. Barold SS. Electrocardiography of rate-adaptive dual-chamber (DDDR) pacemakers: Lower rate behavior. In: Alt E, Barold SS, Stangl K, editors. Rate Adaptive Cardiac Pacing. Berlin: Springer-Verlag, 1993:173.
45. Brandt J, Fahraeus T, Ogawa T et al. Practical aspects of rate-adaptive atrial (AAIR) pacing. Clinical experiences in 44 patients. PACE 1991;14:1258.
46. Mabo P, Pouillot C, Kermarrec A et al. Lack of physiological adaptation of the atrioventric-

ular interval to heart rate in patients chronically paced in the AAIR mode. PACE 1991;14:2133.
47. Ruiter J, Burgersdijk C, Zeeders M et al. Atrial Activitrax pacing. The atrioventricular interval during exercise. PACE 1987;10:1226.
48. Edelstam C, Nordlander R, Wallgren E et al. AAIR pacing and exercise. What happens to AV conduction? PACE 1990;13:1193.
49. Haywood GA, Katrisis D, Ward J et al. Atrial adaptive rate pacing in sick sinus syndrome. Effects on exercise capacity and arrhythmias. Br Heart J 1993;69:174.
50. Clarke M, Allen A. Rate responsive atrial pacing resulting in pacemaker syndrome. PACE 1987;10:1209.
51. den Dulk K, Lindemans FW, Brugada P et al. Pacemaker syndrome with AAI rate variable pacing. Importance of atrioventricular conduction properties, medication and pacemaker programmability. PACE 1988;11:1226.
52. Sanders R, Barold SS. Understanding elective replacement indicators and automatic parameter conversion mechanism in DDD pacemakers. In: Barold SS, Mugica J, editors. New Perspectives in Cardiac Pacing. Mount Kisco, NY: Futura, 1988:203.
53. Stierle U, Schmücker G, Potratz J et al. Pacemaker syndrome in dual chamber pacing. Cardiostimolazione 1992;10:300.
54. Sermasi S, Marzaloni M, Marconi M. Is the "pacemaker syndrome" a rare and negligible complication of VVI pacing? In: Santini M, Pistolese M, Alliegro A. Progress in Clinical Pacing. Amsterdam: Excerpta Medica, 1990:190.
55. Barold SS et al. Cardiac pacing update: Guidelines in choosing pacemakers and optimal pacing modes. In: Zipes DP, Rowlands DJ, editors. Progress in Cardiology. Philadelphia: Lea & Febiger, 1992:171.

25. Dual chamber pacemaker therapy in cardiomyopathy

S. SERGE BAROLD, LUKAS KAPPENBERGER,
CLAUDE DAUBERT & GUY FONTAINE

INTRODUCTION

Over the last few years, new and interesting indications for permanent pacing have emerged for the treatment of hypertrophic cardiomyopathy (obstructive and non-obstructive) and end-stage dilated cardiomyopathy. Even in patients without conduction system disease, symptomatic improvement can be achieved by DDD pacing with an appropriate AV interval and rate. In this chapter, we shall discuss the background and clinical results of this new therapy.

PACING IN HYPERTROPHIC CARDIOMYOPATHY

Based on the pioneering work of several centers [1–5], a number of recent studies have shown that dual chamber pacing can be effective therapy for symptomatic relief in patients with obstructive hypertrophic cardiomyopathy (HCM) [5–12]. Right ventricular apical pacing can often reduce the left ventricular outflow tract (LVOT) gradient in HCM partly due to paradoxical movement of the interventricular septum. A reduction in the LVOT gradient by ventricular pacing alone, however, is associated with a drop in the systolic pressure, cardiac output, and stroke volume. Less commonly, ventricular pacing can increase the left ventricular outflow tract gradient [13, 14]. Patients with HCM are critically dependent on AV synchrony because diastolic left ventricular dysfunction results in decreased ventricular filling and increased left atrial and pulmonary capillary wedge pressures (PCWP).

Acute hemodynamic studies have shown that most patients develop a significant drop in the LVOT gradient with DDD pacing with an optimal (short) AV delay [7–9, 12]. Drug-refractory patients with no demonstrable hemodynamic benefit by pacing and those with important mitral incompetence should probably be treated surgically. In most patients with obstructive HCM, DDD pacing with a short AV interval (50–150 ms and often less than 100 ms) reduces symptoms (angina, dyspnea, pre-syncope, and syncope) adequately and on a long-term basis as shown by Jeanrenaud et al. [8] and improves exercise capacity according to McDonald and Maurer [10]. In most patients, the LVOT gradient diminishes by approximately 50% during DDD pacing without significant alteration in the blood pressure or cardiac output. Elderly patients with obstructive HCM also benefit from DDD pacing [15].

Fananapazir et al. [7] recently reported the benefit of dual chamber pacing in 44 patients with HCM who had failed treatment with verapamil and large doses of beta-blocker agents. Five patients had undergone previous unsuccessful surgery. Twenty-one patients received a Siemens-Pacesetter DDDR Synchrony pacemaker with an AV interval programmed at 125 ms with a rate-adaptive shortening of the AV interval, and 23 patients received a Medtronic Synergyst II DDDR pacemaker (programmed with an AV interval of 125 ms in 11 patients, 100 ms in 7, and 75 ms in 5). All pulse generators were programmed to the DDD mode. The AV intervals were the longest that allowed maximal pre-excitation (widest paced QRS duration). The patients received no drugs after pacemaker implantation.

The patients in the study of Fananapazir et al. [7] were evaluated at follow-up visits 1.5 months (first 24 patients) and 3 months (the remaining 20 patients) after pacemaker implantation. The frequency and severity of effort-induced dyspnea, orthopnea, paroxysmal nocturnal dyspnea, chest discomfort, palpitations, and pre-syncope were all significantly reduced. DDD pacing also appeared to prevent syncope in 15 patients who had previously had a history of effort or postural syncope with a frequency of more than one episode per month (one patient had more than one episode per week) [6]. During a mean follow-up period of 9 months (maximum of 13 months), only one of the 15 patients had further syncope.

The mean New York Heart Association (NYHA) functional status decreased from 3.4 ± 0.5 to 1.7 ± 0.7 ($p < 0.0001$). This correlates with the long-term data reported in 13 patients in the Swiss group [8]. Treadmill exercise durations were significantly greater than those achieved in sinus rhythm before pacing. Patients were evaluated in detail with echocardiography in normal sinus rhythm during the baseline study before pacemaker implantation, at the follow-up visits during DDD pacing, and when the pacemaker was switched off so that the patient was returned to normal sinus rhythm with spontaneous AV conduction. Indices of LVOT obstruction (severity of systolic anterior motion of the mitral valve and Doppler LVOT velocities) were significantly reduced during DDD pacing compared with those recorded during normal sinus rhythm both during the baseline study and at follow-up when the DDD pacemaker was switched off. The baseline LVOT gradient (echo) in normal sinus rhythm was 64 ± 7 mmHg. At the time of follow-up in the DDD mode, the LVOT (echo) gradient was 27 ± 5 mmHg ($p < 0.0001$ compared with baseline study), and in normal sinus rhythm when the pacemaker was switched off, the LVOT gradient (echo) was 43 ± 7 mmHg ($p < 0.01$ compared with baseline study).

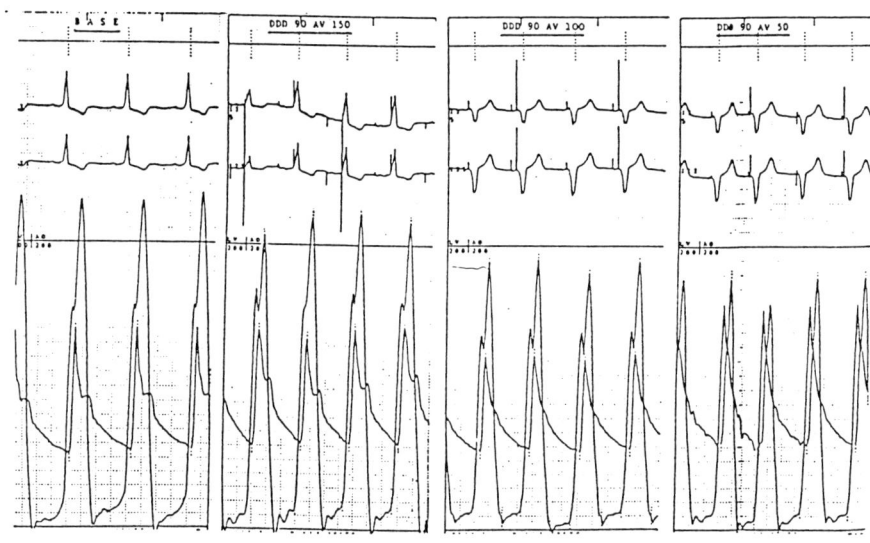

Figure 1. ECG leads II and III with simultaneous recording of left ventricular and aortic pressure in the control state on the left, and during DDD pacing with various AV delays as indicated. Note the reduction of the systolic gradient and the stability of the aortic pressure (LV and AO 200 = 200 mmHg scale).

Apparently, when the DDD pulse generator was temporally switched off at the follow-up visits, measurements in normal sinus rhythm revealed significantly lower pulmonary arterial pressure and LVOT gradient (decreased to about 50 mmHg) compared with the data obtained during sinus rhythm in the baseline study before pacemaker implantation [7]. The mechanism for these observations is unknown, but they may be related to changes secondary to altered depolarization and reduced diastolic pressures.

Jeanrenaud et al. [8] reported virtually the same observations in an earlier acute and long-term hemodynamic and echocardiographic study in patients with HCM refractory to drugs. Acute hemodynamic effects were studied in 13 patients. During DDD pacing at a rate of 90 per minute with varying AV intervals, there was a significant drop in the LVOT gradient compared with the measurements taken during AAI pacing at the same rate. An example of acute hemodynamic measurements is shown in Figure 1. Only patients with severe mitral valve incompetence showed no change and subsequently underwent surgical therapy. The reduction in the LVOT pressure gradient with pacing was shown to depend greatly on the programmed AV delay. The gradient dropped progressively from 82 ± 41 mmHg during AAI pacing at 90/min to 61 ± 37 mmHg during DDD pacing with AV interval 50 ms ($p < 0.002$), then to 52 ± 35 mmHg DDD pacing with an AV interval of

100 ms ($p < 0.0002$), and rose slightly to 62 ± 46 mmHg during DDD pacing with an AV interval of 150 ms ($p < 0.01$). At the optimum AV interval, the LVOT fell by 43% from 82 ± 41 mmHg during AAI pacing at a rate of 90/min to 47 ± 34 mmHg during DDD pacing at the same rate ($p < 0.002$). In this study 8 patients who were still being treated with verapamil and beta-blockers received a permanent pacemaker programmed to the individually optimized AV interval of 50–90 ms. The mean AV interval was 63 ± 18 ms. Observations were made at mid-term (11 ± 10 months) and long-term (after 44 ± 11 months) follow-up. In all 8 patients there was a striking symptomatic improvement, particularly with angina. Dyspnea also improved, and the 2 patients who had suffered previous syncope reported no further episodes after pacemaker implantation. At the mid-term assessment, the LVOT gradient at rest during DDD pacing was 40 ± 31 mmHg, rising to 65 ± 34 mmHg when the pacemaker was switched off. These values were similar to those obtained during the baseline acute hemodynamic study. In contrast, Fananapazir et al. [7] observed a reduction of the LVOT gradient during normal sinus rhythm when the DDD pacemaker was switched off only 6 weeks after implantation [7]. However, with long-term follow-up (reached by 7 patients) [8], the resting LVOT gradient dropped to 17 ± 10 mmHg and was at that time significantly lower than at the mid-term follow-up. When the pacemaker was switched off, the LVOT gradient rose only to 31 ± 36 mmHg, a significantly lower value than at the start of the study or at the mid-term follow-up [8]. In a few cases, however, when pacing was switched off for several hours, a gradual reappearance of an outflow tract obstruction was reported by Aliot [16].

Considerations concerning the use of pacemakers in hypertrophic cardiomyopathy

At present, patients with HCM resistant to standard therapy or those not suitable for surgery should be considered for permanent pacing. The implantation of a dual chamber pacemaker is relatively simple and seems to offer the same benefits as surgery with less cost and fewer risks. Indeed, permanent pacing may soon become first-line therapy for HCM. Often, patients can discontinue drug therapy because pacing alone may produce striking clinical improvement [7]. Most patients improve clinically to a degree comparable to that achieved with myomectomy and the favorable response to pacing is closely tied to optimization of the AV interval. The individual benefit of AV sequential pacing should be determined with a temporary pacing system before considering a permanent pacemaker. A small number of patients in most series demonstrated no hemodynamic improvement with temporary pacing, and they should probably not receive a permanent pacemaker. A noninvasive approach is needed to identify patients unsuitable for pacing. It is emerging from ongoing studies that patients with severe mitral regurgitation do not improve with pacing. Dual chamber pacemakers must be programmed with a short AV interval to avoid spontaneous ventricular depolarization and to ensure ventricular capture at all times to provide apical pre-excitation. The AV delay initiated by atrial sensing should be shorter than the one initiated by pacing and programmable to a large number of values in the 50–150 ms range. The AV delay should be optimized at rest (and at several faster rates) and with effort. On the other hand, the atrial contribution to ventricular filling remains essential, especially in the non-compliant hypertrophic left ventricle, and too short AV intervals may be deleterious. AV ablation or drugs may be useful to achieve the optimal AV interval associated with pacemaker-controlled ventricular depolarization. An autoadaptive AV interval that shortens automatically with an acceleration of sinus node frequency might be another important feature to ensure ventricular depolarization by the pacemaker during exercise [17, 18]. All patients must undergo a treadmill stress test to determine the optimal AV delay on exercise and whether they can maintain a paced ventricular rhythm at all times. Atrial sensing is extremely important, and meticulous care must be taken at the time of implantation to ensure a good atrial signal. Atrial sensing should also be evaluated during exercise. The maximal rate of the pacemaker should be programmed above the maximal sinus rate of the patient, and this may require a short postventricular atrial refractory period. Brinker [19] pointed out that the hypertrophied ventricle is susceptible to ischemia even in the absence of coronary artery disease. Too high a pacing rate (greater than 130) may result in subendocardial ischemia in patients with outflow tract obstruction [20]. Brinker [19] advocates establishing an upper rate limit that avoids ischemia. Perhaps a thallium stress test might be useful in that regard.

Unresolved questions about the benefit of pacing

The use of pacing in HCM has raised a number of questions. (1) How long will it take for the original condition of LVOT gradient to return after discontinuation pacing? (2) Do the patients continue to benefit in the long term with DDD pacing? (3) Can the acute hemodynamic response during pacing studies predict which patients will benefit the most from DDD pacing? (4) Does pacing cause permanent improvement due to structural changes in the ventricular myocardium? (5) Is the combination of pacing with drugs better than pacing alone? (6) Should patients be studied with temporary pacing while taking their drug therapy or when they are not?

Possible mechanism of beneficial effect

The effect of DDD pacing is optimal only when right ventricular apical stimulation is synchronized to atrial systole, producing optimal filling and activation of the LV apex before septal contraction, a mechanism called apical pre-excitation. The beneficial response may be related to paradoxical motion of the ventricular septum, i.e. moving the septum away from the posterior LV wall in systole, resulting in widening of the LVOT. This mechanism results in reduction of the LVOT gradient associated with an increase in LV filling and eventually reduced contractility due to pacing. At the same time, diastolic function improves, and LV filling tends to normalize [21, 22]. A significant reduction in LVOT velocity is also associated with a diminution of systolic anterior movement of the mitral valve. However, the reduction in the LVOT gradient persists in sinus rhythm after the cessation of pacing [7, 8]. Thus, a reduction in the LVOT gradient is not solely due to the mechanical effect of pacemaker-induced ventricular pre-excitation. We might hypothesize that a reduction of the LVOT gradient reduces one of the stimuli responsible for ventricular hypertrophy.

Jeanrenaud et al. [8] showed with biplane ventriculography that ventricular stimulation had a favorable effect on the left ventricular contraction sequence, with abolition of the early systolic obstruction and emptying of the apical portion of the LV before septal contraction. The question arises as to whether there is a correlation between complete or partial left bundle branch block (LBBB) after successful surgery for HCM and the altered ventricular activation sequence from right ventricular pacing which causes a similar pattern of septal depolarization and contraction. In this respect, McAreavey et al. [23] studied 15 patients with obstructive HCM and preexistent LBBB who received DDD devices for the relief of LVOT obstruction. All patients had drug-refractory symptoms. At follow-up after 3.5 ± 0.7 months of pacing, the NYHA class improved from 3.0 ± 0.4 at baseline to 1.6 ± 0.6 following chronic DDD pacing (LVOT baseline = 95 ± 38, follow-up 26 ± 25 during DDD pacing, and 44 ± 22 mmHg in sinus rhythm). Thus, preexisting LBBB does not preclude receiving benefit from DDD pacing. Choi et al. [24] evaluated HCM patients during exercise and found that there was no change in the ejection fraction 1 month before pacemaker implantation compared to the situation during DDD pacing with the pacemaker turned on or off, allowing the patient to function in normal sinus rhythm. However, with DDD pacing there was a statistically significant increase in end-diastolic volume (determined by radionuclide angiography). The symptomatic improvement of patients with obstructive HCM with DDD pacing may in part be due to an increase in end-diastolic volume (thereby decreasing the LVOT gradient) rather than a change in the ejection fraction. Electrocardiographic changes involving the spontaneous QRS complex can occur after a period of DDD pacing, but their significance is unknown, and they do not correlate with changes in the LVOT gradient [25].

NONOBSTRUCTIVE HYPERTROPHIC CARDIOMYOPATHY

Recent work from the NIH [26] in patients with *nonobstructive* hypertrophic cardiomyopathy demonstrated that DDD pacing improved symptoms, functional status, and treadmill exercise duration and lowered the PCWP significantly (33 ± 9 to 27 ± 9 mmHg) with exercise. Thallium scintigraphic evidence of myocardial ischemia during matched levels of exercise was improved or eliminated in four of five patients [25]. At rest and during exercise, the LV ejection fractions were unchanged by chronic DDD pacing. Seidelin et al. [27] also reported the beneficial effect of DDD pacing with a short AV interval in a patient with HCM and no LVOT obstruction. The improvement may be related to an as yet undefined influence on contractility with a resultant improved myocardial diastolic function without LVOT obstruction. Seidelin et al. [27] recommended that a trial of pacing in HCM patients should be performed. McDonald et al. [5] reported a single patient who benefitted from DDD pacing despite the absence of a resting outflow gradient (no physiologic maneuvers were performed to determine whether a provokable gradient was present in this case). The improvement of patients without an LVOT gradient at rest may be due to a reduction of an intermittent undetected LVOT gradient during exercise in the same way as myomectomy or mitral valve replacement benefits patients with a provokable LVOT gradient but none at rest.

PACING IN DILATED CARDIOMYOPATHY

Hochleitner et al. [28] in 1990 reported the beneficial effects of DDD pacing (short AV interval of 100 ms) in the treatment of end-stage idiopathic dilated cardiomyopathy in 16 patients without AV block in whom conventional drug therapy had failed. There was a striking improvement in the symptoms such as dyspnea at rest and pulmonary edema, as well as a significant decrease in the NYHA functional class. Furthermore, DDD pacing actually increased the LV ejection fraction, reduced the left atrial and right atrial sizes, and reduced the cardiothoracic ratio. The short AV interval appeared to reduce mitral regurgitation and improve LV filling [28, 29]. Kataoka [30] described a similar observation of improvement in LV function with the use of an implanted DDD pulse generator and a short AV interval in a patient with first-degree AV block and end-stage dilated cardiomyopathy.

Mechanisms of beneficial effect

Hochleitner et al. [31] postulated that in a dilated heart, prolonged depolarization may create an unfavorable relationship between the atrial and ventricular systole. Pacing may be beneficial by pre-excitation of the apical area to overcome the exaggerated delay in apical activation caused by the massive dilatation of the LV (the latter results in an abnormal coordination of wall motion and increased wall stress in the apical area).

Brecker et al. [32] studied the acute effect of DDD pacing with a short AV interval on ventricular filling time and exercise capacity in 12 patients with dilated cardiomyopathy (3 with ischemic etiology). The duration of both mitral and tricuspid regurgitation was shorter with short AV intervals, and both LV and right ventricular filling times were longer. Short AV delays were associated with greater cardiac output at rest and striking improvement in exercise duration. Brecker et al. [32] also observed that DDD pacing with a short AV interval eliminated presystolic mitral regurgitation (known to occur in patients with complete or first-degree AV block and in patients with severe ventricular disease even when the PR interval is normal) and found that patients with a long QRS duration (≥ 0.12 s) and those with narrow QRS complexes all improved with adapted short AV delay pacing, thereby questioning the role of pacing-induced QRS prolongation as the mechanism of the hemodynamic benefit [33].

Long-term efficacy of DDD pacing

Hochleitner et al. [34] recently reported the long-term efficacy of physiologic dual chamber (DDD) pacing in the treatment of end-stage idiopathic dilated cardiomyopathy as evaluated in a longitudinal study of up to 5 years in 17 patients. The considerable clinical improvement achieved after implantation of a pacemaker programmed for DDD pacing at an AV delay of 100 ms, was maintained throughout the follow-up period or until death and was associated with a consistent decrease in NYHA class and an increase in LV ejection fraction. The cardiothoracic ratio, resting heart rate, and echocardiographic dimensions progressively decreased, and the systolic and diastolic blood pressure increased, excluding the 4 patients who received a heart transplant. The median survival time from pacemaker implantation was 22 months. Three patients refused cardiac transplantation owing to the dramatic clinical improvement in response to DDD pacing. Nine succumbed to undefined sudden death or after a thromboembolic event, and one died from carcinoma. No patient required rehospitalization owing to worsening heart failure after pacemaker implantation. Three patients were evaluated after the interruption of pacing for 2-4 h by programming the pacemaker to the OOO mode. Within the first 2 weeks after pacemaker implantation and, to a lesser extent, after 6 and 12 months; the cardiac function decreased with withdrawal of the

DDD function of the pacemaker. The LV ejection fraction upon acute interruption of DDD pacing decreased during the follow-up from $32 \pm 3\%$ to $18 \pm 3\%$ and from $30 \pm 4\%$ to $23 \pm 5\%$, 2 weeks and 1 year, respectively, after the commencement of DDD pacing ($n = 9$), whereas after 5 years the response to DDD pacing withdrawal was not significant ($40 \pm 2\%$ to $39 \pm 2\%$; $n = 3$). However, the decrease in diastolic blood pressure and the increase in heart rate in response to the change of DDD to OOO mode persisted throughout the observation period. The left atrium still reacted 6 months after pacemaker implantation to the withdrawal of DDD pacing with a significant increase in size (41 ± 2 to 44 ± 2 mm; $p < 0.001$; $n = 9$). All other echocardiographic parameters remained unchanged. Two years after beginning DDD pacing, the dimensions of the left atrium and LV during systole still increased (41 ± 4 to 43 ± 4 mm, and 56 ± 5 to 57 ± 5 mm, respectively; $p < 0.005$; $n = 5$), whereas after 5 years of DDD pacing, the interruption of pacing did not change the echocardiographic dimensions. The considerable deterioration in cardiac function after the short-term removal of DDD pacing in the early stages eventually disappeared. This observation suggests that DDD pacing also has a beneficial impact on the damaged myocardium.

CONCLUSION

The effective treatment of obstructive hypertrophic cardiomyopathy (with or without a LVOT gradient) and dilated cardiomyopathy with DDD pacemakers has ushered in a new set of indications for pacing in the absence of conduction system disease. Pacing for these conditions is still in its infancy, but preliminary results suggest that it might play an important role in the future. It is puzzling that DDD pacing is equally effective in two dissimilar cardiomyopathies with completely different conventional medical and surgical treatments and etiologies. The beneficial effect of pacing persists temporarily upon the cessation of pacing in patients with HCM as well as dilated cardiomyopathy. One might hypothesize that this benefit results from as yet unknown effects of altered myocardial function with electrical stimulation. In hypertrophic cardiomyopathy, hypercontractility is the problem. The different spread of depolarization with pacing might, together with other factors, be a clue to explain the reduction of contractility and obstruction. In contrast to HCM in dilated cardiomyopathy, electric activation appears superior to spontaneous activation because contractility seems to be improved. If there is a real improvement in contractility, the impact of electric stimulation of the heart in patients without conduction system disease might be enormous.

ACKNOWLEDGEMENTS

The authors thank Sharon Sampson (Oklahoma) and Geneviève Werlen (Lausanne) for their generous assistance in the preparation of this manuscript.

REFERENCES

1. Duck HJ, Hutschenreiter W, Pankau H et al. Vorhofsynchrone ventrikelstimulation mit verkurtzter AV Verzogerungszeit als Therapieprinzip der hypertrophen obstruktiven Kardiomyopathie. Z Gesamte Inn Med 1984;39:437.
2. Duport G, Valeix B, Lefevre J et al. Intérêt de la stimulation ventriculaire droite permanente dans la cardiomyopathie obstructive. Nouv Presse Med 1978;32:2868.
3. Gardiner P, Gold RG, Williams DO. Beneficial effects of acute and chronic atrially triggered ventricular pacing in hypertrophic cardiomyopathy. PACE 1983;6:A38.
4. Hassenstein P, Storch H, Schmitz W. Erfahrungen mit der Schrittmacher dauer Behandlung bei Patienten mit obstruktiver Kardiomyopathie. Thoraxchirurgie 1975;23:496.
5. McDonald K, McWilliams E, O'Keefe B et al. Functional assessment of patients treated with permanent dual chamber pacing as a primary treatment for hypertrophic cardiomyopathy. Eur Heart J 1988;9:893.
6. Fananapazir L, Cannon RO III, Tripoli D. Ability of dual chamber pacing to relieve syncope and presyncope associated with left ventricular outflow tract obstruction in patients with hypertrophic cardiomyopathy. J. Am Coll Cardiol 1992;19:224A.
7. Fananapazir L, Cannon RO III, Tripoli D et al. Impact of dual-chamber permanent pacing in patients with obstructive hypertrophic cardiomyopathy with symptoms refractory to Verapamil and B-adrenergic blocker therapy. Circulation 1992;85:2149.
8. Jeanrenaud X, Goy JJ, Kappenberger L. Effects of dual-chamber pacing in hypertrophic obstructive cardiomyopathy. Lancet 1992;339:1318.
9. Sadoul N, Simon JP, Beurrier D et al. Stimulation double chambre et cardiomyopathies hypertrophiques avec obstruction ventriculaire gauche: intérêts et limites. Stimucoeur 1992;20:141.
10. McDonald KM, Maurer B. Permanent pacing as treatment for hypertrophic cardiomyopathy. Am J Cardiol 1991;68:108.
11. Gras D, Guillo P, Mabo P et al. Primary treatment of hypertrophic obstructive cardiomyopathy by permanent DDD pacing with complete ventricular capture. PACE 1992;15:574.
12. Richter T, Cserhalmi M, Lengyel M et al. Changes in left ventricular hemodynamics of hypertrophic obstructive cardiomyopathy (HOCM) patients treated with VAT pacing. In: Baroldi G, Camerini F, Goodwin JF, editors. Advances in Cardiomyopathies. New York: Springer-Verlag, 1990:168.
13. Gambhir DS, Arora R, Khalilullah M. Beneficial effects of dual chamber pacing on hemodynamics of hypertrophic obstructive cardiomyopathy. PACE 1992;15:546.
14. Gross J, Cooper J, Keltz T et al. Profound 'pacemaker syndrome' in hypertrophic cardiomyopathy. PACE 1991;14:698.
15. McAreavey D, Fananapazir L. Ventricular pre-excitation is highly effective for elderly patients with obstructive hypertrophic cardiomyopathy and symptoms refractory to medication. J Am Coll Cardiol 1993;21:354A.
16. Aliot E. European Cardiac Society Annual Meeting, Barcelona 1992, personal communication.
17. Daubert C, Ritter P, Mabo P et al. AV delay optimization in DDD and DDDR pacing. In: Barold SS, Mugica J, editors. New Perspectives in Cardiac Pacing. 3, Mount Kisco, NY: Futura 1993:259.

18. Ritter P, Vai F, Bonnet JL et al. Rate adaptive atrio-ventricular delay improves cardiopulmonary performance in patients implanted with a dual chamber pacemaker for complete heart block. Eur J Cardiac Pacing Electrophysiol 1991;1:31.
19. Brinker JA. Permanent pacemakers: Optimal choices for specific clinical scenarios. Intelligence Reports in Cardiac Pacing and Electrophysiology 1992;II:1.
20. Cannon RO III, Schenke WH, Maron BJ et al. Differences in coronary flow and myocardial metabolism at rest and during pacing between patients with obstructive and patients with non-obstructive hypertrophic cardiomyopathy. J Am Coll Cardiol 1987;10:53.
21. Erwin J, McWilliams E, Gearty G et al. Hemodynamic assessment of dual chamber pacing in hypertrophic cardiomyopathy using radionuclide angiography. Br Heart J. 1986;55:507.
22. McDonald K, O'Sullivan JJ, King C et al. Dual chamber pacing improves left ventricular filling in patients with hypertrophic cardiomyopathy. Eur Heart J 1989;10 (Suppl): 401.
23. McAreavey D, Tripoli D, Epstein N et al. Dual chamber pacing relieves outflow tract obstruction in hypertrophic cardiomyopathy despite pre-existing left bundle branch block. J Am Coll Cardiol 1993;21:123A.
24. Choi BW, Tripoldi D, Fananapazir L. Exercise induced and diastolic volume changes in obstructive hypertrophic cardiomyopathy with dual chamber pacing. J Am Coll Cardiol 1992;19:306A.
25. McAreavey D, Fananapazir L. Altered cardiac hemodynamic and electrical state in normal sinus rhythm after chronic dual-chamber pacing for relief of left ventricular outflow obstruction in hypertrophic cardiomyopathy. Am J. Cardiol 1992;70:651–6.
26. Cannon RO III, Dilsiziam V, Bonow RO et al. Symptom, hemodynamic, and myocardial benefit of atrial synchronized ventricular pacing in non-obstructive hypertrophic cardiomyopathy. J Am Coll Cardiol 1992;19:120A.
27. Seidelin PH, Jones GA, Boon NA. Effects of dual-chamber pacing in hypertrophic cardiomyopathy without obstruction. Lancet 1992;340:369.
28. Hochleitner M, Hörtnagl H, Ng CK et al. Usefulness of physiologic dual chamber pacing in drug-resistant idiopathic dilated cardiomyopathy. Am J Cardiol 1990;66:198.
29. Iskandrian A. Pacemaker therapy in congestive heart failure. Am J Cardiol 1990;66:223.
30. Kataoka H. Hemodynamic effect of physiological dual chamber pacing in a patient with end-stage dilated cardiomyopathy: A case report. PACE 1991;14:1330.
31. Hochleitner M, Hörtnagl H, Hörtnagel H et al. Letter to the editor. Lancet 1992;340:369.
32. Brecker SJD, Xiao HB, Sparrow J et al. Effects of dual-chamber pacing with short atrioventricular delay in dilated cardiomyopathy, Lancet 1992;40:1308.
33. Xiao HB, Lee CH, Gibson DG. Effect of left bundle branch block on diastolic function in dilated cardiomyopathy. Br Heart J 1991;66:443.
34. Hochleitner M, Hörtnagl H, Fridrich L et al. Long-term efficacy of physiologic dual-chamber pacing in the treatment of end-stage idiopathic dilated cardiomyopathy. Am J Cardiol 1992;70:1320–5.

26. DDD rate-responsive pacing: state of the art

MASSIMO SANTINI, G. ANSALONE & G. CACCIATORE

INTRODUCTION

Previous studies with pacemaker patients have documented the significant contributions of heart rate and atrioventricular (AV) synchrony to an increase in cardiac output during exercise [1–3]. Several authors have hypothesized that the heart rate is the dominant factor [4–7]. In fact, it is well-known that before the advent of rate-responsive pacing, many patients were limited by fixed rate pacing (VVI) or by minimal increases in heart rate during physical or emotional stress. As comparable hemodynamics can be achieved at maximum exercise through the increase in rate without maintaining AV synchrony [7–11], single chamber ventricular rate-adaptive (VVIR) pacing has been advocated alternative approach to dual chamber pacing (DDD).

However, recent studies [12–15] have shown the additional advantages of AV synchrony at rest and at low levels of exercise over VVIR pacing, particularly if the AV interval is also rate adaptive [16,17]. In addition, single chamber rate-responsive pacing (VVIR) is also not immune from the development of the pacemaker syndrome [15,18,19], which results from the loss of AV synchrony and the presence of ventriculoatrial conduction. Dual chamber rate-adaptive (DDDR) pacing thus combines the advantage of a sensor-driven rate response as well as AV synchronization, providing the opportunity for optimizing functional capacity and minimizing adverse effects (e.g. pacemaker syndrome).

The currently approved sensors in common use are those responsive to motion and thoracic impedance [20,21]. Both sensors have strengths and weaknesses. Currently, a variety of additional physiologic sensors are being investigated as a means to provide the rate response [20–22]. Activity sensing is the one most widely used for rate-adaptive pacing. Its advantages lie in the case of implementation minimum current drainage and excellent speed of rate response, although the main drawback is the relatively low sensor proportionality to workload [23]. Another dual chamber rate-responsive device recently approved by the US Food and Drug Administration (FDA) assesses minute ventilation by measuring the transthoracic impedance. Previous studies have shown that this system closely matches metabolic demand [24,25].

However, there is concern that the clinical benefit of sensor-driven rate-responsive dual chamber pacing with regard to increased patient physical endurance has not been objectively demonstrated through comparative exercise tests. Instead of a mere quantification of changes in cardiac output during exercise, evaluation of the functional capacity was done by direct measurement of oxygen uptake (VO_2) and carbon dioxide production (VCO_2) [26].

Furthermore, because DDDR systems are in many respects designed for use in patients with abnormal sinoatrial function, the susceptibility of these patients to increased atrial pacing thresholds, inadequate atrial sensing, or atrial tachyarrhythmias may be an important potential limitation to the long-term effectiveness of dual chamber rate-adaptive pacing modes. In fact, there is concern that clinical and programming complexities may necessitate a frequent reprogramming of pacemakers from the DDDR mode to less physiologic pacing modes, in particular VVI or VVIR. To date, the duration of the clinical performance assessments of DDDR devices has been brief [13,14,20,27–31], and only one study [32] assessed the clinical course over a longer term of a group of patients who had received an activity-based, DDDR-capable pacemaker.

In spite of these disadvantages, there is general agreement that the quality of life of DDDR-paced patients is better [12,14,33,34], according to the capability for a greater and longer muscular workload compared with fixed-rate paced patients and also with DDDR effectiveness in preventing atrial arrhythmias both in bradycardiac patients and in those suffering from brady-tachy syndrome.

Finally, it must be emphasized that definitive results about the effects on survival are not yet available.

PREVIOUS STUDIES

In 1986, Kappenberger and Herbers [27] reported for the first time two patients with chronotropic incompetence and atrioventricular block who were successfully paced with dual chamber rate-adaptive pacing mode. Afterwards, many authors described the hemodynamic benefits of DDDR pacing, suggesting that this pacing modality can provide a rise of cardiac output under effort to a greater extent than DDD or VVIR [14,35].

Batey et al. [33] found that in very selected patients with marked chronotropic incompetence, the exercise tolerance was greater with VVI rate-responsive pacing than with DDD fixed-rate pacing; but when the heart rate could spontaneously reach at least 100 bpm, this superiority of ventricular rate-responsive pacing was not found.

Jutzy et al. [14] compared the DDDR, DDD, and VVIR pacing modes in 14 patients using paired cardiopulmonary exercise treadmill testing. In comparison with VVIR, they found in DDDR patients a 10% greater exercise duration and a 69% greater increment of cardiac output. In the subset of patients with chronotropic incompetence, the DDDR mode was also associated with a better performance than was the DDD mode. In particular, DDDR pacing compared with the DDD mode resulted in a 4% greater exercise duration and a 68% greater increment of cardiac output.

Sulke et al. [30] also compared DDDR with DDD and VVIR pacing using a double-blind crossover design. Twenty-two patients with activity sensor DDDR pacemakers were evaluated using scheduled reprogramming to the various modes to be tested. Of these, 59% strongly preferred the DDDR mode, whereas 73% found single chamber rate-adaptive pacing to be the least acceptable because of a remarkable worsening of symptoms. This finding was in agreement with the greater increase of stroke volume during dual chamber pacing than during single chamber pacing at rest.

Previous investigators [36], evaluating aerobic capacity in rate-modulated pacing, have described a 27% improvement in O_2 uptake at the anaerobic threshold with the DDDR mode as compared with the DDD stimulation in patients who are chronotropic incompetent, whereas Lemke et al. [37] found an overall improvement in functional capacity of only 12% for DDDR versus DDD pacing.

In Lemke et al.'s study [37], the overall work capacity in the DDDR mode compared with VVIR was improved by 17%. Considering only patients with isolated sinus node disease the increase of VO_2 and work capacity at the anaerobic threshold during the DDDR mode was more pronounced than during VVIR (20% and 16%, respectively). Conversely, in patients with AV block, the difference between the two pacing modalities was not significant. The authors suggested that this might be due to a lesser degree of chronotropic incompetence in this subgroup. Therefore, only the association of heart rate increase and preservation of AV synchrony provides a significant improvement in aerobic capacity during exercise.

Using the same evaluation methods, that is the cardiopulmonary exercise test with DDDR versus DDD pacing, Capucci et al. [38] found that DDDR pacing was associated with higher maximal heart rates, higher VO_2 max, and higher VO_2 at the anaerobic threshold, without significant differences in the mean exercise time. The increase VO_2 max, obtained in DDDR over DDD, was significantly related to the increase in maximal heart rate, and the increase in VO_2 at the anaerobic threshold was similarly related to the increase in heart rate at the anaerobic threshold. In patients with chronotropic incompetence, the improvement obtained in DDDR versus DDD was even more significant. This objective enhancement in exercise capacity in subjects with chronotropic incompetence was associated with a better subjective tolerance as demonstrated by the symptom questionnaire. These results show that the achievement by DDDR pacing of submaximal heart rates (120–140 min), which are in the range of heart rates reached during daily activities by elderly patients [39], represents a substantial increment in exercise capacity, particularly evident in subjects with chronotropic incompetence.

To study if during DDDR pacing competitive atrial pacing due to the sensor-triggered rate response may tend to aggravate atrial tachyarrhythmia susceptibility, Spencer et al. [40] evaluated 10 patients with ambulatory electrocardiographic monitoring. The authors did not find any significant difference between pacing modes with respect to atrial arrhythmia events (DDDR 1.25 versus DDD 1.75 atrial events/24 h). However, the patients preferred the DDDR mode. Other authors [32] also confirmed that the DDDR mode is not associated with a high incidence of new-onset symptomatic atrial tachyarrhythmias. When atrial tachyarrhythmia recurrences occurred, they tended to be restricted to patients in whom such arrhythmias had been known to occur spontaneously before pacemaker implantation. Furthermore, in patients with a history of atrial tachyarrhytmias, less than half (8 of 23; 35%) had evident arrhythmia recurrence during the follow-up. In such cases, careful antiarrhythmic drug therapy associated with dual chamber pacing can diminish the risk of atrial tachyarrhythmias.

To verify the stability of the pacing mode programming and the factors affecting pacing mode selection in patients with the DDDR pacing system, Benditt et al. [32] assessed the clinical status in 75 patients during a follow-up of 18.2 ± 6.7 months. Twenty-three patients had a history of atrial tachyarrhythmias. At implantation, 66 devices (88%) were programmed to DDDR mode, 7 (9%) to DDD, and 2 (3%) to DVIR. At the end of the follow-up period, the respective distribution of programmed modes was 83% DDDR, 10% DDD, 4% DVIR and 3% VVIR. The initial pacing mode remained unchanged in 54 patients (72%) and needed modification in 21 (28%). Atrial tachycardia was the cause of the programming change in 11 (52%) of whom 8 had a history of atrial tachycardias. The remaining reprogrammings were primarily to optimize the hemodynamic benefits.

The implantable sensor can be used to judge the appropriateness of the P wave rate. Should the rate be considered faster than the patient's current physiological requirement, pacemaker-mediated tachycardia can be diagnosed so that pacemakers respond either by a mode shift from DDDR to ventricular rate adaptive (VVIR) pacing or by the limitation of the maximum ventricular response rate to an interim level to ameliorate the adverse hemodynamic consequences of the tachycardia.

The role of implantable sensors to control pacemaker-mediated tachycardias was investigated by Lau et al. [41] in 16 patients with two different dual chamber rate-adaptive (DDDR) pacemakers, which sensed either minute ventilation or body acceleration. In the unipolar atrial sensing mode, myopotential sensing and external chest wall stimulation at 250 beats/min were induced to be preferentially sensed by the atrial channel to simulate the conditions of atrial arrhythmias. In the DDD mode, these maneuvers resulted in ventricular responses of 88 ± 3 beats/min and 110 ± 3 beats/min for myopotential sensing and chest wall stimulation, respectively. The pacing rate

Table 1. Results of exercise testing in DDI and DDIR mode

	DDI	DDIR	%	p
VO_2 max (ml/min)	1242 ± 425	1451 ± 410	17	<0.001
VO_2 AT (ml/min)	984 ± 358	1225 ± 413	24	<0.001
Total work (min)	9.16 ± 2.2	10.4 ± 2.1	13	<0.0001
AT work (min)	6.66 ± 2.6	8.38 ± 2.2	26	<0.0001
Peak HR (bpm)	109 ± 10	131 ± 8	20	<0.0001

was significantly reduced in the DDDR mode, with the sensor correctly detecting and responding to the sensed abnormal atrial signals (68 ± 5 beats/min during myopotential sensing and 71 ± 5 beats/min during chest wall stimulation; $p < 0.005$ compared with the corresponding DDD rate). One patient developed spontaneous atrial flutter, and the ventricular tracking responses were 140 and 85 beats/min in the DDD and DDDR pacing modes, respectively. Thus, the use of implantable sensors to judge the appropriateness of the atrial rate is a new approach to the management of pacemaker-mediated tachycardias.

Based on the reported experiences, at this time it must be accepted in carefully selected patients that there is a greater efficacy of DDDR pacing than VVIR and DDD in guaranteeing a better quality of life, an improved hemodynamic setting, and a smaller incidence of complications. In our opinion, this will probably also be reflected in an improvement of survival when controlled studies become available.

HEMODYNAMIC BENEFITS OF DDIR PACING MODALITY: AN ITALIAN MULTICENTER TRIAL

Fifty-two patients, 34 male and 18 female, mean age 70 ± 9 years, suffering from sick sinus syndrome (SSS) with chronotropic incompetence and impaired AV conduction, were treated with a DDDR pacemaker, Medtronic Elite 7075–77 [42]. To evaluate the hemodynamic benefits of DDIR pacing, all patients underwent symptoms-limited exercise testing before and after the implant. The peak heart rate increased from 97 ± 19 beats/min to 117 ± 17 beats/min ($p < 0.00001$); the work length increased from 7.1 ± 3.7 min to 8.8 ± 4.3 ($p < 0.0001$); the symptoms score significantly improved for dyspnea (< 0.001) and dizziness ($p < 0.05$).

Eighteen patients, 15 male and 3 female, mean age 72 ± 8 years, performed sequential treadmill exercise testing (Bruce protocol) in DDI and DDIR mode with expired gas analysis. Their peak oxygen uptake (VO_2 max), anaerobic threshold (VO_2 AT), total work, work at anaerobic threshold, and peak heart rate were measured. The frequency trend during ergometric test in DDI and DDIR were matched with the theoretical frequency trend calculated by the Wilkoff mathematical model (Table 1).

The DDIR trend was superimposed on the theoretical trend up to 6th min, with a lower rise between the 6 and 12th min. At all work loads, the DDI trend was significantly lower than either the DDIR or theoretical trends.

In conclusion, the results suggest that the DDIR pacing system improves the physical working capacity in patients with SSS and chronotropic incompetence.

REFERENCES

1. Karlöf I. Haemodynamic effect of atrial triggered versus fixed rate pacing at rest and during exercise in complete heart block. Acta Med Scand 1975;197:195–206.
2. Kappenberger L, Gloor HO, Babotai I et al. Hemodynamic effects of atrial synchronisation in acute and long-term ventricular pacing. PACE 1982;5:639–45.
3. Lemke B, Gude J, Von Driander S et al. Effects of AV-synchrony and rate increase on hemodynamic and atrial natriuretic peptide in patients with complete AV-block. Z Kardiol 1990;79:547–56.
4. Fananapazir L, Bennett DH, Monks P. Atrial synchronized pacing: Contribution of the chronotropic response to improved exercise performance. PACE 1983;6:601–8.
5. Pehrsson SK. Influence of heart rate and atrioventricular synchronisation of maximal work tolerance in patients treated with artificial pacemakers. Acta Med Scand 1983;214:311–5.
6. Munteanu J, Wirtzfeld A, Stangl K et al. Is the hemodynamic benefit of VDD pacing due to AV synchrony or to rate responsiveness? In: Gomez FP, editor. Cardiac Pacing. Madrid: Editorial Grouz, 1985;893–7.
7. Kristensson BE, Arnman K, Ryden L. The hemodynamic importance of atrioventricular synchrony and rate increase at rest and during exercise. Eur Heart J 1985;6:773–8.
8. Nordlander R, Pehrsson SK, Astrom H et al. Myocardial demands of atrial-triggered versus fixed rate ventricular pacing in patients with complete heart block. PACE 1987;10:1154.
9. Pehrsson SK, Hjelmdahl P, Nordlander R et al. A comparison of sympathoadrenal activity and cardiac performance at rest and during exercise in patients with ventricular demand or atrial synchronous pacing. Br Heart J 1988; 60:212.
10. Hedman A, Hjelmdahl P, Nordlander R et al. Effects of mental and physical stress on central hemodynamics and cardiac sympathetic nerve activity during QT interval sensing rate responsive and fixed rate ventricular inhibited pacing. Eur Heart J 1990;11:903.
11. Linde-Edelstam C, Nordlander R, Pehrsson SK et al. A double-blind study of submaximal exercise tolerance and variation in paced rate in atrial synchronous compared to activity sensor modulated ventricular pacing. PACE 1992; 15:905.
12. Higano ST, Hayes DL. Hemodynamic importance of atrio-ventricular synchrony during low levels of exercise (abstract). PACE 1990;13:509.
13. Lau CP, Wong CK, Leung WH, Liu WX. Superior cardiac haemodynamics of atrioventricular synchrony over rate responsive pacing at submaximal exercise: Observations in activity-sensing DDDR pacemakers. PACE 1990;13:1832–7.
14. Jutzy RV, Florio J, Isaeff DM et al. Comparative evaluation of rate modulated dual chamber and VVIR pacing. PACE 1990;13:1838–46.
15. Oldoyd KG, Rae AP, Carter R et al. Double blind crossover comparison of the effects of dual chamber pacing (DDD) and ventricular rate adaptive (VVIR) pacing on neuroendocrine variables, exercise performance, and symptoms in complete heart block. Br Heart J 1991;65:188–93.
16. Mehta D, Gilmour S, Ward DE et al. Optimal atrioventricular delay at rest and during exercise in patients with dual chamber pacemakers: A non-invasive assessment by continuous wave Doppler. Br Heart J 1989;61:161–6.
17. Ritter PH, Vai F, Bonnet JL et al. Rate adaptive atrioventricular delay improves cardiopul-

monary performance in patients implanted with a dual chamber pacemaker for complete heart block. Eur J Cardiac Pacing Electrophysiol 1991;1:31–8.
18. den Dulk K, Lindemans FW, Smeets JLRM et al. Pacemaker syndrome with AAI rate variable pacing: Importance of atrioventricular conduction properties, medication and pacemaker programmability. PACE 1988;11:1226–33.
19. Ruiter J, Burgersdijk, Zenders M et al. Atrial activitrax pacing: The atrioventricular interval during exercise (abstract). PACE 1987;10:1226.
20. Proctor EE, Leman RB, Mann DL, Kaiser J, Kratz J, Gillette D. Single versus dual-chamber sensor-driven pacing: comparison of cardiac outputs. Am Heart J 1991;122:728–32.
21. Benditt DG, Milstein S, Buetikofer J, Gormick CG, Mianulli M, Fetter J. Sensor-triggered, rate variable cardiac pacing. Ann Intern Med 1987;107:714–24.
22. Rossi P. Rate-responsive pacing: biosensor reliability and physiologic sensitivity. PACE 1987;10:454–66.
23. Lau CP, Metha D, Toff W et al. Limitations of rate response of activity sensing rate responsive pacing to different forms of activity. PACE 1988;11:141–50.
24. Lau CP, Antoniou A, Ward D et al. Initial clinical experience with a minute ventilation sensing rate modulated pacemaker: Improvements in exercise capacity and symptomatology. PACE 1988;11:1815–22.
25. Mond H, Strathmore N, Kertes P et al. Rate responsive pacing using a minute ventilation sensor. PACE 1988;11:1866–74.
26. Wasserman K, Beaver WL, Whipp BJ. Gas exchange and the lactic acidosis (anaerobic) threshold. Circulation 1990;81(Suppl II):14–30.
27. Kappenberger LJ, Herbers L. Rate responsive dual chamber pacing. PACE 1986;9:987–91.
28. Jutzy RV, Isaeff DM, Bansal RC, Florio J, Marsa RJ, Jutzy KR. Comparison of VVIR, DDD and DDDR pacing. J Electrophysiol 1989;3:194–201.
29. Mukharji J, Rehr RB, Hastillo A et al. Comparison of atrial contribution to cardiac haemodynamics in patients with normal and severely compromised cardiac function. Clin Cardiol 1990;13:639–43.
30. Sulke N, Chambers J, Dritas A, Sowton E. A randomized double-blind cross-over comparison of four rate-responsive pacing modes. J Am Coll Cardiol 1991;17:696–706.
31. Griffin JC. VVIR or DDD(R): does it matter? Clin Cardiol 1991;14:257–60.
32. Benditt DG, Wilbert L, Hansen R et al. Late follow-up of dual-chamber rate-adaptive pacing. Am J Cardiol 1993;71:714–9.
33. Batey LR, Sweesy MW, Scala G, Forney RC. Comparison of low rate dual chamber pacing to activity responsive rate variable ventricular pacing. PACE 1990;13:646–52.
34. Bubien RS, Kay GN. A randomized comparison of quality life and exercise capacity with DDD and VVIR pacing modes. PACE 1990;13:524.
35. Capucci A, Boriani G. La stimolazione DDDR. Considerazioni critiche sull'impiego clinico. Cardiostimolazione 1991;19:107–13.
36. META DDDR. Clinical Study Summary. Telectronics Pacing Systems. Englewood, Colorado, April 1992.
37. Lemke B, Dryander SV, Jager D, Machraoui A, Mac Carter D, Barmeyer J. Aerobic capacity in rate modulated pacing. PACE 1992;15:1914–8.
38. Capucci A, Boriani G, Specchia S, Marinelli M, Santarelli A, Magnani B. Evaluation by cardiopulmonary exercise test of DDDR versus DDD pacing. PACE 1992;15:1908–13.
39. Camm AJ, Evans KE, Ward DE et al. The rhythm of the heart in active elderly subjects. Am Heart J 1980;99:598–603.
40. Spencer WH III, Markowitz T, Alagona P. Rate augmentation and atrial arrhythmias in DDDR pacing. PACE 1990;13:1847–51.
41. Lau CP, Tai YT, Fong PC et al. Clinical experience with an activity sensing DDDR pacemaker using an accelerometer sensor. PACE 1992;15:334–43.
42. Ricci R, Azzolini P, Puglisi A et al. Hemodynamic benefits of DDIR pacing modality. An Italian multicenter trial (abstract). PACE 1993;16:1194.

27. Heart rate response based on changes in central venous oxygen saturation, minute ventilation and body activity

OLE-JÖRGEN OHM, SVEIN FŒRESTRAND
& FINN HEGBOM

INTRODUCTION

Although the research has been going on much longer, the clinical use of pacemakers which can change their stimulation rate on the basis of physiological parameters other than atrial rate only started on a significant scale around 1983. This new mode of stimulation was named rate-variable or rate-responsive pacing. With the introduction of the rate-responsive pulse generators, pacemaker treatment entered a new era [1–3]. The importance of rate-variable pacing for clinical practice is evident from the fact that the most frequently implanted pacemaker model today is a rate-responsive system.

A number of artificial sensors have been developed to mimic the normal sinus node function [4,5]. Several of the sensors have demonstrated long-term reliability. Of the clinically proven sensors, the one which responds to body activity has been the most successful, together with the sensor which is based on minute ventilation [3,6–8]. An advantage with these two sensors is also that standard pacemaker leads can be applied. Recently, these two systems have in addition proved efficient in dual chamber systems. Several new sensors which respond to various physiological parameters are under development, for central venous oxygen saturation, relative right ventricular pressure, relative right ventricular stroke volume, relative right ventricular contractility, the preejection interval and evoked ventricular depolarization gradient. Several combined sensors are under evaluation, including activity + temperature, QT interval + activity and activity + minute ventilation.

One major limitation with some available sensors is that their rate response is not proportional to physiological demand [6,9]. In recent models programmable heart rate acceleration and deceleration algorithms have been incorporated to compensate for this shortcoming. Therefore, there has been a continuous search to find an optimal sensor to meet the physiological demand. In this presentation two pacemaker systems currently under development have been studied. One system is based on changes in central venous oxygen saturation [10,11]. The second system can be controlled either by an activity or minute ventilation sensor or their combination [12].

CENTRAL VENOUS OXYGEN SATURATION CONTROLLED PACING

Most of the oxygen in the blood is bound to haemoglobin. Oxygenated haemoglobin reflects certain wavelengths in the red portion of the light spectrum better than non-oxygenated haemoglobin. This property is routinely used in clinical chemistry to measure oxygen saturation. An implantable sensor based on this principle has been developed for chronic use, incorporated in a pacemaker lead close to the electrode tip. In order to compensate for the expected fibrin and other deposits on the window which lets the light pass from the sensor housing, two wavelengths are used. Through this sensor the pulse generator emits red and infrared light into the blood in the right ventricle every 4th sensed or paced ventricular beat. The infrared light with a wavelength of 880 nM is reflected independent of the oxygen saturation, while less red light (which has a wavelength of 660 nM) is reflected when oxygen saturation drops. The reflection of the light of the red wavelength depends strongly on the state of oxygenation of the haemoglobin, while the infrared light reflection is almost independent of the oxygen saturation. Measurement of oxygen saturation is based on the ratio of reflected infrared and red light. Thus, the oxygen saturation is less influenced by the total amount of light reflection, which affects both the infrared and red reflection.

When the pacemaker detects that the oxygen saturation is dropping, the pacing rate is increased. Various relationships between pacing rate and measured oxygen saturation can be realized by the pacemaker circuits, and non-invasive programmability allows selection of the most appropriate response setting for the individual patient.

Methods for evaluation of the heart rate response

Acute testing
We have used this system on a temporary basis in 12 patients [10]. Similarly to other rate-responsive pacemakers, this system can be programmed to different rate-response settings. In the supine position the patients performed a 3-min arm exercise of 25 watts using an electrically braked bicycle. During rate-responsive ventricular pacing, there was an immediate and significant increase in heart rate of 31 ± 5 bpm from rest to peak exercise compared with a minor increase of 4 ± 5 bpm during spontaneous rhythm.

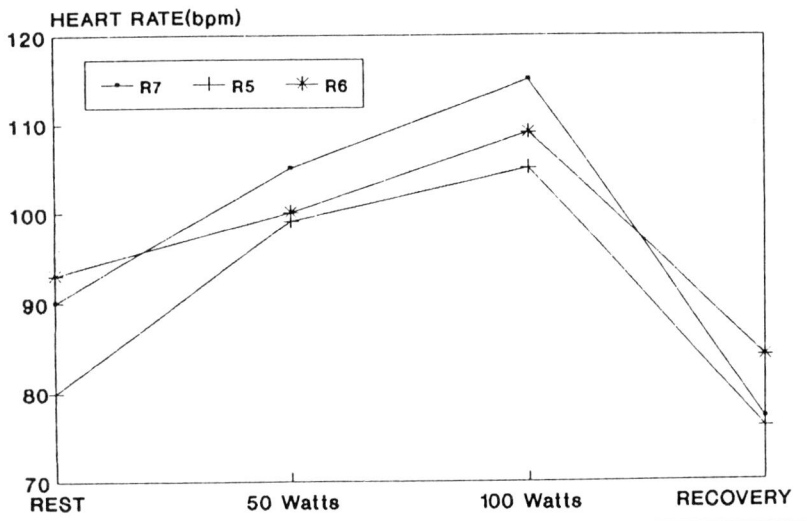

Figure 1. Pacing rates during bicycle exercise testing in three different response settings (R5-7 indicate increased sensitivity).

Testing during follow-up
During follow-up the optimal programming was obtained after repeated exercise tests on bicycle and treadmill as well as repeated 24-h Holter recordings. The system has been implanted in a total of 14 patients with a mean follow-up of 39 months (longest 55 months) and a total device experience of 547 months or 45 years [11].

Results

In Figure 1 is shown the heart rate response during bicycle exercise testing in the same patient at three different rate-response settings. It is clearly demonstrated that when the rate-response setting is increased, both the pacing rates at rest and during exercise are increased. In this same patient bicycle exercise tests were repeated on six different occasions from 1 to 30 months after implantation, always at a rate-response setting of 6. There is good conformity of the different exercise tests, indicating sensor stability (Figure 2).

Figure 3 elucidates the time course of the dynamics of telemetered oxygen saturation at the 1-year follow-up from a representative patient during supine bicycle exercise tests. The average ($n = 12$) time delay of 14 ± 2 s, the time constant of 47 ± 6 s and the response time of 93 ± 9 s are all quite satisfactory.

Figure 4 demonstrates changes in telemetered oxygen saturation and pac-

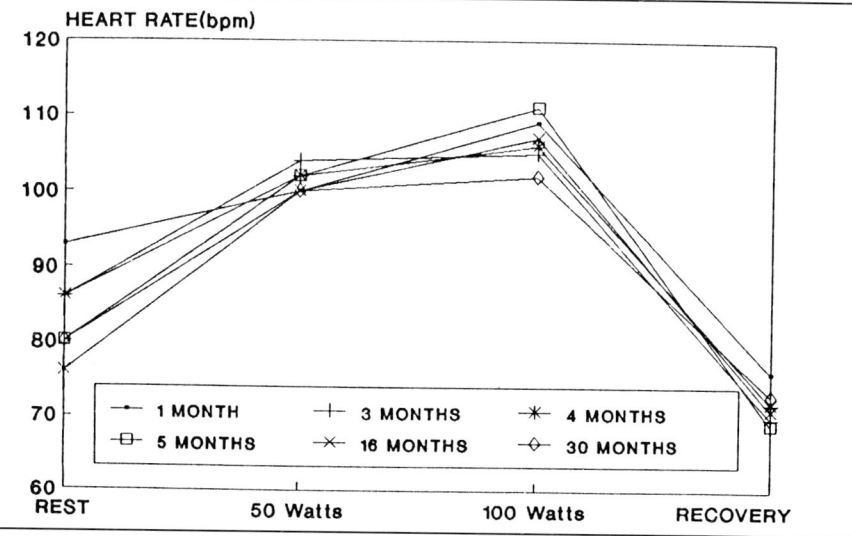

Figure 2. Bicycle exercise progression study.

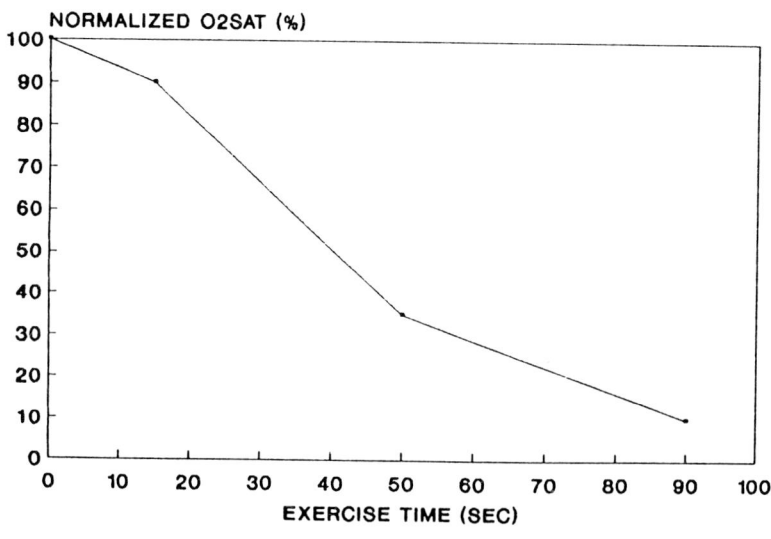

Figure 3. Time delay to 10%, 65% and 90% reduction of oxygen saturation (O_2Sat) during bicycle exercise testing from one representative patient.

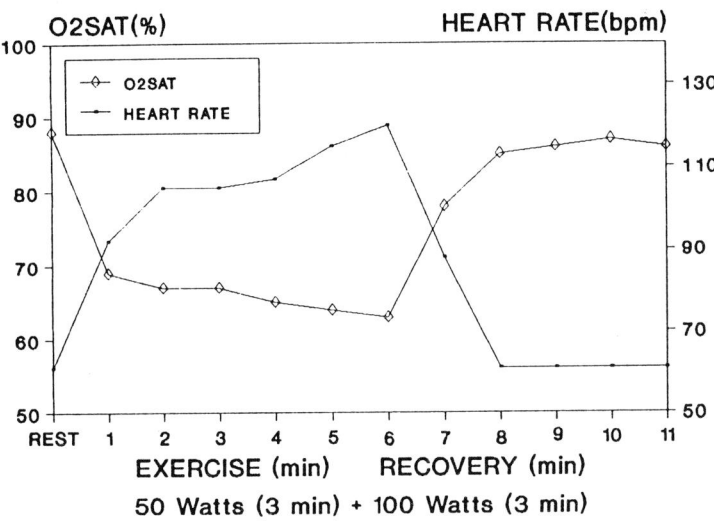

Figure 4. Heart rates and telemetered oxygen saturations (O$_2$Sat) during bicycle exercise from one representative patient.

ing rate during bicycle exercise testing in a representative patient. On average ($n = 13$) the oxygen saturation dropped about 20% and the heart rate increased 37 bpm after 3 min of exercise at 50 watts, with a further decrease in oxygen saturation of 4% to a minimum of 36% and a simultaneous increase in heart rate of 9 bpm to a maximum of 122 bpm after a load of 100 watts over 3 min.

One patient caught pneumonia 4 years after pacemaker implantation. The telemetered oxygen saturation demonstrated a decrease in saturation of 20% with a concomitant 26 bpm increase of the pacing rate. At recovery the oxygen saturation increased and pacing rate decreased to baseline values (Figure 5). A similar response was observed in another of our patients with verified pneumonia.

In one patient with coronary artery disease, a significant drop in oxygen saturation and a concomitant increase in pacing rate were observed during two episodes of angina pectoris. The patient also had aortic regurgitation. After implantation of an aortic valve prosthesis and bypass grafting, no new episodes of inappropriate pacing rate have been observed.

Conclusion

From these data we have seen that a rate-responsive system based on an oxygen saturation sensor which changes the pacing rate depending on changes in the central venous oxygen saturation has a fast and physiological rate response at the onset of exercise. In 50% of individuals, the system has

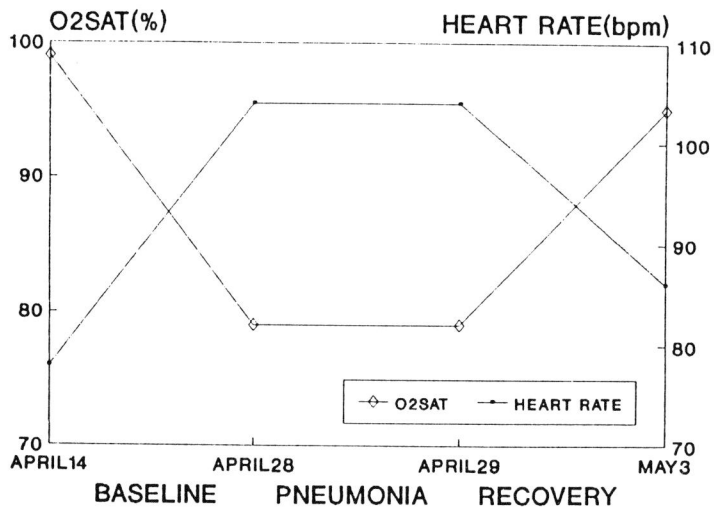

Figure 5. Oxygen saturation (O$_2$Sat) and heart rate before, during and in the recovery phase of pneumonia.

term stability (Figure 2). However, in patients with symptomatic coronary artery disease, the pacemaker system may lead to undesirable fast pacing rates during episodes of angina pectoris. Myocardial ischaemia may reduce the oxygen saturation and contribute to the persistence of a high pacing rate. Also, the maximum heart rate (Figures 1, 2, 4) which can be achieved with an individual optimal programming is at best between 120 and 130 bpm. On the other hand, the system has responded physiologically in two of our patients with lung infection.

PACEMAKERS CONTROLLED BY MINUTE VENTILATION AND BODY ACTIVITY

When a person is physically active, movements cause mechanical vibrations in the body. Forces on an implanted pacemaker which can be detected by means of a piezo-electric crystal bound to the inside of the pulse generator housing are thus able to increase the pacing rate. Although clinically successful, early objections arose to this principle because both the rate acceleration during exercise and the rate deceleration during recovery occurred in a non-physiological way [6]. Furthermore, it has been shown that this pacemaker is not able to increase the maximum heart rate to more than 110–120 bpm if a reasonable resting heart rate is to be obtained. Although a setting giving a maximal heart rate of 110 bpm may be adequate for most of the patients during daily activities, this system will give an inadequate response if heavy physical activity is attempted.

This has led to a search for more physiological signals that have a more direct relation to the body's oxygen demand. An early development was the respiratory rate pacemaker [2]. One drawback with this system is that it requires an additional lead implanted underneath the skin of the chest to measure the electrical impedance changes in the thorax.

The body's oxygen consumption and heart rate are almost linearly related to the amount of physical work performed. The volume of air inspired per minute (the respiratory minute volume = respiratory rate × tidal volume) correlates better with oxygen consumption than the respiratory rate. By applying more sophisticated processing techniques to the same thoracic impedance signal described for the respiratory rate pacemaker, an estimate can be obtained of the respiratory minute volume. This value can be used to control the pacing rate [7,8].

We have tested a pacemaker system which has two separately single mode programmable rate-responsive functions: activity rate response and minute ventilation rate response or their combination. This pacemaker can measure physical activity by means of a piezo-ceramic sensor in the pulse generator can and also the patient's minute ventilation by measuring changes in transthoracic impedance. If both functions are programmed at the same time, they each calculate the pacing rate as a result of variations in body vibration and minute ventilation, respectively. The pacemaker stimulates the heart at the highest calculated pacing rate. Theoretically, one can thus take advantage of the more rapid initial rate response of the piezo-ceramic sensor and the slower minute ventilation sensor which correlates better with oxygen uptake during exercise at higher workload levels.

The pacemaker system uses a standard bipolar lead which is required for the thoracic impedance measurement (Figure 6). It is possible to program the device to both unipolar and bipolar pacing and sensing, but a bipolar lead is always required for the impedance measurement.

The 'rough' unfiltered minute ventilation electrograms can be transferred via telemetry (Figure 7). The impedance signal is filtered by a low pass -0.8 Hz filter (corresponding to a respiratory rate of 48 per minute) before it is processed by the pacemaker circuit. Therefore, the cardiac component (typically 1 Hz) which is dominant in Figure 7B is not taken into consideration for the determination of the pacing rate.

The theoretical considerations of the response of the multisensor rate-adaptive pacemaker is shown in Figure 8. The algorithm of this system lets the fastest of the two sensors determine the pacing rate. If, for example, the minute ventilation is set too conservatively, this could result in an unnecessary delay in sensor response and thereby cause subjective symptoms of exhaustion. Thus far, this has not been a problem.

The body's minute ventilation and heart rate are almost linearly related

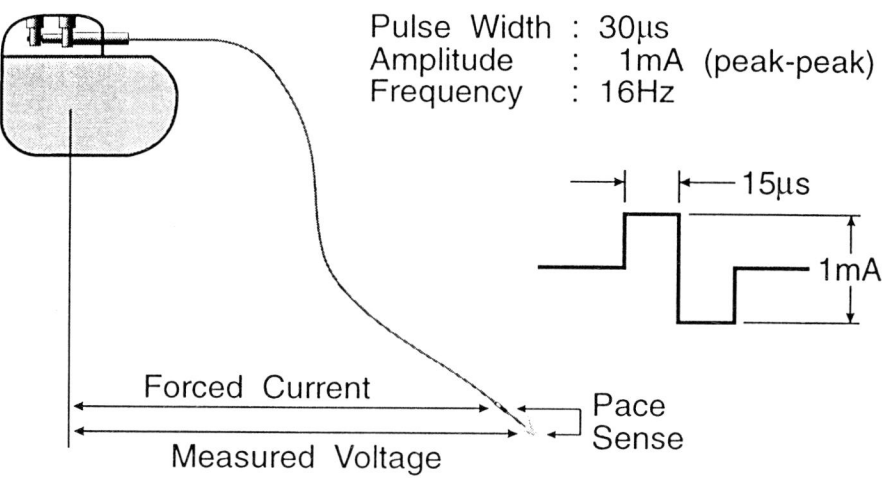

Figure 6. Multisensor pacemaker system (Medtronic Legend Plus). The figure indicates that the device is programmed to bipolar pacing and sensing (between ring and tip of lead). A biphasic current (upper right part) is forced between the pulse generator case and lead ring. The measured voltage between the pulse generator case and lead tip forms the basis for the thoracic impedance measurement.

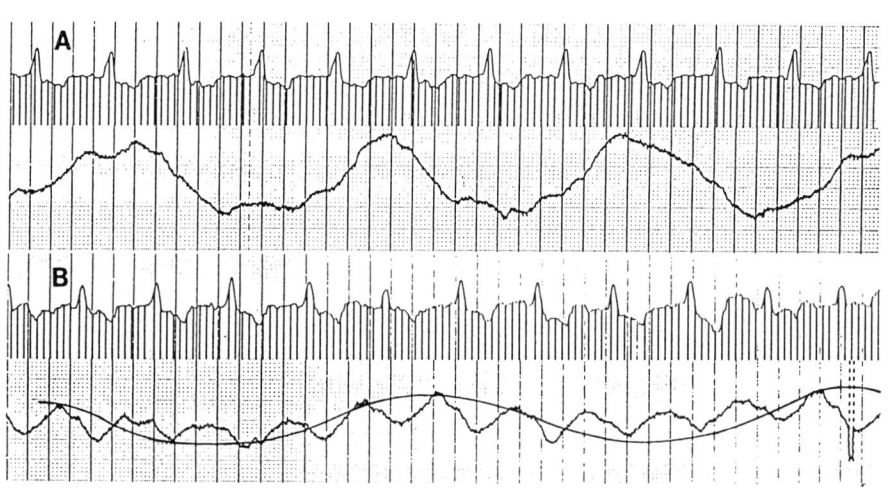

Figure 7. Telemetered unfiltered minute ventilation electrograms from two different patients, A and B. In (A) the respiratory cycles are most pronounced, and in (B) the cardiac component is most distinctive (respiratory cycles superimposed). These differences can be caused by variation in lead position or the implant site (i.e. right or left).

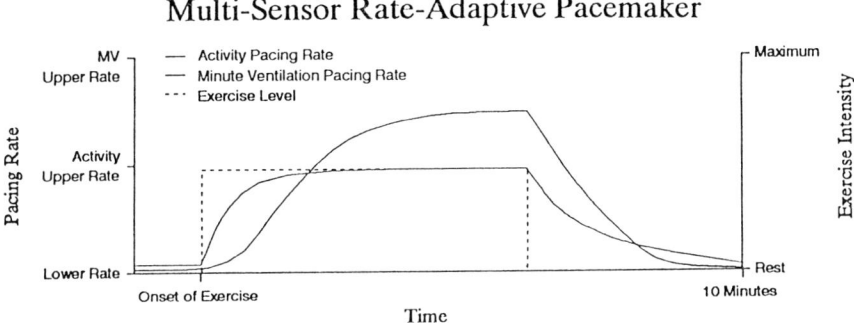

Figure 8. The theoretical rate response during dual sensor pacing. The activity sensor has a quick onset but also an upper rate limit which is compensated for with the workload response of minute ventilation.

(Figure 9). The system also shows a close relationship between minute ventilation and heart rate during exercise (Figure 10).

Methods for evaluation of the heart rate response

The pacemaker has been implanted in a total of eight patients who have been followed for an observation period of 6–12 months and a total device experience of 72 months. During evaluation of this pacemaker, the patients performed repeated treadmill step tests and exercise tests (Figure 11). One step test and one exercise test were done on the same day with 1 h rest between the tests. The step test lasted for 5 min at a constant speed of 4.8 km/h and a slope of 6 degrees. The exercise test was performed according to the Chronotropic Assessment Exercise Protocol (CAEP) to the maximum of the patient's exercise capacity. This protocol has a staged increase in speed and inclination with a slope increase of 2 degrees every 2nd minute.

Results

It has been demonstrated that in most patients the rate response is initially slower with the minute ventilation sensor than with the activity sensor. In our patients we did not find the difference to be as large as expected during

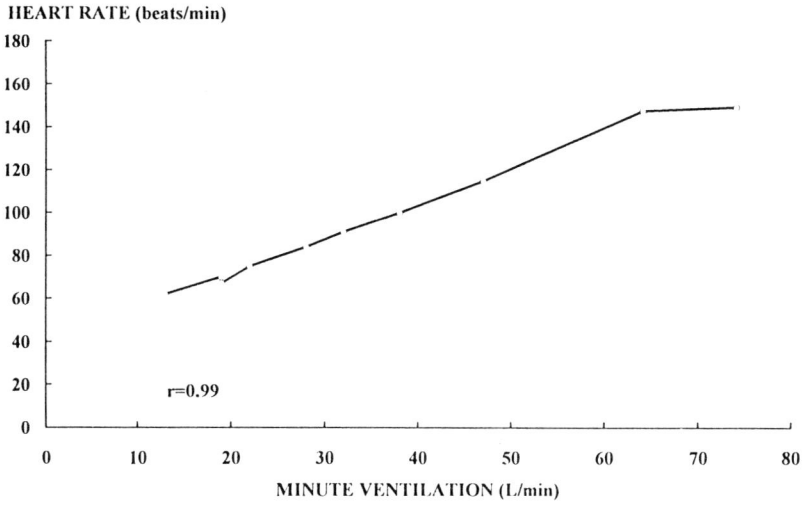

Figure 9. Example of relationship between heart rate and minute ventilation during a treadmill exercise test.

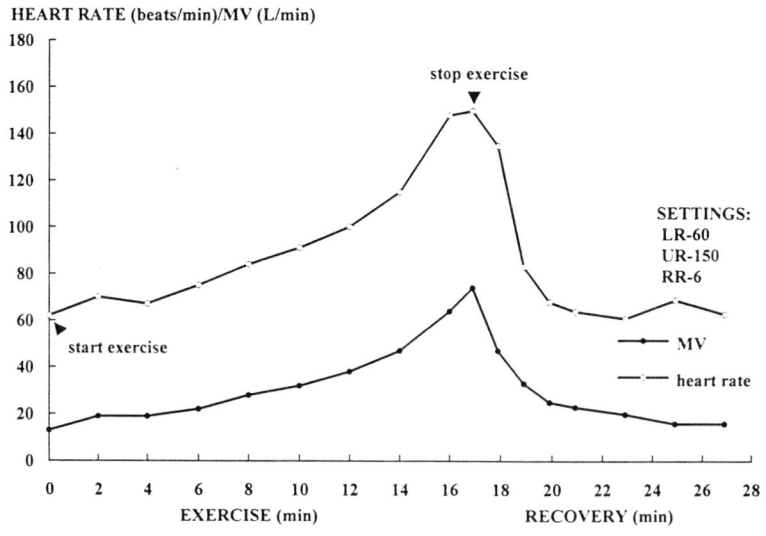

Figure 10. Treadmill exercise test with pacemaker programmed in minute ventilation (MV) mode in one patient. Pacemaker settings: lower rate (LR) = 60 bpm; upper rate (UR) = 150 bpm; rate response (RR) = 6. Acceleration and deceleration were programmed to nominal values.

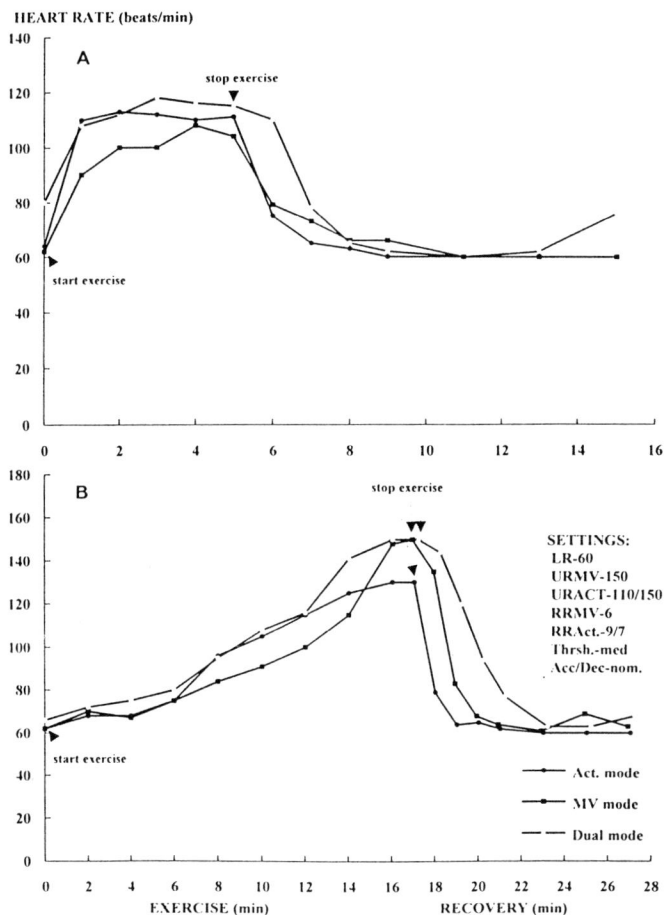

Figure 11. Treadmill step test (A) and treadmill exercise test using the CAEP protocol (B) during activity (Act), minute ventilation (MV) and dual modes in the same patient. The pacemaker settings were identical during the step and exercise tests. URMV-150 = upper rate 150 bpm in single mode; URAct-110/150 = activity sensor upper rate 110 bpm in dual mode and 150 bpm in single activity sensor mode; RRAct.-9/7 = rate response in dual and single modes, respectively; Thrsh.-med = medium threshold; Acc/Dec-nom. = nominal acceleration and deceleration. For additional abbreviations, see Figure 10.

the exercise test, but it became more marked during the step test (Figure 11). This reflects the higher initial activity during the step test. After 12–15 min of exercise, the pacing rate is determined by the minute ventilation sensor. In the activity sensor mode the pacemaker does not reach the pre-programmed upper rate of 150 bpm. However, there is really no difference in exercise capacity in these three situations.

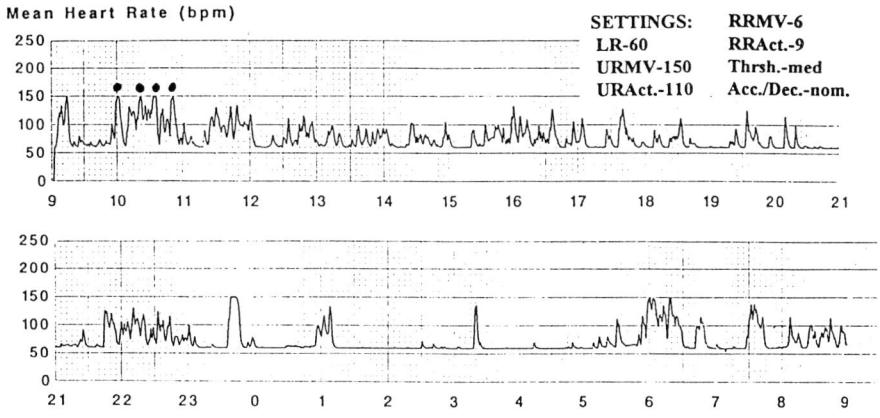

Figure 12. A 24-h Holter recording taken from the same patient as in Figure 11. The pacemaker was programmed in the dual mode. The patient tested the system during rapid stair climbing over six floors within 1 h between 10 and 11 a.m. The pacemaker's programmed maximum rate of 150 bpm (·) was reached on all four occasions. For abbreviations, see Figures 10 and 11.

The heart rate deceleration appears most physiological when the pacemaker is programmed in the minute ventilation or dual modes. In the clinical study the heart rate deceleration controlled by the minute ventilation sensor was positively correlated to the workload performed by the patient [13]. A typical heart rate deceleration time after the symptom-limited exercise test is around 6–8 min and after a step test, between 4–6 min (Figure 11).

In Figure 12 is shown a Holter recording from a 55-year-old woman. After radiofrequency ablation of the atrioventricular node, she was chronotropic incompetent. The recording demonstrated concordance between the patient's physical activity and heart rate based on her diary.

In the example given in Figure 13 the heart rate response during recovery after the treadmill exercise demonstrated a persistent fast pacing rate when the pacemaker was programmed in the minute ventilation mode. A possible explanation for this sensor behaviour was that the patient was convalescing after a pulmonary infectious disease. This probably resulted in a higher ventilatory drive which increases the thoracic impedance changes, thereby increasing the heart rate changes. This sensor behaviour suggests the need for cross-checking of the sensor signal to avoid inappropriate non-physiological rate responses. An activity sensor would not be influenced by such conditions.

Conclusion

Based on these studies involving a limited number of patients over a short period of time, this new combined sensor system has functioned satisfactorily

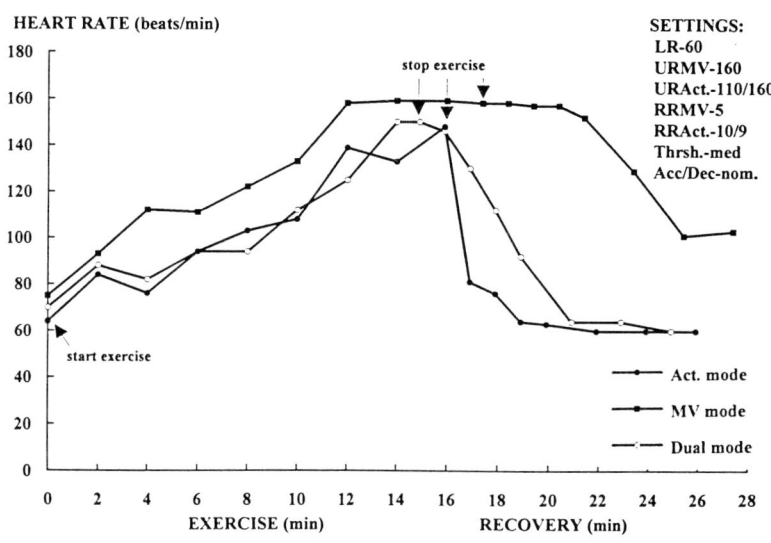

Figure 13. Exercise tests performed in the same patient in three different pacing modes at different follow-up periods. The rate response was fastest when the pacemaker was programmed in the minute ventilation mode and continued to stimulate at the upper rate for about 3 min before rate deceleration started in the recovery period. The pacing rate was still above 100 bpm 10 min after exercise. See text for explanation. For abbreviations, see Figures 10 and 11.

during daily activities. When the patients exhibited their maximum exercise capacity, the minute ventilation and dual sensor functioned most adequately both during the period of maximal heart rate and during the recovery phase. However, the dual sensor was not found to be advantageous compared with the single sensor with respect to oxygen uptake and work capacity.

ACKNOWLEDGEMENT

This study was supported by L. Meltzers Höyskolefond to the University of Bergen, and the Norwegian Council on Cardiovascular Diseases.

REFERENCES

1. Wirtzfeld A, Goedel-Meinen L, Bock T, Heinze R, Liess HD, Munteanu J. Central venous oxygen saturation for the control of automatic rate-responsive pacing. PACE 1982;5:829–35.
2. Rossi P, Plicchi G, Canducci G, Rognioni G, Aina F. Respiratory rate as a determinant of optimal pacing rate. PACE 1983;6:502–7.
3. Rydén L, Smedgård P, Kruse I, Anderson K. Rate responsive pacing by means of activity sensing. Stimucoer 1984;12:181–4.

4. Furman S. Rate-modulated pacing. Circulation 1990;82:1081–94.
5. Lau CP. The range of sensors and algorithms used in rate adaptive cardiac pacing. PACE 1992;15:1177–1211.
6. Færestrand S, Breivik K, Ohm O-J. Assessment of the work capacity and relationship between rate response and exercise tolerance associated with activity-sensing rate-responsive ventricular pacing. PACE 1987;10:1277–90.
7. Alt E, Heinz M, Hirgstetter C, Emslander H-P, Daum S, Blömer H. Control of pacemaker rate by impedance-based respiratory minute ventilation. Chest 1987;92:247–52.
8. Lau CP, Antoniou A, Ward DE, Camm AJ. Initial clinical experience with a minute ventilation sensing rate modulated pacemaker: Improvements in exercise capacity and symptomatology. PACE 1988;11:1815–22.
9. Lau CP, Butrous GS, Ward DE, Camm AJ. Comparative assessment of exercise performance of six different rate adaptive right ventricular cardiac pacemakers. Am J Cardiol 1989;63:833–9.
10. Færestrand S, Skadberg BT, Anderson K, Ohm O-J. Acute clinical testing and follow-up of a rate variable pacemaker controlled by central venous oxygen saturation. J Am Coll Cardiol 1989;13:112A.
11. Færestrand S, Ohm O-J. Long-term follow-up of a rate-variable pacemaker controlled by central venous oxygen saturation. J Am Coll Cardiol 1991;17:289A.
12. Slade A, Pee S, Jones S, Murgatroyd F, Camm AJ, Ward D. Clinical experience with a new dual sensor rate responsive pacemaker generator. PACE 1993;16:178A.
13. Medtronic. Report on the clinical evaluation of the Medtronic Legend Plus[TM] pacemaker system models 8446/8448, 1993 (FDA report, PMA submission).

28. DDDR and atrial arrhythmia

VÉRONIQUE MAHAUX

INTRODUCTION

Since the introduction of atrial synchronous pacing, several reports have pointed out the interest of preserving atrial stimulation and AV synchrony [1,2]. The incidence of thromboembolism and atrial fibrillation has been reduced and the general well-being improved. Nevertheless, atrial fibrillation still occurs in 5–10% of patients during long-term DDD pacing [3] and may be an indication for reprogramming to a nonatrial tracking mode, either the DDI [4] pacing mode when the arrhythmia is paroxysmal or VVI/VVIR when it is permanent. However, DDI does not provide rate adaptation with exercise, and VVIR does not ensure an AV synchronization which might be hemodynamically important at rest and at low levels of exercise [5] and which might indirectly further reduce atrial fibrillation episodes [6]. The ideal solution would be a DDDR mode implemented with algorithms protecting the ventricles against high atrial pacing rates during supraventricular arrhythmia. To permit a better understanding of the non-chronotropically related benefits of the DDDR mode, a critical review of the interactions between dual chamber stimulators and atrial rhythm disturbances is provided.

The DDDR pacing mode was first considered as associated with a theoretical increased risk of atrial arrhythmia induction. During sensor-driven stimulation, a short coupling interval might occur between an atrial extrasystole falling in the PVARP and the next atrial paced event and possibly lead to atrial fibrillation. The reported incidence of atrial arrhythmias in DDDR pacing during a United States Food and Drug Administration trial ranged from 8 to 10% [7]. Nonetheless, acute Holter recordings performed in a series of 10 patients alternatively paced in the DDD and DDDR mode did not disclose any proarrhythmic effect of the rate-adaptive mode [8].

Furthermore, analysis of the timing intervals of dual chamber rate-adaptive devices points out potential benefits over the conventional DDD mode. The following aspects are discussed: (a) the escape interval, (b) the sensor-related shortening of the atrial channel refractoriness, (c) the programming of dis-

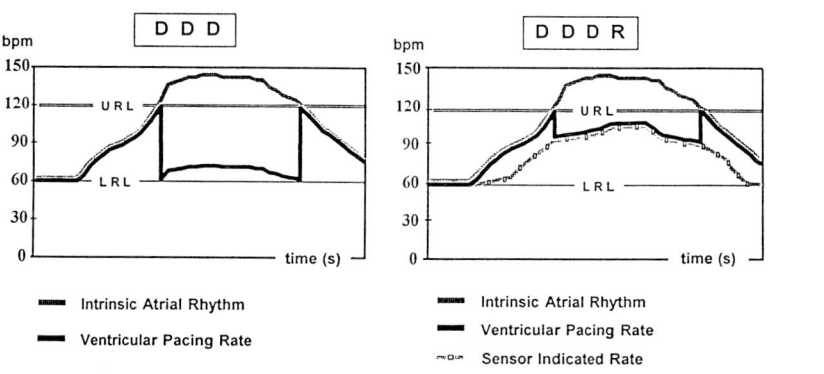

Figure 1. Upper rate behaviour in dual chamber pacing. In DDD (left panel), atrial tracking occurs up to the programmed maximum pacing rate. When the PP intervals are shorter than the total atrial refractory period (AV delay + PVARP), the 2:1 blocking ratio allows the ventricular pacing rate to fall to half the atrial rate or to the programmed lower rate. In DDDR (right panel), atrial tracking occurs up to the programmed maximum pacing rate. When the PP intervals are shorter than the total atrial refractory period (AV delay + PVARP), the 2:1 blocking ratio allows the ventricular pacing rate to fall to half the atrial rate or to the sensor rate, producing a 'sensor smoothing' when exercise is detected.

tinct exercise and non-exercise related upper rates and, most importantly, (d) the inclusion of the sensor signal in algorithms aimed at checking the adequacy of high atrial rates.

UPPER RATE BEHAVIOUR AND ATRIAL ESCAPE INTERVAL

The easiest way to determine the upper rate of DDD pacemakers involves the programming of the components of atrial channel refractoriness: AV delay and PVARP. P waves occurring during those periods do not initiate an AV interval and are not followed by paced ventricular complexes. As the number of unsensed P waves increases proportionally to the atrial rate, the maximum achievable tracking rate finally and indirectly becomes a function of the programmed AV delay and PVARP. At this upper rate limit, a sudden fall in ventricular rate occurs with the development of Mobitz II block. The paced ventricular rate is half of the atrial rate or equal to the lower rate (Figure 1, left panel). This abrupt rate change is quite often acutely felt by the patient, particularly during exercise [9].

An alternative solution is to control the ventricular upper rate behaviour according to the programmed maximum rate: in the presence of high atrial rates, the ventricular stimulus is released only at the completion of the upper rate limit interval. The AV delay becomes progressively longer as the ventricular channel waits to deliver its stimulus until the upper rate limit interval is over. In other words, Wenckebach periods limit the paced ventricular rate by extending the AV interval and produce an intermittent block, whose ratio depends on the atrial rate [10–12]. This avoids a sudden reduction of the paced ventricular rate and maintains some degree of AV synchrony. However, at the highest atrial rates, the P waves again fall in the PVARP, and the 2:1 block occurs. The Wenckebach upper rate response should therefore be considered as a way of providing a smoother transition from a 1:1 ventricular response to a fixed ratio.

Some specific mechanisms have been proposed to further limit the variations of ventricular pacing rate. The 'fallback' is intended to limit the length of time during which the ventricular rate remains at the programmed upper rate and might be useful in patients who cannot tolerate sustained high rates. The algorithm is activated by the detection of an atrial rate faster than the programmed upper rate. The ventricular pacing rate gradually decreases to more tolerable programmable rate levels than the upper rate of the pulse generator. During the response, the generator continues to monitor the atrial activity, and as soon as the detected atrial rate falls below the upper rate, fallback terminates, and atrial synchronous pacing resumes. To avoid a sudden rate jump during the AV resynchronization, some stimulators also provide a 'rate smoothing' feature which prevents rate changes by more than a certain percentage from one cardiac cycle to another.

Refined, recently available fallback algorithms also screen supraventricular arrhythmia which is slower than the programmed maximum tracking rate by detecting sudden atrial rate accelerations. The DDDR mode automatically provides a 'sensor smoothing' (Figure 1, right panel). Indeed, as the atrial escape interval is sensor related, sudden rate drops at the upper rate limit behaviour will be reduced.

SENSOR-RELATED SHORTENING OF THE ATRIAL REFRACTORY PERIOD

To reduce the theoretical risk of competitive atrial pacing and arrhythmia induction, recent dual chamber rate-adaptive stimulators include sensor-rate related shortening(s) of component(s) of the total atrial refractory period. Those algorithms improve atrial sensing during exercise, avoiding atrial competition and ensuring a maximum tracking of native P waves. The point corresponding to a 2/1 upper rate blocking ratio is improved and becomes a function of the sensor level (Figure 2).

Rate-adaptive AV delay mimicks the physiological PR behaviour with promising clinical effectiveness [13,14]. Rate-adaptive PVARP allows to choose a long resting PVARP, thereby providing added protection to retrograde conduction without compromising the maximum upper rate attained.

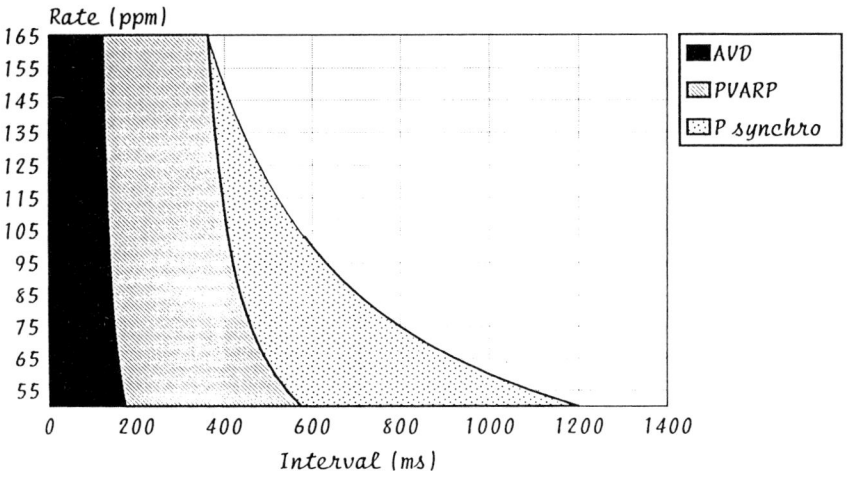

Figure 2. Rate-adaptive atrial refractoriness. Rate-related shortening of the AV delay (AVD) and PVARP preserves an atrial sensing window (P synchro) during exercise and avoids atrial competition. In this example, shortening of both components of the atrial refractory period allows atrial synchronous pacing up to 165 bpm, whereas fixed values would have limited atrial tracking to 105 bpm.

MAXIMUM SENSOR RATE AND MAXIMUM TRACKING RATE

The first DDDR device (Synergyst™ II, Medtronic Inc.) had no ability to automatically prevent rapid ventricular tracking of atrial arrhythmias. Thus, in the presence of supraventricular tachycardia, a reprogramming to a non-tracking mode (DVIR) was necessary. In a 16-month follow-up study of 37 patients, episodes of atrial tachyarrhythmias required temporary or definitive pacing mode alterations in 30% of the cases [15].

In Synchrony™ (Siemens Pacesetter) and Elite™ II (Medtronic Inc.), improved behaviours were associated with separate programming of the maximum tracking rate and maximum sensor rate. When the programmed maximum sensor rate is higher than the programmed maximum tracking rate, the following situations can occur: (a) when the sensor rate is higher than the sinus rate, the device stimulates both chambers at the sensor-indicated rate (b) when the sinus rate is faster than the sensor rate, the ventricular spike will occur at a variable AV interval with respect to the termination of the sensor-indicated rate interval. This behaviour is in effect similar to DDIR pacing with a lower rate equal to the sensor-indicated rate.

SENSOR-DRIVEN ALGORITHMS CHECKING SINUS RATE ADEQUACY

Today's dual chamber rate-adaptive generators offer many methods to limit the ventricular response to physiological or pathological atrial high rates and use the implantable sensor signals to judge the appropriateness of the atrial rate [16]. This approach was designed to prevent excessive tracking of atrial arrhythmias and to detect and indirectly correct pacemaker-mediated tachycardia. The currently available algorithms act either via an automatic temporary mode switching to VVIR, DDIR or by a limitation of the maximum ventricular response to a specific rate when the sensor does not detect activity [17–20]. The clinical benefit and effectiveness of those devices will be extensively discussed further in this volume.

CONCLUSION

The present chapter is intended to stress the potential non-chronotropically related benefits of dual chamber rate-adaptive devices. The DDDR mode is automatically associated with a smoothing of the atrial escape interval, thus providing improved upper rate behavior. Rate-adaptive atrial refractoriness reduces the risk of competitive atrial pacing and improves the point corresponding to the 2:1 blocking ratio.

With the advent of rate-adaptive pacing, an additional input could be used to check the adequacy of high atrial rates and eventually lead to an automatic temporary mode reprogramming. The applications of sensors for non-rate-adaptive purposes will broaden the indications of DDDR pacing to patients requiring dual chamber pacing but showing paroxysmal supraventricular rhythm disturbances and in whom dual chamber pacing would otherwise have been precluded.

ACKNOWLEDGEMENTS

I am grateful to Mr. J.M. Hottois and Mr. R. Willems for their technical support.

REFERENCES

1. Rosenqvist M, Brandt J, Schüller H. Long-term pacing in sinus node disease. Effects of stimulation mode on cardiovascular morbidity and mortality. Am Heart J 1988;116:16–22.
2. Mitsuoka T, Kenny RA, Yeung TA, Chan IS, Perrins JE, Sutton R. Benefits of dual chamber pacing in sick sinus syndrome. Br Heart J 1988;60:338–47.
3. Gross J, Moser S, Benedek M, Andrews C, Furman S. Clinical predictors and natural history of atrial fibrillation in patients with DDD pacemakers. PACE 1990;3:1828–31.

4. Floro J, Castellanet M, Florio J, Messenger J. DDI: a new mode for cardiac pacing. Clin Prog Pacing Electrophysiol 1984;2:255.
5. Lau CP, Wong CK, Leung WH, Liu WX. Superior cardiac hemodynamics of atrioventricular synchrony over rate responsive pacing at submaximal exercise: observations in activity sensing DDDR pacemakers. PACE 1990;13:1832–7.
6. Sutton R. Pacing in atrial arrhythmias. PACE 1990;13:1823–7.
7. Circulatory System Devices Panel of the Food and Drug Administration. Transcript. June 30, 1989:90–123 ⌀160–72.
8. Spencer WH, Markowitz T, Alagona P. Rate augmentation and atrial arrhythmias in DDDR pacing. PACE 1990;13:1847–51.
9. Barold SS, Falkoff MD, Ong LS. Electrocardiography of contemporary DDD pacemakers. A. Basic concepts, upper rate response, retrograde ventriculoatrial conduction, and differential diagnosis of pacemaker tachycardias. In: Saskena S, Goldschlager N, Editors. Electrical therapy for cardiac arrhythmias. Pacing, antitachycardia devices, catheter ablation. Philadelphia: Saunders, 1990: 225–64.
10. Barold S, Mugica J, Falkoff MD. Multiprogrammability in cardiac pacing. In: Barold S, Mugica J, editors. The Third Decade of Cardiac Pacing. Mount Kisco: Futura, 1982:16.
11. Hauser RG. The electrocardiography of AV universal DDD pacemaker. PACE 1983;6:399.
12. Furman S. Retreat from Wenckebach. PACE 1984;7:1.
13. Daubert C, Ritter P, Mabo P, Ollitrault J, Descaves C, Gouffault J. Physiological relationship between AV interval and heart rate in healthy subjects: applications to dual chamber pacing. PACE 1986;9:1032–9.
14. Ritter P, Daubert C, Mabo P, Descaves C, Gouffault J. Hemodynamic benefit of a rate-adapted A-V delay in dual chamber pacing. Eur Heart J 1989;10:637–46.
15. Benditt DG, Alagona P, Spencer WH et al. Dual-chamber rate-adaptive (DDDR) pacing: a stable pacing mode during sixteen months follow-up (abstract). PACE 1992;15:511.
16. Lau CP, Tai YT, Fong PC, Chung FLW. Rate adaptive dual chamber pacing (DDDR) using a minute ventilation sensor (abstract). PACE 1991;14:699.
17. Lau CP, Camm AJ. Rate responsive pacing: Technical and clinical aspects. In: El-Sherif N, Samet P, editors. Cardiac pacing and electrophysiology, Philadelphia: Saunders, 1991;524–44.
18. Ilvento J, Fee J, Shewmaker S. Automatic mode switching from DDDR to VVIR: A management algorithm for atrial arrythmias in patients with dual chamber pacemakers (abstract). PACE 1990;13:1199.
19. Lau CP, Tai YT, Fong PC, Li JPS, Chung FLW, Song S. The use of implantable sensors for the control of pacemaker mediated tachycardias: A comparative evaluation between minute ventilation sensing and acceleration sensing dual chamber rate adaptive pacemakers. PACE 1992;15:34–44.
20. Lee MT, Adkins A, Woodson D, Vandegriff J. A new feature for control of inappropriate high tracking in DDDR pacemakers. PACE 1990;13:1852–5.

29. Holter and pacemaker diagnostics

PAUL A. LEVINE

INTRODUCTION

The introduction of Holter monitoring almost 30 years ago was a major advance with respect to arrhythmia diagnosis and management, permitting medical personnel to identify transient arrhythmias, correlate symptoms with a multiplicity of rhythm disorders, and assess the effectiveness of any therapeutic interventions. Holter studies have also been used to evaluate pacing system function, often identifying a multiplicity of abnormalities, commonly transient and commonly not associated with symptoms. Thus, some physicians have recommended that Holter studies should be a routine component of a pacing system evaluation [1–4]. The Holter study commonly provides a variety of different formats for the same data. An individual study may comprise a continuous display of the rhythm at a compressed format, often showing 1 h of rhythm on a single page, an expansion of the rhythm for symptomatic events, counts of the number of ectopic beats which may be further separated by morphology and rhythm sequences, as well as heart rate trends. For all the elegance of the current Holter recordings, knowledgeable personnel need to review the final result and often relabel individual complexes which are misinterpreted by the automatic recognition algorithms.

As pacing systems increase in complexity, assessing pacing system function requires more time and effort and even then may miss intermittent problems, spontaneous but infrequent arrhythmias, or the fact that the pacing system may not be optimally programmed for the patient. Bidirectional telemetry has allowed for the transmission of a variety of real-time data from the pacing system, including programmed parameters, lead and battery status, endocardial electrograms, and annotated event markers [5–12]. These have enhanced the physician's ability to assess the pacing system function while the patient is in the office. If a problem is present during that evaluation, real-time telemetric features which have virtually eliminated a multiplicity of ancillary tests allow a precise diagnosis to be made immediately. However, this capability cannot retrospectively identify an intermittent problem, assess the overall function of the pacing system, nor provide clues as to the etiology of an episode of palpitations or near-syncope that occurred prior to the office evaluation. Thus, Holter studies are often a valuable adjunct to the evaluation of the implanted paging system.

The utilization of Holter monitors to assess the implanted pacing system is associated with some major limitations. Many recording systems utilize special filters to minimize baseline noise which may render recognition of the pacing stimulus difficult, if not impossible in the case of some bipolar pacing systems. In addition, the sensor signal used to modulate the function of an increasing number of pacemakers is electrocardiographically invisible. Perhaps the major limitations are that the recording period is commonly limited to 24 h, that the staff who process these recordings are not knowledgeable with respect to pacing system timing, and that the patient has to come in one day to have the monitoring system applied and return the next day to have the unit removed. In addition, Holter recording systems are usually prescribed after the patient experiences a symptomatic episode which, if infrequent, results in a nondiagnostic study.

Concomitant with the enhanced real-time diagnostic capabilities of the modern pacemaker, technologic advances with respect to random access memory (RAM) and read only memory (ROM) systems capable of functioning in a low-power environment and bidirectional telemetry have allowed memory to be incorporated in the implanted pacemaker and cardioverter-defibrillator. Devices are now capable of providing the medical staff caring for the patient with a variety of data concerning the system's performance over a variable period of time. This capability, generically termed event counter telemetry, has also been described as an implantable Holter system since it can provide data similar to that available with the external Holter studies even though it lacks the ECG rhythm strips that are the hallmark of a Holter recording.

Relatively simple memory storage systems were first utilized to allow the physician to enter administrative data into the implanted device, including the date of implantation, threshold and impedance measurements made at the implant procedure, and lead configuration. Whenever the pacemaker is read, these data would be reported along with the programmed parameters.

EVENT COUNTER CAPABILITY

As the memory capacity increased, manufacturers included the ability to report the percent of time the pacemaker was either inhibited or pacing. Further refinements of these algorithms allowed the pacemaker to report episodes of bradycardia defined as very slow rates for a period of time. If the bradycardia persists for a defined length of time, then pacing at a faster rate is initiated, a form of hysteresis function, with additional details being provided by the event counter such as the number of times this feature was activated [13].

Single chamber pacing utilizes only two pacing states. Either a pacemaker pulse is emitted or a native complex is sensed, thus resetting the timing circuits of the pacemaker prior to completion of the timing period. Since pacemakers function by a series of timing circuits, the system will know the interval from the start of the timing period to the moment when it is reset. Within a series of ranges, these data can also be stored, allowing the event counters to report not only the number of paced and sensed events, but the number of beats occurring within a series of rate bins during the time period being monitored.

Dual chamber pacemakers, specifically the DDD mode, function in one of five pacing states, including the following. An atrial sensed event followed by a ventricular sensed event is most commonly a native sinus complex and may be designated PR or AsVs depending upon the system. An atrial sensed event followed by a ventricular paced event is P wave synchronous ventricular pacing and will be identified by the notation PV or AsVp. An atrial paced complex followed by a sensed ventricular event would reflect functional single chamber atrial pacing with intact AV nodal conduction. It would be identified by the cryptic notation AR or ApVs. An atrial paced event followed by a ventricular paced event represents AV sequential pacing and would be labeled AV or ApVp. A sensed ventricular complex, an R wave, that is not preceded by any atrial activity as far as the pacemaker is concerned would be a premature ventricular event, abbreviated PVE.

Interpreting event counter data is similar to interpreting event marker data. This diagnostic feature reports the pacemaker's perception of what is happening. Namely, the pacemaker effectively knows when it releases an output pulse and when it inhibits or resets a timing circuit based upon a sensed event. It is not yet sufficiently sophisticated to know whether the output pulse was clinically appropriate or effective. For example, oversensing of myopotentials on the atrial channel will trigger a ventricular output, and the system will report one or more PV events. The system has no way of ascertaining that the atrial sensed event was not a true P wave. By the same token, the implanted pacemaker cannot determine that the released output pulse was effective in causing a depolarization. The released pulse could have occurred in a physiologic refractory period due to a primary undersensing problem, or it could have been ineffective but the patient was asymptomatic because there was a native complex shortly after the ineffective pacing stimulus. This native complex might not be sensed because it coincides with the pacemaker's refractory period. Without an independent evaluation of the pacing system performance and clinical knowledge of the patient, the ability to interpret the event counter data will be limited.

SYSTEM PERFORMANCE COUNTERS

This subset of event counter capability is similar to the tabular summary reports in many Holter systems, providing total counts of sinus, atrial, and ventricular ectopic beats, number of runs of supraventricular and ventricular tachycardia, etc. The system performance counters in a pacemaker will provide an overview of the system performance either during a finite monitoring period or since the last time the counters were cleared. The amount of data capable of being collected is directly dependent upon the memory capacity of the pacemaker.

Each data point (sensed or paced event) is stored as a bit represented in a binary system using '1's' and '0's'. If the memory capacity has 8 bits, there will be 256 potential combinations of '1's' and '0's' allowing the system to store 256 data points. In practice, this is not very much memory if each paced or native beat is considered one sequence of 8 bits. At a rate of 60 bpm, a little over 4 min of data will be collected to fill the memory. However, increasing the number of bits results in a geometric increase in memory capacity. Twenty-four bits or 3 bytes (1 byte equals 8 bits) allows for the collection of approximately 17 million data points which will provide 6 months of data when every complex is stored. The Pacesetter Synchrony® series of pacemakers assign over 4000 bytes of memory to event counter functions. Progressively increased memory will allow for the storage of even larger amounts of data.

Event counter telemetry in a first generation DDD pacemaker, the Intermedics Cosmos® series, reported the number of counts in each of the five pacing states, the percent of time pacing occurred in the atrium and the ventricle, the number of times the pacemaker reached the programmed upper rate limit up to a maximum of 255 times, and the largest number of sensed peaks in a given complex [14, 15]. On subsequent iterations of the software controlling this system, no limit was placed on the number of times that the pacemaker reached its upper rate limit that could be reported, and in place of the number of peaks in a sensed event, they reported the number of times the tachycardia termination algorithm was utilized (Figure 1).

The Intermedics event counters were very helpful in providing an overview of the pacing system performance. A large percentage of AR or AV pacing reflected base rate pacing. A large percentage of PV pacing reflected either AV block or too short a programmed AV delay. These counters, without the ability to also report the rates that were achieved, became limiting with the advent of rate modulation. While a patient with sinus node dysfunction with or without concomitant AV block would be expected to be predominantly atrially paced, either AR or AV, one cannot assess the appropriateness of the sensor parameters without knowing the actual distribution of the rates within the AR and AV pacing states. By the same token, knowing that a majority of the complexes are atrial sensed, either PV or PR, does not allow the physician to assess the chronotropic function of the sinus node. One needs to know also the actual rates which have been achieved in each of these pacing states.

The report of pacing state and rate data is included in the Event Histogram [16] feature of the Siemens Pacesetter series of rate-modulated pacemakers.

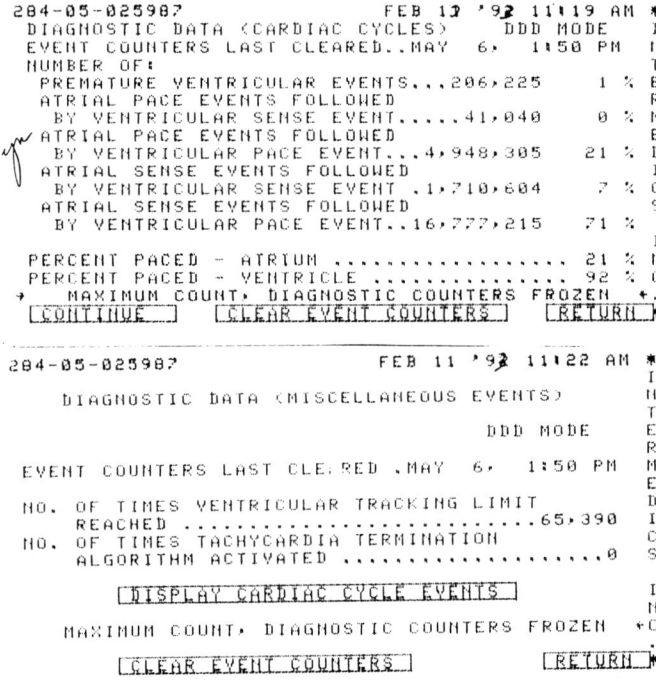

Figure 1. Printout from the event counters in an Intermedics Cosmos II model 284–05. Total number of counts in each of the five pacing states are reported along with the percent paced in atrium and ventricle, number of times the maximum tracking rate was reached, and number of times the PMT algorithm was activated. The counters were frozen after accumulating 16 777 215 counts in one of the pacing state bins. The distribution of counts in each of the pacing states is retained until the counters are cleared.

This feature utilizes 192 bytes of memory and has been documented to record over 400 days of data while monitoring every event and without having reached the maximum storage capacity. It has been calculated that if the system were set to a sampling rate of every 26 s and all the complexes were at the identical rate and pacing state, it would take at least 13 years before the counters would be full.

This capability allows the physician to assess the distribution of rates in each of the pacing states that occurred over a period of time, the effect of various programming changes on pacing system behavior, as well as the percentage pacing in both the atrial and ventricular channels (Figure 2). If the AV delay is increased and AV nodal conduction is intact, one should see an increased percentage of ventricular sensed events (PR and AR) with a concomitant reduction in the percent of ventricular paced events. If the

EVENT HISTOGRAM

Total Time Sampled 69d 8h 37m 33s
Sampling Rate EVERY EVENT

```
Mode _____ DDD
Sensor _____ PASSIVE
Rate _____ 50 ppm
Max Track _____ 143 ppm
Maximum Sensor Rate _____ 135 ppm
A-V Delay _____ 250 msec
Rate Resp. A-V Delay _____ ENABLE
```

Note: The above values were obtained
when the histogram was interrogated.

Rate ppm	PV	PR	AV	AR	PVE
0-60	50,839	665,860	73,137	24,227	0
61-67	117,617	1,009,981	8	14	409
68-75	22,925	1,498,991	0	0	820
76-85	3,957	1,814,918	0	0	693
86-100	352	1,510,115	0	0	12,287
101-119	35	374,277	0	0	39,037
120-149	101	94,198	0	0	15,081
> 149	0	3,359	0	0	1,095
Total:	195,826	6,971,699	73,145	24,241	69,422

Total Event Count: 7,334,333

Percent Paced in Atrium _____ 1%
Percent Paced in Ventricle _____ 4%
Total Time at Max Track Rate _____ 0d 0h 0m 0s

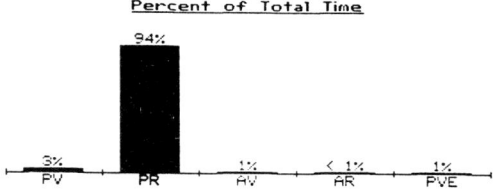

Figure 2. The event histogram from a Siemens Pacesetter Synchrony 2022 showing both the total number of counts and percent pacing in each pacing state. In addition, the distribution of complexes in a series of 8 rate bins allows the physician to assess chronotropic function and if the sensor had been enabled, the actual number of AV and AR pacing complexes above the base rate that would have been due to the sensor.

sensor is enabled one would expect to see AR and AV paced complexes up to the programmed maximum sensor rate. Further, since the majority of individuals spend most of their time in relatively sedentary activity, one would expect to see the largest number of complexes at the lower rates, with progressively smaller numbers in the higher rate bins. If this is not the case, one might suspect that the sensor was not set appropriately.

The effect of enabling the sensor or adjusting a pharmacologic regimen according to the frequency of premature ventricular events, most commonly ventricular ectopic beats or accelerated junctional rhythms, can also be assessed by taking advantage of this feature at the time of the routine follow-up pacing system evaluations without having to repeatedly perform true Holter studies.

The Event Histogram has also been used to help determine whether the patient even needs the rate-modulated features of the pacemaker. One approach is to not enable the sensor parameters of the pacemaker at the time of initial implantation, even in those patients who are known to be chronotropically incompetent. It is preferable that the pocket first heal and the patient acclimate to the higher base rates associated with pacing. The sensor is programmed to PASSIVE, which will provide access to the event counters. When the patient is seen at the 1 month follow-up visit, the counter data is retrieved. This provides an overview of the system function during that 1-month period of time. If there is a limitation to the chronotropic reserve, the sensor is then enabled. If chronotropic function is normal, one can either continue to monitor the system performance by leaving the sensor PASSIVE or further reduce the battery current drain by programming the sensor to OFF. When the sensor is OFF, the system will not acquire and store the event counter data. On an annual basis, the sensor is programmed to PASSIVE to take advantage of the event counters for a period of approximately 1 month to determine if chronotropic function continues to be normal or has been compromised, warranting activation of the sensor at that follow-up visit. Similarly, the counters can be utilized to assess the effect of changing the patient's pharmacologic regimen on heart rate performance and AV conduction.

The major limitation of system performance counters with respect to the rate-modulated function of the implanted pacemaker is that they do not report the direct behavior of the sensor unless the sensor is totally controlling the pacing rates. If the single chamber system is being inhibited by the native rhythm or the dual chamber system is tracking native P waves, the counters described above will report the various rates and pacing states that actually occurred.

SENSOR-INDICATED RATE COUNTERS

Sensor-indicated rate counters allow the system to monitor and report the rates that would have occurred had the sensor been driving the pacemaker even when the pacemaker was being controlled by sensed native events [17, 18]. In the Pacesetter series of rate-modulated pacemakers, the data is obtainable with the sensor either ON and potentially controlling the pacemaker or simply being set to collect data, namely PASSIVE. Medtronic® also allows data collection with respect to the sensor function, but the system cannot be in the rate-modulated mode, and the counter must be specifically programmed to monitor the sensor behavior.

Being able to monitor the sensor behavior as reflected in the rates that would have resulted had the sensor been controlling the pacemaker allows the medical staff caring for the patient to set the sensor parameters even when the pacemaker is being inhibited. If data can be collected over a protracted period of time, one can also acquire an overview of the sensor performance based upon the distribution of rates (Figure 3). If these rate distributions are reasonable and rate modulation is desired based upon the system performance event counter data (i.e. chronotropic incompetence), one might simply enable the sensor (ON) without having to do any additional testing. If the sensor behavior is not optimal based upon the sensor-indicated rate counter data, then a formal testing series would be indicated if rate modulation is desired.

Sensor-indicated rate counters also allow the medical staff to determine the system response to a variety of activities of daily living in an electrocardiographically unmonitored environment, whether this be in the physician's office, walking outside, taking a shower, or swimming in the ocean. The response to specific activities can be assessed by clearing the counters, allowing the patient to do the activity, and then reading the counters upon completion of the activity.

The major strength of the sensor-indicated rate counters is also its major limitation. It reports the rates that would have occurred had the sensor been totally controlling the pacing rate. It does not report the actual rates which were achieved which might have been a combination of the sensor and native rhythms or totally controlled by the native rhythm. Thus, the system performance and sensor-indicated rate counters complement one another.

Both these counters suffer from a common limitation. Their data regarding rates are stored in rate bins. Even during short periods of monitoring providing data with respect to one specific activity, each rate is simply stored in its respective bin. One does not know when one complex represented by a pacing state and rate occurred with respect to another complex. There is yet a third counter capability which might be generically identified as a time-based system performance counter.

TIME-BASED SYSTEM PERFORMANCE COUNTERS

Time-based system performance counters acquire and store data with respect to rate, pacing state, and time. Placing each pacing complex in a time sequence requires a significant increase in memory capacity. By way of example, the Event Histogram in the Pacesetter rate-modulated pacemakers utilizes 192 bytes of memory capable of accumulating upwards of 1 year of data when sampling every event. The Event Record, which is a time-based system performance counter, utilizes 4096 bytes of memory and then, sam-

SENSOR INDICATED RATE HISTOGRAM

Total Time Sampled: 53d 19h 25m 46s
Sampling Rate: 1.6 seconds

```
Sensor _____ PASSIVE
Rate _____ 50 ppm
Maximum Sensor Rate _____ 135 ppm
Slope _____ 8 (Normal)
Threshold _____ AUTO (+0.5)
Reaction Time _____ FAST
Recovery Time _____ MEDIUM
   Measured Average Sensor _____ 4.0
```

Note: The above values were obtained when the histogram was interrogated.

Bin Number	Range (ppm)	Time				Sample Counts
1	45 – 57	42d	8h	19m	29s	2,251,550
2	57 – 69	6d	8h	19m	37s	337,463
3	69 – 81	2d	16h	9m	34s	142,138
4	81 – 93	1d	10h	30m	12s	76,438
5	93 – 105	0d	18h	18m	14s	40,550
6	105 – 117	0d	4h	30m	13s	9,977
7	117 – 129	0d	1h	9m	56s	2,582
8	129 – 141	0d	0h	8m	32s	315
					Total:	2,861,013

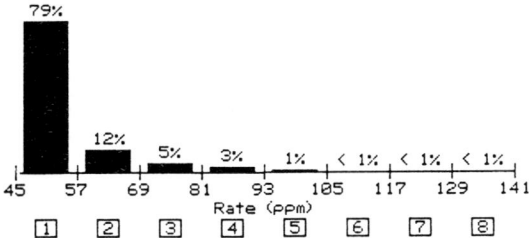

Figure 3. The sensor-indicated rate histogram reporting on the behavior of the sensor over the preceding 53 days. This shows an appropriate distribution of rates as if the sensor had been totally controlling the system. As it was, the sensor was PASSIVE and thus disengaged from any control of the actual pacing rate. Had the patient required rate-modulated support, the sensor could have been enabled at these parameters as there was an appropriate distribution of rates.

pling every event, will acquire roughly 1 h of data. Less frequent sampling rates can increase the monitoring period to 30 h.

There are two ways of processing these data. One is to provide a fixed amount of data storage capability which is frozen when all the counters are full. Interpreting the stored data will be difficult if it is months old since the patient will not remember the activities or symptoms that occurred while the data was being collected. A more effective means of using these data is analogous to a transient arrhythmia monitor. Once the counters are full, the oldest data is deleted to make room for the newest data. This capability has been termed LIFO (last in, first out). In some cases, specific symptoms can be marked as with placement of a magnet over the pacemaker, but this then requires that the patient either hold the magnet in place until the data can be downloaded into the programmer or the patient goes to the physician's office before the data are effectively erased by the continued acquisition of new data. In the future, the system capability will allow the patient to activate a special device which will cause the pacemaker to store and not erase a symptomatic episode until the data can be retrieved at a later date.

At the present time, real-time system performance counters have proven very effective in assessing symptoms and system behavior, screening for chronotropic incompetence, and determining if the sensor is responding appropriately. I prefer to leave the monitoring frequency at every event. Prior to coming into the office, the patient is asked to perform a standard series of activities that would be done in the course of a normal day. These same activities are repeated each time the patient comes for a follow-up evaluation. During the initial evaluation, the real-time system performance counter data is acquired via telemetry. A clinical judgment can be made as to whether the level of increase in rate was appropriate or inappropriate for the given activity that was performed just prior to entering the office (Figure 4). Indeed, if it is appropriate, the rate response of the patient, whether due to the intrinsic sinus mechanism or the sensor, has been effectively assessed without taking additional time during the office evaluation. Further, the data can be displayed in a number of different formats reflecting actual pacing state distributions, atrial sensed vs. atrial paced rates, or the scale for a specific section can be expanded, allowing an examination of each and every complex that was recorded.

This has proven to be extremely helpful when the patient presents with an episode of palpitations in that it reports the pacemaker's perspective of the symptomatic event which, either alone or in combination with the surface ECG [16], may give a further insight in to the rhythm (Figures 4, 5 and 6).

Another real-time counter that is proving effective in programming the system is the 'redraw' feature included in the Intermedics rate-modulated series of pacemakers. The system monitors the ventricular rates which have been achieved over a period of time while the patient performs various activities. When the patient returns, a graph of the rates that have been achieved is displayed. Also monitored and transmitted to the programmer is

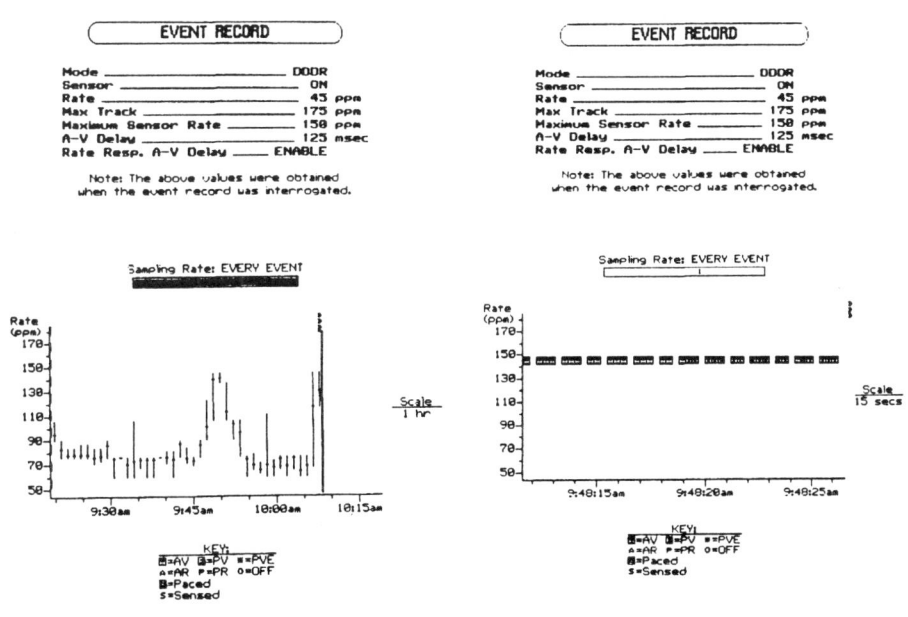

Figure 4. Time-based system performance counter called an event record in a patient with a Siemens Pacesetter Synchrony 2020. The sensor parameters were too responsive, resulting in an increase in the sensor-controlled rate to 140–150 bpm during a normal walk. (Reprinted with permission from Siemens Pacesetter [16]).

the sensor-input signal data acquired by the pacemaker during this exercise period. By entering different rate response factors into the programmer, the rates that would have developed based upon the sensor signals' response to the new sensor parameters at the various points in time during the exercise are displayed in graphic form. The medical staff caring for the patient can then determine which sensor rate-response parameter provides the best response for that patient. It is noteworthy that the rates which are displayed may be due to either sensor drive or endogenous rhythms. This feature is a combination of the time-based system performance and sensor-indicated rate counters.

ANTITACHYCARDIA SYSTEMS

The foregoing discussion focused on bradycardia and rate-modulated pacing systems and how the various counters have been and could be used to better understand and assess the effectiveness of any programming of the implanted system. Devices implanted specifically for the management of tachycardias

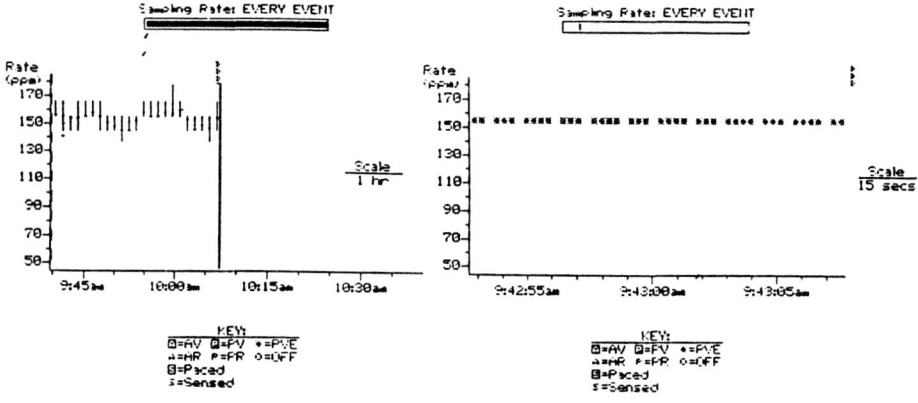

Figure 5. Time-based system performance counter recorded during a sustained tachycardia. While each of the complexes is identified by the pacemaker as a PVE, further evaluation demonstrated AV nodal reentrant tachycardia with each of the P waves occurring in the terminal portion of the QRS and, thus, coinciding with the PVARP. Although a brief rhythm strip as represented by the 15 s of data shown on the right was absolutely stable, the rate can be seen to fluctuate on the 30 min of compressed data shown in the printout on the left.

require additional capabilities to enable the physician to assess system performance and determine if therapy had been delivered and if it was appropriate [19–23].

The third-generation tiered therapy devices capable of providing both antitachycardia pacing as well as low-energy and high-energy shocks incorporate a multiplicity of counters in conjunction with real-time clocks. The system continuously monitors its performance. When a tachycardia is identified and therapy initiated, many systems will report the time, the system's diagnosis, the rates or intervals that occurred, the therapy that was delivered, and the response to that therapy (Figure 7). Some systems will store the actual intervals between a consecutive number of sensed complexes preceding and a similar number of complexes following delivery of therapy, whether it be antitachycardia pacing or a shock.

Some systems also store the actual electrograms (Figure 8) rather than just intervals (Ventritex Cadence®) or a snapshot of the various morphology complexes within the tachycardia and following delivery of therapy (Telec-

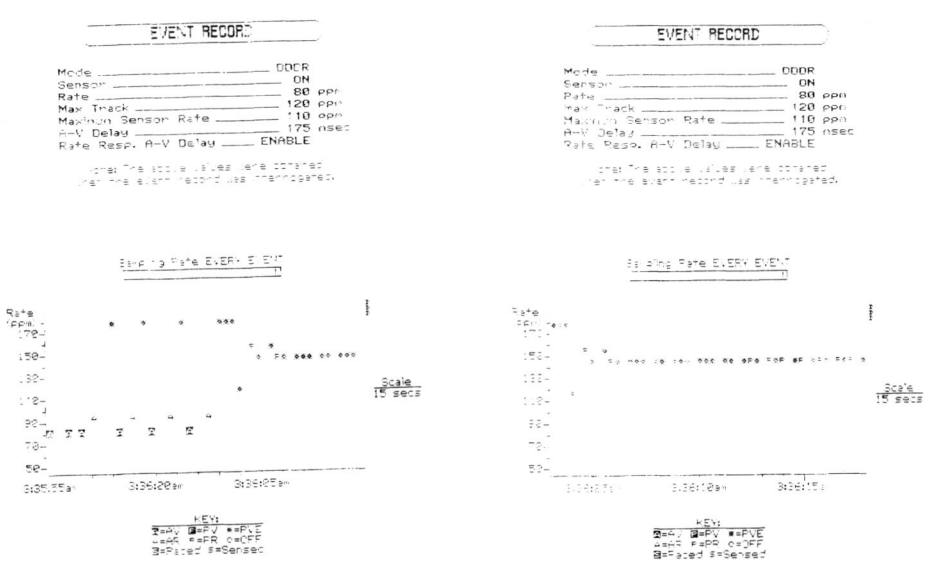

Figure 6. Time-based system performance counter showing the onset and early portion of a sustained monomophic ventricular tachycardia. The early portion of the pacing system behavior is shown on the left. There is AV pacing identified by the letter A within the black box and frequent PVEs which were true PVCs. Those PVCs which followed an atrial output were identified as AR by the pacemaker and shown by the letter A. The patient developed a sustained monomorphic ventricular tachycardia with 2:1 retrograde VA conduction. The retrograde P wave was sensed, and when this was followed by the ventricular tachycardia beat, the pacemaker labeled it a PR complex and noted this with an isolated P label.

tronics Guardian®). Storage of continuous electrograms requires a significant amount of memory, and thus, electrograms for only the last three episodes are retained. At the moment, the instructions to the device to store this information is based upon the determination of a tachycardia and the delivery of therapy. Many manufacturers are working on the ability to store electrograms, possibly from both the atrial and ventricular channels in the case of dual chamber systems, with automatic storage occurring in response to either specified events or patient initiated based upon symptoms. Extensive electrogram storage will require a marked expansion of the device's memory capacity. Work is actively proceeding in this area by many manufacturers.

IMPLANTABLE MONITORS

The data storage capabilities that have been discussed above have been recognized by many investigators as forming the basis for a fully-implanted rhythm monitoring device [24]. If there is sufficient memory, the electrocar-

| Episodes |

```
            1992 Aug 5 07:16        Therapy Successful

Detection Rate ............ 179 bpm  Term. Coupling Int:  S1 ... 229 ms
Predetection Rate .......... 97 bpm                       S2 ... 229 ms
Cycle Length Stability ..... 33 ms                        S3 ... 229 ms
                                                          S4 ... 279 ms
                                                          S5 ... 279 ms
No of Extra Stim Attempts .... 1
No of Stim in Last Attempt ... 5



            1992 Jul 10 06:48       Therapy Successful

Detection Rate ............ 187 bpm  Term. Coupling Int:  S1 ... 219 ms
Predetection Rate ......... 121 bpm                       S2 ... 219 ms
Cycle Length Stability .... 189 ms                        S3 ... 219 ms
                                                          S4 ... 270 ms
                                                          S5 ... 270 ms
No of Extra Stim Attempts .... 2
No of Stim in Last Attempt ... 5
```

Figure 7. Summary of two episodes of ventricular tachycardia identified and treated by a Siemens Pacesetter Siecure 2120 ICD using antitachycardia pacing therapy. The tachycardia rate and stability are identified. The native rate preceding the tachycardia is also reported, as are the number of ATP attempts that were required, the number of extra stimuli in each attempt, and the cycle lengths of the successful ATP sequence. The actual time and date are also recorded by the implanted system.

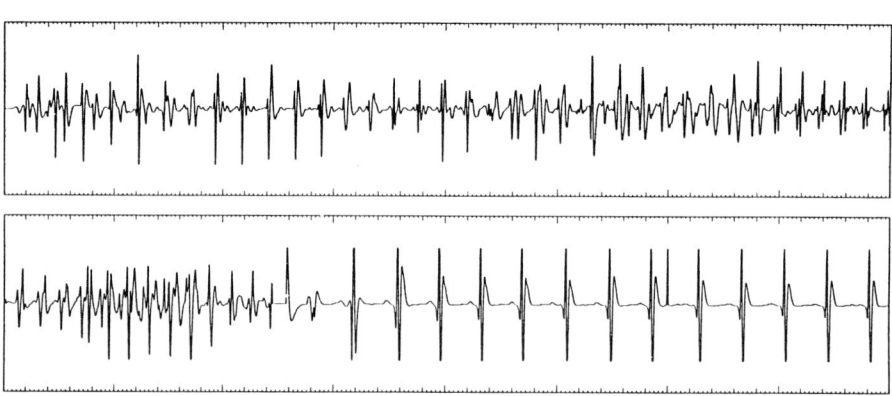

Figure 8. Stored electrograms from a Ventritex Cadence documenting an episode of either ventricular fibrillation or polymorphic ventricular tachycardia successfully terminated by a single shock. Contributed by Dr. Eric Fein, Ventritex Inc.

diogram as recorded from subcutaneous electrodes located on the housing of the implanted device will permit long-term monitoring in high-risk patients. This is a direct outgrowth of the experience with implantable pacemakers and antitachycardia systems. These will be true implanted Holter monitors, eliminating the need for the placement of special leads or visits to place and remove a Holter monitor and allowing the recording of rhythm data during activities such as swimming which are currently precluded with an external device. Further refinements in technology will allow physiologic parameters other than rhythm (i.e. oxygen saturation, temperature, pH, blood glucose) to be monitored over protracted periods of time. These data will be available for retrieval at the time of a routine office visit assuming that the physician has the appropriate receiver to communicate with the implanted monitor and, possibly, transtelephonically.

CONCLUSION

The diagnostic features incorporated in the modern pacemaker greatly facilitate the ability of medical staff in caring for the patient to assess the pacing system and to better understand the interaction between the patient and the implanted pacemaker. The multiple capabilities, while not required for all patients at each follow-up visit, complement one another and provide a valuable baseline for future evaluations should a problem with the system be either suspected or actually present. An integral part of these diagnostic features include extensive event counter monitoring and electrogram storage capability. This technology will continue to grow until fully-implantable Holter and other physiologic monitors which are on the horizon can greatly facilitate the physician's ability to care for all patients.

REFERENCES

1. Famularo MA, Kennedy HL. Ambulatory electrocardiography in the assessment of pacemaker function. Am Heart J 1982;104:1086–94.
2. Janosik DL, Redd RM, Buckingham TA et al. Utility of ambulatory electrocardiography in detecting pacemaker dysfunction in the early postimplantation period. Am J Cardiol 1987;60:1030–5.
3. Ursell S, El-Sherif N. Electrocardiography of single chamber pacemakers. Value of Holter monitoring for follow-up of pacemaker patients. In: Saksena S, Goldschalger N, editors. Electrical Therapy for Cardiac Arrhythmias. Philadelphia: Saunders, 1990:220–4.
4. Van Gelder LM, Bracke FALE, El Gamal MIH. Fusion or confusion on Holter recording. PACE 1991;14:760–3.
5. Kruse I, Markowitz T, Ryden L. Timing markers showing pacemaker behavior to aid in the follow-up of a physiologic pacemaker. PACE 1983;6:801–5.
6. Olson W, McConnell M, Sah R et al. Pacemaker diagnostic diagrams. PACE 1985;8:691–700.

7. Levine PA, Schüller H, Lindgren A. Pacemaker ECG. Utilization of pulse generator telemetry. Solna, Sweden: Siemens Elema AB, 1988.
8. Levine PA, Sholder J, Duncan JL. Clinical benefits of telemetered electrograms in the assessment of DDD function. PACE 1984;7:1170-7.
9. Clarke M, Allen A. Use of telemetered electrograms in the assessment of normal pacemaker function. J Electrophysiol 1987;1:388-95.
10. Sarmiento JJ. Clinical utility of telemetered intracardiac electrograms in diagnosing a design dependent lead malfunction. PACE 1990;13:188-95.
11. Luceri RM, Castellanos A, Thurer RJ. Telemetry of intracardiac electrograms; Applications in spontaneous and induced arrhythmias. J Electrophysiol 1987;1:417-24.
12. Levine PA. The complementary role of electrogram, event marker and measured data telemetry in the assessment of pacing system function. J Electrophysiol 1987;1:404-16.
13. Stangl K, Wirtzfeld A, Sichart U et al. The combined use of hysteresis and Holter functions improves diagnosis and therapy in patients with sick sinus syndrome. PACE 1988;11:1698-702.
14. Sanders R, Martin R, Frumin H et al, Data storage and retrieval by implantable pacemakers for diagnostic purposes. PACE 1984;7:1228-33.
15. Levine PA, Lindenberg BS. Diagnostic data: An aid to the follow-up and assessment of the pacing system. J Electrophysiol 1987;1:396-403.
16. Levine PA. Utility and clinical benefits of extensive event counter telemetry in the follow-up and management of the rate-modulated pacemaker patient. Sylmar, CA: Siemens Pacesetter, 1992.
17. Hayes DL, Higano ST, Eisinger G. Utility of rate histograms in programming and follow-up of a DDDR pacemaker. Mayo Clin Proc 1989;64:495-502.
18. Levine PA, Sholder JA, Florio J. Obtaining maximal benefit from a DDDR pacing system: A reliable yet simple method for programming the sensor parameters of Synchrony. Sylmar, CA: Siemens Pacesetter, 1990.
19. Newman D, Dorian P, Downar E et al. Use of telemetry functions in the assessment of implanted antitachycardia device efficiency. Am J Cardiol 1992;70:616-21.
20. Wang PJ, Mandalakas N, Clyne C et al, Accuracy of rhythm classification using a data log system in implantable cardioverter defibrillators. PACE 1991;14:1911-6.
21. Luceri RM, Puchferran RL, Brownstein SL et al. Improved patient surveillance and data acquisition with a third generation implantable cardioverter defibrillator. PACE 1991;14:1870-4.
22. Hurwitz JL, Hook BG, Flores BT, Marchlinski FE. Importance of abortive shock capability with electrogram storage in cardioverter-defibrillator devices. J Am Coll Cardiol 1993;21:895-900.
23. Almeida HF, Buckingham TA. Inappropriate implantable cardioverter defibrillator shocks secondary to sensing lead failure: Utility of stored electrograms. PACE 1993;116:407-11.
24. Leitch J, Klein G, Yee R et al. Feasibility of an implantable arrhythmia monitor. PACE 1992;15:2232-5.

30. Clinical relevance of histograms in the follow-up of DDDR pacemakers

MARC M.J. BERKHOF, JOZEF P. SNOECK, MARNIX P.N. GOETHALS & MARC J. CLAEYS

INTRODUCTION

As technology has improved over the years, implanted devices designed for pacing therapy have become more and more sophisticated. Due to the development of dual chamber pacemakers with rate-response systems, the treatment of bradyarrhythmia has become more 'physiological'. Appropriate individualized programming of the pacemaker is both possible and necessary. Information about the intrinsic heart rate and the sensor rate-response of the pacemaker is obligatory for optimal adjustment of the rate-modulated pacemaker. An accurate detection of atrial tachyarrhythmia is mandatory to program the response of the pacemaker to a pathological rate-excess (e.g. by using automatic mode switching). Until now, exercise tests and external telemetry (24-h Holter recording) were the main tools available to obtain this information. Both techniques are time consuming and rather expensive. Moreover, exercise tests do not represent normal daily activity and have a rather low sensitivity for the detection of atrial arrhythmias. Holter recording has the disadvantage of evaluating the heart rhythm during a limited period and can be difficult to interpret because of low P wave signals.

Therefore, telemetry pacing systems have recently been expanded with internal diagnostic databases. These systems store both the native heart rhythm and the activity of the internal sensor. This information can be reproduced and presented by means of histograms. Both numeric and graphic information on the intrinsic heart rate and the sensor-driven pacing-rate distribution over time is thus available. The histogram provides a conveniently arranged summary of data stored over a long period of time. In the following paragraphs the different kinds of histograms will be discussed. Special attention will be drawn to the clinical relevance of histograms in follow-up of DDD(R) pacemakers.

HISTOGRAM FOLLOW-UP PROCEDURE OF A DDDR PACEMAKER

Patients with chronotropic incompetence with or without normal AV conduction are candidates for a sensor-driven device (AAIR or DDDR) [1]. In order to choose the correct device, one should investigate the patient's chronotropic (in)competence before implanting the device. This is, however, not always possible in daily practice. Therefore, we suggest implanting only DDD or VVI pacemakers in patients with manifest chronotropic competence. In case of doubt, a rate-adaptive system is chosen, and the chronotropic competence can be evaluated after implantation. After implantation, the pacemaker is programmed in DDD mode and, if available, with PASSIVE sensing. From the first day after implantation, the atrial rate and the sensor-indicated rate (SIR) are stored without affecting the patient's basic stimulation rate [2]. This information can be obtained as histograms, providing graphic representation by rate bins over time. During subsequent days, the pacemakers basic DDD functions are carefully observed. Only when these are operating appropriately [3], is the following DDDR follow-up procedure started. This procedure encompasses the evaluation of:

1. P wave amplitude
2. Sinus node function
3. AV node function
4. Lower and upper rate behavior
5. Mode switching
6. Long-term ventricular rate

To obtain the full benefit from a sophisticated DDDR device, we suggest proceeding systematically through this follow-up schedule by using the appropriate histograms. If the interrogation of these histograms are too time-consuming for the cardiologist, he or she might delegate this function to a senior engineer or senior nurse. The senior can put the print-outs into the medical file for review by the cardiologist at a later time. Not every manufacturer or DDDR pacemaker allows the retrieval of all the diagnostic data mentioned, however. Nevertheless, the follow-up procedure can be a guideline for the follow-up of a DDDR pacemaker.

CLINICAL BENEFITS OF HISTOGRAMS

The P wave amplitude histogram

A P wave histogram as measured in the Vitatron model 800 type Diamond (DDDR QT + ACT) is shown in Figure 1. The graph represents data of the sensed peak-to-peak amplitude for different mV ranges. The P wave amplitude histogram is upgraded only for sensed beats. Therefore, these data can only be obtained if the programmed lower rate limit (LRL) is below the patient's intrinsic heart rate. Figure 1A shows that a majority of sensed P

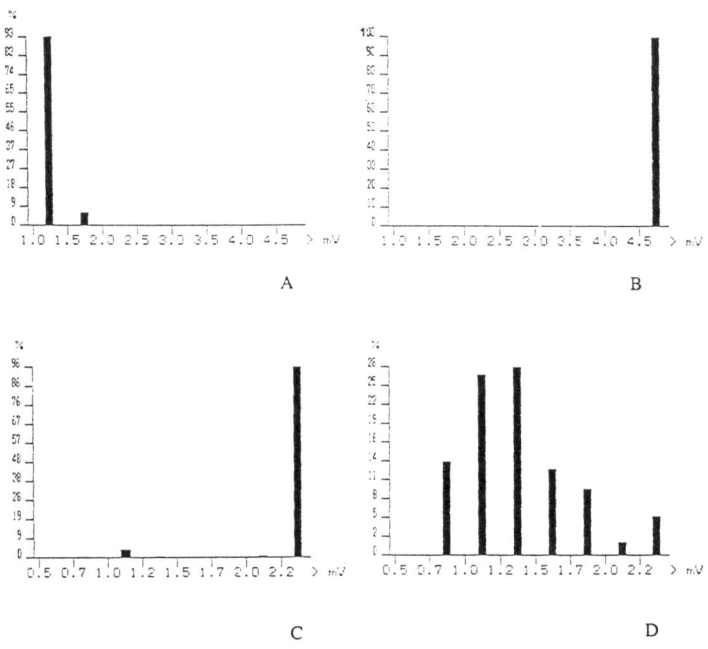

Figure 1. Different P wave amplitude histograms in % over mV bin ranges. (A) A low P wave amplitude. (B) A high P wave amplitude. (C) The presence of atrial arrhythmias. (D) The P wave amplitude of an atrial screw-in during the acute phase, or the suggestion of an unstable lead position in the chronic phase.

wave amplitudes lies in the bin range of 1.0–1.5 mV. These results indicate that the device should be programmed to an atrial sensitivity of less than 1.0 mV to achieve a good atrial sensing. Figure 1B illustrates an instance of much higher P wave amplitudes. Here the atrial sensitivity can be programmed up to a maximum of 2.5 mV with an acceptable sensing safety margin. Figure 1C shows a histogram with P-wave amplitudes of 2.5 mV, but at the same time some P waves of low amplitude (±1 mV). A clear gap is thus present between the two measured bin ranges. This suggests the presence of atrial arrhythmias. A wide, spread of sampled P wave bin ranges, such as shown in Figure 1D, can be observed in the acute phase post-implantation of an atrial screw-in lead. In the chronic phase it suggests an unstable lead tip position.

Sinus node function: Atrial rate, event and SIR histogram

During the programming and follow-up of DDDR devices, there is a need for data concerning the atrial response to daily life activities in order to

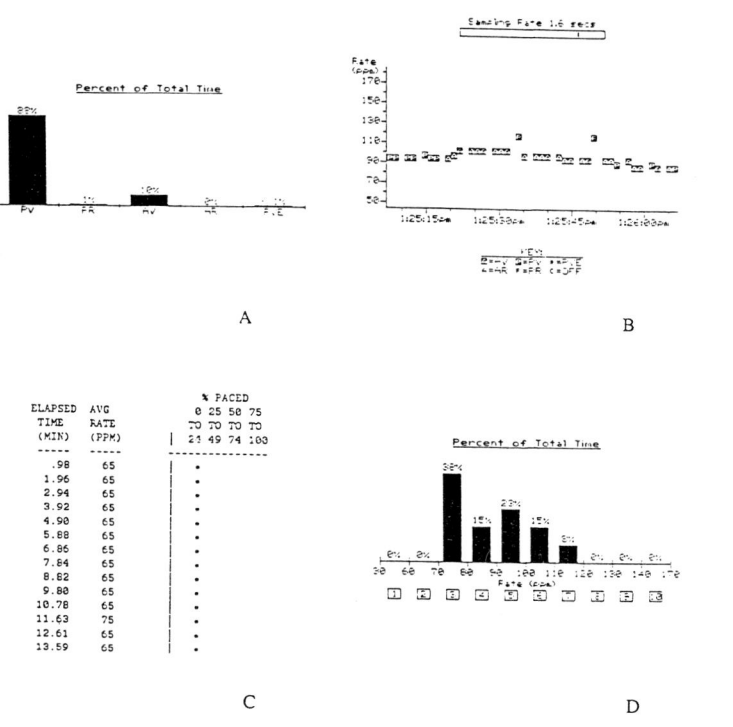

Figure 2. Histograms which can be used to investigate chronotropic (in)competence. (A) Data on the number of atrial and ventricular sensed (P and R) and paced (A and V) beats in DDD mode. (B) Rate of sensed and paced beats. (C) Percentage of paced beats as well as the average heart rate in a 'rolling trend'. (D) The sensor-indicated rate histogram (SIR) which can be used to define the sensor response 'in relation to activity.

adjust the rate-adaptation parameters. This can be obtained from exercise tests and repeated 24-h Holter recordings. These procedures are time-consuming and in many cases difficult to achieve, especially in elderly patients. We therefore propose using the *atrial rate and event histograms* in order to define the patient's chronotropic status.

An *atrial rate histogram* displays the atrial rate bin ranges over time in DDD mode (for example in the Vitatron Diamond). This histogram has to be programmed and cleared before an observation period.

An *event histogram* contains data on the number of atrial and ventricular sensed (P and R) and paced (A and V) beats in DDD mode (see Figure 2A obtained in a Siemens DDDR + ACT, model 2022, type Synchrony II). The rate of sensed and paced atrial beats allows an evaluation of chronotropic competence (Figure 2B) [4–6]. Data can also be obtained on the timing of the sensed P waves (e.g. during refractory period, alert period. etc.). An alternative presentation is provided by the Medtronic DDDR + ACT, model 7086, type Legend II Event Counter. The printout comprises the percentage of paced beats as well as the average heart rate in a 'rolling trend' (Figure 2C).

In addition, simultaneously the sensor-indicated rate is stored into the *SIR* histogram (Figure 2D). The SIR histogram provides numeric and graphic data of the sensor rate distribution pattern over a long period of time. The printout shows the absolute number of counts per bin, total sampling time, sampling rate, and a graphic representation of the percentage of time that the sensor rate has been in the various ranges.

If during the follow-up a patient complains that he or she cannot do a certain exercise and the SIR histogram demonstrates only data in the lower rate bins, then the sensor threshold should be adapted. When the performance remains low, the other rate-adaptive parameters can be adjusted. Evaluation of the patient after some time and comparing his or her subjective impression with the SIR histogram allows careful adjustment of the rate-adaptive sensor parameters. The SIR histograms also permits the evaluation of a false-positive responsiveness of the sensor. This can be of use if the patient is working in an unstable environment. Testing in the PASSIVE mode avoids unwanted high responses due to environmental sources [7].

AV node function: AV delay vs. rate histogram

Once the sinus node function is well tested and the choice of the option sensor ON or OFF is made, the AV node function should be evaluated. The assessment of the optimal antegrade conduction time needs to be done regardless of the ON or OFF programming of the rate-responsiveness. An optimized AV interval is important for the patient's hemodynamic function [8]. When AV nodal conduction is intact and the native QRS is normal, optimal hemodynamics are usually achieved with an AV interval programmed to a longer value than the native AV interval. The native AV interval results definitely in a better ejection flow pattern [8]. Programming long AV delays can furthermore reduce the current drain up to 50% since the ventricular channel is not pacing. If the native AV conduction is absent or slowed, the patient's hemodynamic status should be optimized by using the algorithm of AV shortening during increasing atrial activity. The PR and AR data provide information concerning the normal antegrade conduction, and the AV, on the microprocessor-controlled AV delay. The Vitatron DDDR QT + ACT, model 800, type Diamond, measures the AV interval versus rate in the form of a histogram. This means that every PR and AR is marked on the graphic display. The clinical relevance is to define the presence of native AV conduction and its relation to rate.

Lower and upper rate behavior: Atrial rate and upper rate limit vs. time Holter

The atrial rate histogram allows adequate programming of the lower rate limit (LRL) as described above. The atrial rate above the upper rate limit (URL) can be monitored by using an URL Holter, which is present e.g. with the VITATRON DDDR QT + ACT, model 800, type Diamond. This Holter measures the time the atrial rate is above the programmed URL and discriminates physiological and pathological rate changes. If these data show physiological pacing above the URL, the URL should be set at a higher rate. If the Holter equals zero, the patient never exceeds the URL. If the data show pathological pacing above the URL, one should investigate the presence of atrial arrhythmias.

Mode switching

One of the major advantages of mode switching is the automatic switch at the start of an atrial arrhythmia from DDD(R) to VVI(R) or DDI(R) and the reversion to DDD(R) after the arrhythmia has stopped. There are at this moment no histograms that show direct data on mode switching. Programming the AV delay versus rate histogram can, however, give information as to whether there has been mode switching: long AV intervals on the histogram indicate the presence of mode switching from DDD(R) to DDI(R). If the AV interval versus rate histogram is not available, as is the case in the Telectronics DDDR + MV, model 1250H, type META, mode switching can be tested during pacemaker follow-up by using ECG markers on the liquid crystal display of the programmer. An indirect event counter for mode switching is present in the ELA Medical pacemaker DDDR + MV, model 7034, type CHORUS RM.

Long-term ventricular rate: SIR and ventricular rate vs. time histogram

After the final setting of the pacemaker parameters, a histogram can also be programmed for ventricular rate versus time. Interrogation of this histogram at follow-up, together with the SIR histogram, gives an indication of the patient's daily life activity [9] and on the presence of ventricular arrhythmias.

CONCLUSION

Little information is currently present in the medical literature on the usefulness and clinical relevance of histograms in pacemaker follow-up. A systematic approach is suggested to evaluate programming of a DDDR pacemaker.

The application of histograms that are obtainable from the devices can help the cardiologist in the management of the patient. Hopefully, in the near future standardisation will allow a user-friendly application of the histograms.

ACKNOWLEDGEMENTS

We would like to express our special thanks to Mrs. Monique Schrooten for her secretarial advice in preparing this manuscript, and to Mr. Marc Roovers for his Macintosh advice. Personally, I am most of all indebted to Prof. Dr. J. Snoeck, Head of the Department of Cardiology, who provided me with the knowledge of cardiac pacing throughout the past 14 years.

REFERENCES

1. Griffin JC. The optimal pacing mode for the individual patient: The role of DDDR. Cardiostim: New Perspect Cardiac Pacing 2 1991;14:325–38.
2. Hayes DL, Higano ST. Utility of rate histograms in programming and follow-up of a DDDR pacemaker. Mayo Clin Proc 1989;64:495–502.
3. Nalos PC, Nyitray W. Benefits of intracardiac electrocardiograms and programmable sensing polarity in preventing pacemaker inhibition due to spurious screw-in leads. PACE 1990;13:1101–4.
4. Throne RD, Jenkins JM, Dicarlo LA. The bin area method: A computationally efficient technique for analysis of atrial and ventricular intracardiac electrocardiograms. PACE 1990;13:1286–96.
5. Mahaux V, Waleffe A, Kulbertus H. Usefulness and adequacy of sensor data and retrieval for rate response simulation. PACE 1992;15:1688–95.
6. Levine PA. Utility and clinical benefits of extensive event counter telemetry in the follow-up and management of the rate-modulated pacemaker patient. Training Centre Siemens-Pacesetter 1992:1–26.
7. Marco D, Elsinger G, Hayes DL. Testing of work environments for electromagnetic interference. PACE 1992;15:2016–22.
8. Daubert JC, Ritter P et al. Physiological relationship between AV interval and heart rate in healthy subjects: Applications to DDD pacing. PACE 1986;9:1032–9.
9. Kostis JB, Moreyra AE, Amendo MT et al. The effect of age on heart rate in subjects free of heart disease. Circulation 1982;65:141–5.

31. Holter and telemetry in pacemakers and ICDs: new developments

ALAIN RIPART

INTRODUCTION

The purpose of this chapter is to explore new developments that go beyond basic Holter function technology in pacemakers and ICDs. The introduction of the microprocessor-based pacemaker in the early 1980s led to the development of the 'software pacemaker'. This in turn, opened the way for the development of multi-programming and telemetry of the main parameters of implantable pulse generators. Soon after, long-term evolutions of the rhythmologic profile of the patient, data concerning the functioning of the prosthesis, the tools to verify both (such as non-invasive programmed stimulation, NIPS), storage of electrograms and pacing thresholds changed in the patient follow-up could all be stored in the random access memory (RAM).

Since the first articles about data storage in the pacemaker memory were published, many improvements have been made: the storage capacity has been multiplied more than ten times, functions more and more complex, e.g. dual chamber DDD pacing with sophisticated algorithms, have been released [1–6]. But the main advantage of an implantable microprocessor is not its ability to manipulate and memorize data, but its capability to incorporate new instructions into the program non-invasively, thereby altering the pacemaker's function [7].

In the Chorus pacemaker, the program can be divided between the passive ROM and the active RAM memories. The program controlling normal pacing functions is stored in the ROM. This program is structured so that it can be connected to the RAM memory and temporarily programmed to perform special routines. Once this ancillary program has been run, the pacemaker automatically reverts to the main program. The dialogue between the RAM 〈〉 ROM programs is controlled and regulated by safety procedures which prevent and/or correct transmission errors.

The introduction of new Holter functions in the pacemaker after implantation allows for more accurate diagnoses. Once the diagnostic results are obtained, a new program can be loaded in the memory of the pacemaker to improve its therapeutic functions.

MEMORY FUNCTION IN MODERN PACEMAKERS

Modern pacemakers must perform sophisticated diagnoses which require expanded memory capabilities in the pulse generator. This 'mini-Holter' function can memorize diverse information about the patient and the pacemaker:

- Historical data such as information on the patient at implant, reasons for implantation, pacemaker and lead models, implant date, post-operative measurements and associated therapy. The essential information requested in the European Pacemaker Registration Card could be easily stored in the pacemaker memory [8].
- Pacemaker follow-up such as lead impedances, pacing thresholds, current consumption, battery impedance and battery depletion, percentage of atrial and ventricular pacing. The monitoring of lead impedance can help detect an insulation defect which could lead to leakage. The follow-up of pacing thresholds may show an early lead dislodgement or a long-term threshold increase. By knowing the percentage of pace/sense beats, lead impedance and thresholds, it is possible to optimize current consumption. Information from the stored battery impedance curve, which directly correlates to the battery depletion curve in the pacemaker, is particularly useful. The discharge curve of a lithium iodine cell shows a linear impedance increase during the useful lifetime of the battery. The curve is steeper when the elective replacement indicator is reached. This point may change from one pacemaker to another due to battery dispersion and circuit variability. Monitoring of the depletion curve or magnetic rate curve is more precise than giving an absolute value for cell impedance and should help to optimize pacemaker replacement.

Other data may be particularly relevant to adjusting pacing parameters: the number of events detected within the safety window (possibly due to the presence of cross-talk and the need to reprogram the blanking period) and the number of PMT detected and stopped (indicating a retrograde conduction and the duration of VA conduction time). The unit will also record the number of self-reprogrammations, indicating an increase of the PVARP and optimization of the AV delay. Arrhythmias detected by the pacemaker, such as premature atrial or ventricular contractions and/or runs, can be stored, as can the number of switches in the fallback mode from the maximum upper rate (which is correlated to the presence of atrial tachycardia). The presence of two leads, one atrial, the other ventricular, should allow a dual-chamber pacemaker with short atrial and ventricular refractory periods to discriminate atrial arrhythmias from ventricular rhythm disturbances.

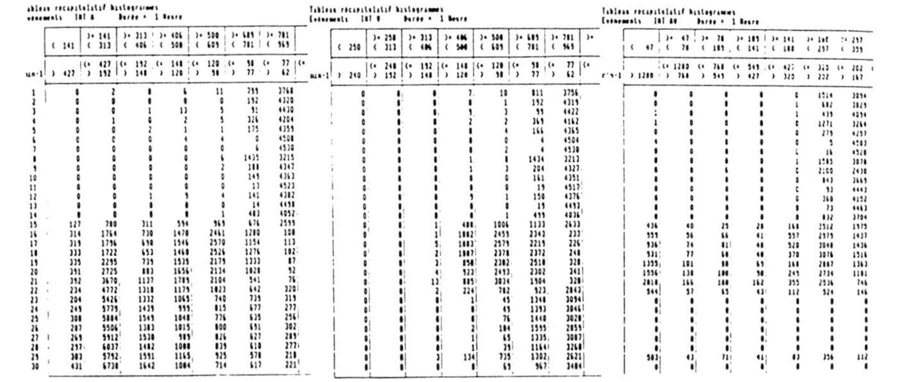

Figure 1. Rate histogramms of A-A-, V-V-, and AV intervals recorded on a 30-h period of a patient implanted with a CHORUS I pacemaker presenting paroxysmal AV block with atrial fibrillation. We note, at hour 15, a chaotic variation of A-A intervals, followed by a wide modulation of AV intervals. Nevertheless the ventricles are almost never depolarized at a rate higher than the programmed upper rate limit.

In patients with sinus node dysfunction (no chronotropic incompetence) and a normal AV conduction, a smart pacemaker programmed initially to AAI can switch automatically to DDD mode if a paroxysmal AV block occurs. The pacemaker continuously monitors the PR interval and stores its mean value. If the PR interval should abruptly lengthen, the pacemaker switches to the DDD mode with an AV delay adjusted to the sinus rate. When the block disappears, the unit returns to the AAI mode after a few pacing cycles and verification of the quality of the AV conduction. This automatic mode commutation (AMC) preserves the maximum hemodynamic benefits obtained with pure atrial pacing [9–12]. The implementation of AMC requires permanent storage and analysis of the pacing interval up to a few dozen cycles.

DATA PRESENTATION

Memorized data can be displayed as:

- Histogram series of A-A, V-V, A-V intervals. The ability to simultaneously store histograms of various intervals, or the same histograms from different time periods) is helpful for the diagnosis as shown by Figure 1 [13].
- The average rate distribution may be stored in periods over 24 h or shorter

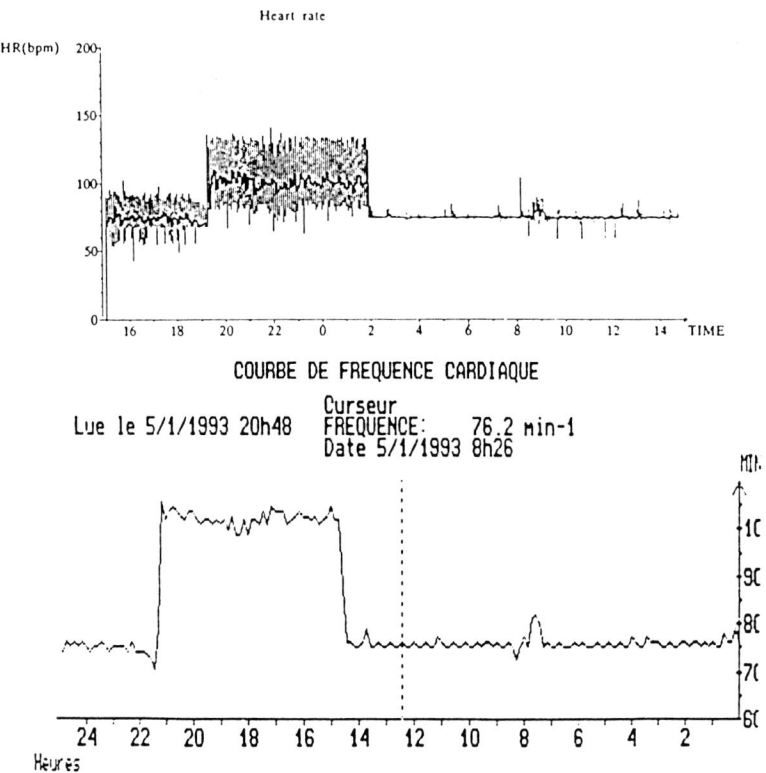

Figure 2. Comparison between the 24-h average rate curve recorded by a conventional holter recorder (upper trace) and the one stored in a software pacemaker CHORUS II-6234. The patient suddenly went from normal sinus rhythm to atrial tachycardia.

if a better resolution is needed. Figure 2 shows such a 24-h average rate curve. Displayed in the upper part of the figure is the mean heart rate recorded on a conventional Holter recorder. The lower trace shows the rate recorded by the implanted pacemaker. Even if the time tables used for recording purposes appear different, the correlation between these two strips is evident: the patient suddenly went from normal sinus rhythm to atrial tachycardia.

Another example of such curves will be shown for rate-modulated pacemakers and for ICDs.

One of the questions addressed with this simplified 'mini-Holter' function is its reliability compared with the standard surface ECG Holter recording. A recent study [14] showed that, in a limited sample of patients, there was a very good correlation between the data stored by the pacemaker and the information continuously monitored on a regular Holter tape and analyzed cycle-by-cycle with an ELATEC (ELA Medical) system analyzer. In this study, the events histograms were ranked according to the boundaries programmed in the implanted unit. The rate profiles were very similar, and the number of V intervals recorded in both systems were closely related ($r = 0.97$; $p < 0.0001$). In fact, because of the reduced level of noise, the information monitored by the implantable Holter had a better signal/noise ratio than the one recorded by the conventional Holter and had almost no analysis banking period. The reliability of these results should also be compared with the preliminary Holter data acquired with implanted recorders connected to small, closely spaced electrodes placed subcutaneously in the upper thorax [15].

STORAGE OF MARKER CHAINS

It has been shown that the telemetry of coded event markers from the pacemaker to the programmer (representing sense/pace sequences) was useful. Complex ECG or electrograms can be clarified by analyzing the timing sequence of the event as displayed by the marker chains.

The storage of particular events sequences in the pacemaker memory may identify the conditions of occurrence, duration and arrest of particular arrhythmias. For example, in the Chorus II pacemaker, sequences of ventricular events occurring under specific conditions can be recorded to elucidate the initiation of tachyarrhythmias:

- Prematurity: the ventricular event should occur within a time interval shorter than the previous 'normal cycle'. This prematurity is programmed as a percentage of the normal cycle.
- Threshold rate: for all the ventricular events after the premature event, the ventricular rate must remain higher than a programmed threshold rate for a number of cycles greater than a programmable value. Once the criteria are satisfied, the pacemaker will store the markers of the eight events following the beginning and the end of this specific cycle (Figure 3).

RATE-MODULATED PACEMAKERS

The follow-up of rate-modulated pacemakers is more complex as it demands the monitoring of one or more additional physiological parameters. The optimization of rate adaptation may require a number of exercise tests with different response curve settings. Repetition of such exercise tests may be difficult for the patient and is time consuming for the medical team.

Modern pacemakers can memorize the frequency curve and the curve of

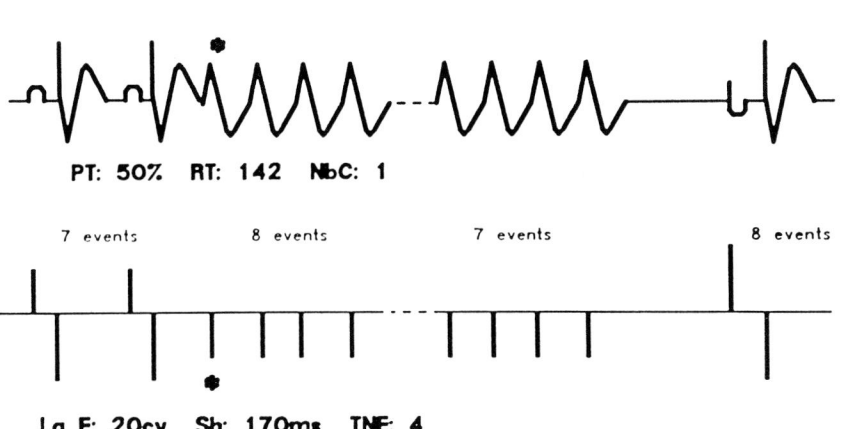

Figure 3. Storage of a sequence of event markers after detection of a V-tach: the prematurity criteria was set at 50%; the threshold rate 142 bpm; the minimum number of cycles following these criterias.

sensory data obtained during exercise tests, which are transmitted by telemetry to the programmer. This programmer, a PC unit, will store and display the data sent via the telemetry link. The physician can simulate a number of response curves in regard to the sensitivity settings and slope. He or she may then adjust the parameters to optimize the rate response (Figure 4) [16].

However, the physiological conditions and the nature and duration of exercise vary during the course of a day, a week or months. The optimum parameter settings chosen during a calibrated exercise test may have no relevance to short duration submaximal efforts.

A smart pacemaker with sophisticated algorithms should be capable of automatic rate adjustment over the short and long term, leading to optimal slope control of the mechanism of rate modulation [17].

In the Chorus RM, a rate-modulated pacemaker driven by minute ventilation, the calibration of the rate-responsiveness is based on the measurement of two values of minute ventilation. One is resting ventilation (resting VE), which corresponds to the patient's resting state and, consequently, the basic rate. The other is exercise ventilation (exercise VE), which corresponds to maximum exercise and thus to the maximum sensor-driven rate.

To calculate the optimal slope, the pacemaker uses the data from the sensor memorized in the active RAM memory and updated continuously

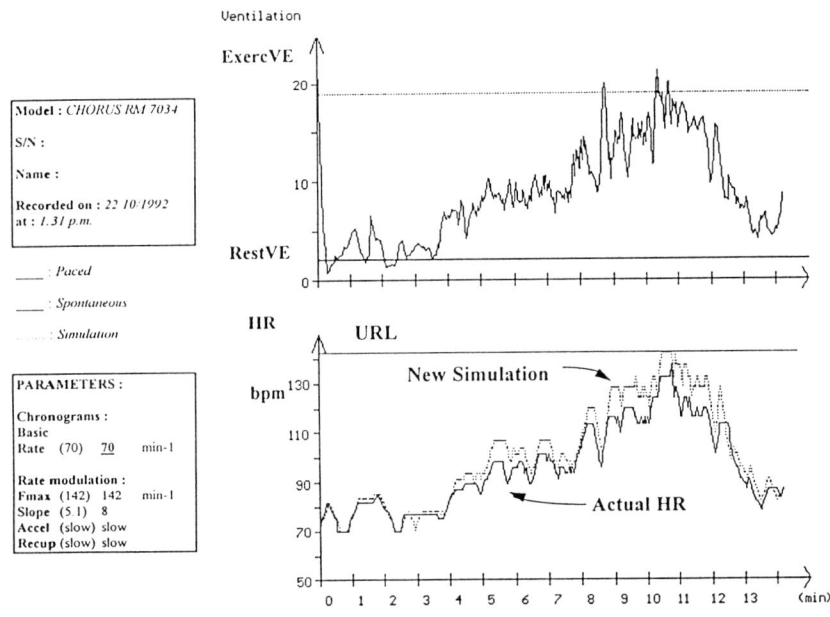

Figure 4. Optimization of the slope of a minute ventilation rate adaptive pacemaker during a standardized exercise test: The minute ventilation VE is recorded and displayed on the upper part of the figure. On the lower part is depicted the corresponding pacing rate. An increase of the slope allows the pacemaker to reach the programmed upper rate limit the maximum of exercise.

(Figure 5). To determine resting VE, the Chorus RM looks at the minimum minute ventilation value and recalculates the resting VE every 32nd respiratory cycle if a change has occurred. To determine exercise VE, the unit monitors the maximum minute ventilation value and recalculates the value of exercise VE every eight cycles if a change has occurred. The sensor-driven rate is given by linear interpolation between these two values.

The Chorus RM records the values of resting VE and exercise VE calculated during the calibration. The unit calculates their mean value on a daily basis and stores the mean value for the last 30 days. The corresponding rate response slope number is calculated for each day. The data can be displayed as three curves corresponding to the resting minute ventilation, exercise minute ventilation, and rate response slope number (Figure 6).

The pacemaker also records the rates calculated from minute ventilation for the last 3 days. The data are displayed on the programmer as three successive rate histograms of 24 h. This allows verification of the correct pacemaker behavior in response to the level of activity of the patient (Figure 7).

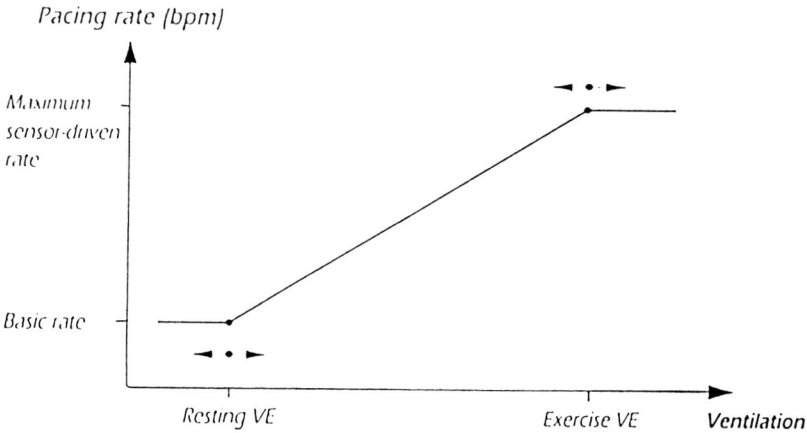

Figure 5. Automatic adjustment of the rate modulation slope for a minute ventilation rate adaptive pacemaker. The unit memorizes the sensor data in the active RAM memory, which is permanently updated and computes the optimal slope. If the pacemaker records too often an upper pacing rate, the value of the VE max is increased. Conversely if the upper rate limit is rarely reached, the value of VE max is decreased. The same kindof sequence is applied to VE min. Consequently, the slope is permanently adjusted.

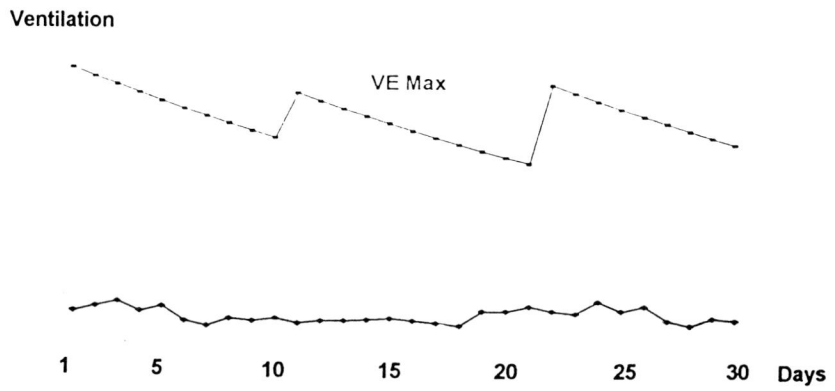

Figure 6. Monitoring of ventilation minute (VE) in a rate adaptive pacemaker. The CHORUS RM computes and then records the values of resting and exercise (VE) on a daily basis and stores their mean values for the last 30 days. The figure shows an increase of VE max, almost every ten days, corresponding to a regular jogging period. No signicant variation of VE was detected atrest (lower curve) during the same period.

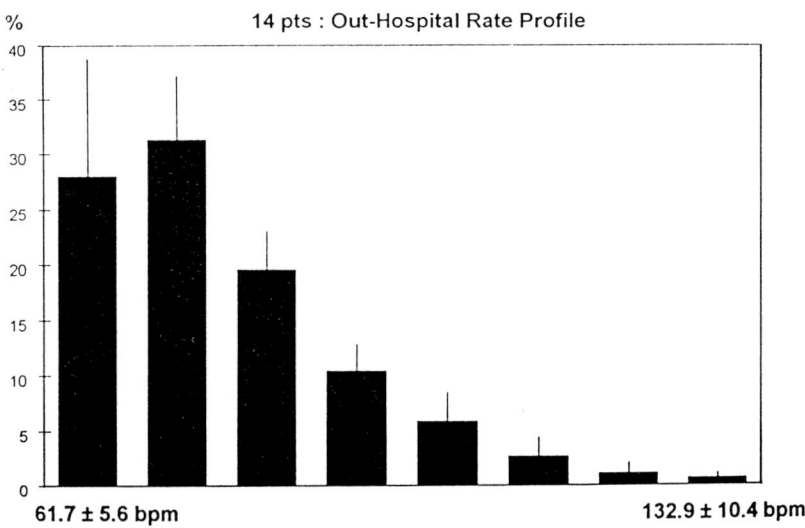

Figure 7. Rate histogram of 14 out of hospital patients implanted with a rate adaptive minute ventilation pacemaker. The mean rate profile seems well adapted to patients' normal behaviour, but has to be verified in every simple patient.

The new generation of pacemakers that uses two or even three sensors will need an enlarged memory capacity and data processing capabilities. Information sent by the sensors will be combined to take into account the physiological specifics of each sensor response in certain situations.

HOLTER IN ICDs

The Holter function is mandatory for ICDs. With such a unit, the physician wants to know which arrhythmia occurs, its characteristics (rate of occurrence, mechanism of initiation), whether it is a supraventricular arrhythmia or a ventricular arrhythmia, the therapy used, ATP cardioversion, defibrillation, the results of this therapy, and if the delivery of shocks is appropriate [18–21].

In addition to the storage of synthetic events displayed by marker chains, the storage of snapshots of electrograms has proven very useful, as it allows verification of the nature and the characteristics of the arrhythmia treated. Reprogramming devices based on analysis of the stored electrograms was associated with a dramatic reduction of false ICD responses for non-VT rhythms [22,23].

The technical constraints tied to reduced memory space and to the necessity of low battery consumption limits the amount of data treated and memorized. As such, the length of storage time of the endocardial electrogram is greatly reduced. To correctly reproduce an electrogram, it should be sampled at a minimum rate of about 200 samples a second.

If we request an accurate amplitude resolution of 1 byte (8 bits), i.e. 256 points full-scale, we can easily compute that 40 s of stored electrogram are contained in a 8 k-bytes static CMOS memory chip, which is the state-of-the-art today. Eight of these chips can be arranged in a suitably sized package to obtain a total storage capacity of between 40 s and 5 min, and this without substantially shortening the lifetime of the defibrillator.

New static CMOS memories of 64 kbytes are in development and should be released soon. Associated with efficient data compression algorithms (>3), we can expect the capacity storage to increase by a factor of 8×3 in the near future. This means that a total electrogram storage time in the range of 16 min to 2 h could be achieved. The current consumption in an elementary memory is due to the charge of parasitic capacitors. As the size of this element decreases, the capacitor, and consequently consumption, are reduced. Therefore, an increase in the number of memory cells should not lead to a large increase in the amount of battery current needed during recording time [24].

The transfer of these memory contents to the programmer may create a problem in transmission duration. Actually, most modern cardioverters-defibrillators only transmit short messages of a few dozen bytes. To obtain the information from the implanted unit, the physician should maintain the position of the programming head to the pacemaker-cardioverter-defibrillator during time lapses of a few minutes. New units should, therefore, have a quicker and safe telemetry system which also maintains acceptable current consumption.

STORAGE OF TEMPORARY PACEMAKER OR ICD FUNCTIONS

With the Chorus pacemakers it is possible to store in the active RAM memory not only Holter function data, but also new temporary or permanent instructions or special routines. The memory space is then divided between the new instructions and the data storage. Safety procedures are included to prevent transmission errors between the microprocessor and the RAM. This additional program can be a new diagnostic function or a new therapy customized for a particular patient. Let us now discuss the capabilities of pacemakers with additional temporary software.

Temporary software for diagnosis

New diagnosic functions may be loaded to better understand patient arrhythmia and to optimize the functioning of the pacemaker. This is illustrated by the following examples.

In some patients exhibiting syncope or presyncope states, the origin of the disease may not be completely defined. The diagnosis of paroxysmal AV block or severe bradycardia may be difficult to determine even with multiple external Holter recordings. In patients who receive a pacemaker, it is interesting to note the nature and the gravity of the arrhythmia.

A diagnostic tool was designed and loaded in the RAM memory of Chorus II. The pacemaker functions then as a VDI pacemaker with multiple programmable escape intervals; for example, a basic rate of 70 bpm and a low diagnosis rate typically programmed around 30 bpm. When the bradycardia occurs, the unit paces at this rate and, after a programmed number of stimulations, returns progressively to the basic rate. The sequence may resume or be deactivated automatically after the diagnosis has been transmitted.

The pacemaker records continuously the atrial (sense) and ventricular (sense and pace) event markers and stores them in the memory each time a sequence has occurred. The presence or absence of atrial detection during bradycardia, visualized on a printout of the markers, determines the diagnosis of either AV block or sinus node dysfunction (Figure 8). When the diagnosis has been transmitted, the program may be downloaded, and the pacemaker functions again as a regular DDD.

Multicenter clinical study has proven the clinical usefulness of such programs which could help improve our knowledge of the epidemiology of some bradyarrhythmias [25].

Unexpected functioning of a pacemaker

In November 1991 the clinical evaluation was started of Chorus II which integrates among its new functions a sophisticated algorithm allowing the automatic switching from AAI to DDD when paroxysmal AV block is detected. When the arrhythmia ends, the unit reverts automatically to DDD after a short ventricular pacing.

After a few months, pacemakers programmed in this new mode showed abnormal atrial premature beats in a few patients. Conventional investigations conducted at the patient's bedside as well as in the catheter laboratory failed to provide any explanation. Standard Holter recordings were normal. It was therefore decided to load a temporary program into the pacemaker memory with telemetry. This 'spy' program was substituted for the Holter data storage program and was used to track abnormal pacing and save the variables involved in computation of the escape interval. The memory, which

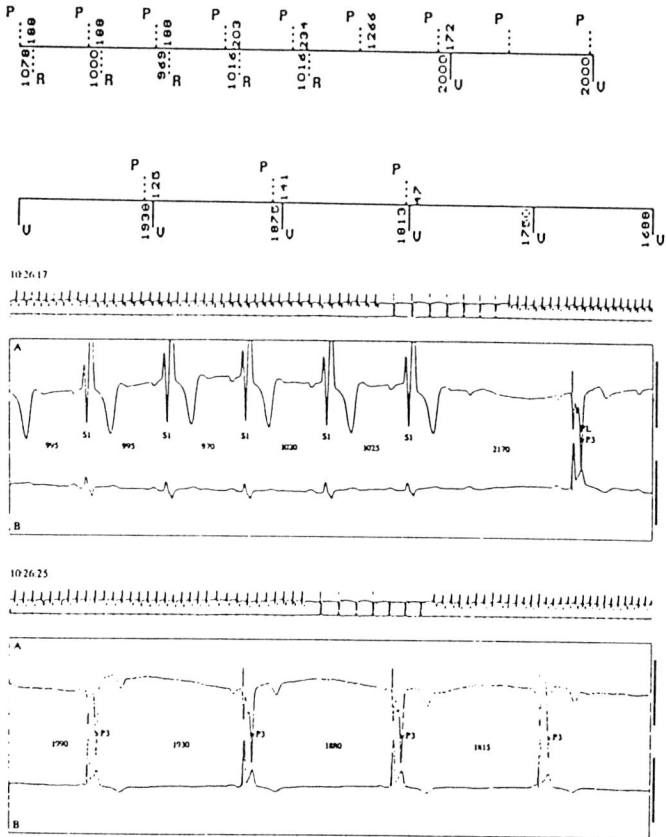

Figure 8. Diagnosis of AV block by analysis of continuously recorded and stored atrial (sense) and ventricular (sense and pace) event markers. We note, that after diagnosis of preprogrammed too seconds ventricular pauses the pacemaker progressively shortens the pacing interval to the basic preprogrammed on (850 m).

was read and analysed a few days later, helped us to understand the performance of the pacemaker. We determined the appropriate variables, modified one of the program's instructions and loaded it in the RAM of the pacemakers involved. The ROM memory content was modified later [26].

Temporary software for therapy

Some atrial and ventricular arrhythmias are induced by a short cycle/long cycle sequence after a premature beat. A temporary program was designed to reduce the long cycle and slightly overdrive the rate in the event of multiple premature beats. This program, designed to prevent arrhythmias, was loaded temporarily in the RAM memory of patients implanted previously (in some cases, more than 1 year before) with a Chorus I 6033 for bradyarrhythmia. In selected patients, the multicenter study has shown a dramatic reduction of the number of VPBs or APBs.

As pacemaker functions are becoming more and more sophisticated, careful evaluation is needed to determine their advantages and disadvantages. Unfortunately, most of the clinical data can only be acquired and validated after implantation. The possibility of later modifying the pacemaker's functions insures the safe implementation of complex algorithms. These new functions are programmed by the physician when the patient needs them and can be effected by transmitting instructions non-invasively to the pacemaker, in some cases years after implantation [27].

Analysis of the data gathered by the pacemaker or the ICD will be facilitated by the presence of a pseudo 'Expert System' between the physician and the pacemaker. The 'Assistant Program' will help programming by translating medical choices into pacing functions and parameter settings [28]. It should also, after analysis of the recorded data and underlying pathology, suggest recommendations for optimum programming of the Holter function.

The physician can therefore dedicate his or her time to reviewing the choices and verifying that the prothesis is well adapted to the patient's needs.

REFERENCES

1. Edhag O, Vallin H. An implantable bradycardia indicating pacer. 1st European Symposium on Cardiac Pacing. London, May, 1978.
2. Attuel P, Mugica J, Buffet J. The diagnostic pacemaker. 1st European Symposium of Cardiac Pacing. London, May, 1978:83.
3. Ripart A, Jacobson P. Memory technology and implantable Holter systems. In: Barold S, Mugica J, editors. The Third Decade of Cardiac Pacing. Mount Kisco, NY: Futura, 1982.
4. Mugica J, Coumel P, Attuel P. Holter implantable, concept de stimulation cardiaque avec fonction Holter incorporée. Arguments cliniques. In: Mugica J, editor. Cardiostim 80-SEPFI, Paris, 1981.
5. Fletcher RD et al. Noninvasive serial electrophysiologic testing using an implanted pacemaker. In: Feruglio GA, editor. Cardiac Pacing. Padova, Italy: Piccin Medical Books, 1982.
6. Ripart A, Jacobson P, Dalmolin R. Clinical value of a microcomputer in an implantable pacemaker. In: Quetglas GM et al., editors. The Applications of Computers in Cardiology. Amsterdam: Elsevier Science Publishers, 1984.
7. Ripart A, Fontaine G, Mugica J. How should the software pacemaker be programmed during manufacturing and after implantation? PACE 1984;7:1202–6.
8. Chorus II, Physicians' Manual. ELA Medical, 1991.
9. Girodo S et al. Improved dual chamber pacing mode in paroxysmal atrioventricular conduction disorders. PACE 1990;13:2059A.
10. Rosenquist M, Obel IWP. Atrial pacing and the risk for A-V block: Is there a time for change in attitude? PACE 1989;12:97–101.
11. Pouillot C. La Stimulation Atriale à Fréquence Asservie. Thése de doctorat en médecine, Rennes, June 1989.

12. Delay M et al. Automatic mode commutation: first clinical results. Europace Abstract 1991;42:8.
13. Lascault G, Frank R, Barnay C et al. Diagnosis of ventricular tachycardia using the Holter function of a dual chamber pacemaker. PACE 1993;16:918A.
14. Cazeau S, Ritter P, Limousin M et al. What is the reliability of the Holter function of a new DDD pacemaker compared to the gold standard surface ECG Holter recording? PACE 1993;16:931 A.
15. Lee BB et al. First results using an implantable arrhythmia monitor. PACE 1993;16:893 A.
16. Chorus RM, Physicians' Manual. ELA Medical, 1992.
17. Cazeau S, Bonnet JL, Ritter P et al. Is it possible to simplify the programming of sensor-driven pacemakers using a continuous self-adaptation of the rate-modulation slope? PACE 1993;16:918 A.
18. Fogoros RN, Elson JJ, Bonet CA. Actuarial incidence and pattern of occurrence of shocks following implantation of the automatic implantable cardioverter defibrillator. PACE 1989;12:1465–73.
19. Maloney J, Masteron M, Khoury D et al. Clinical performance of the implantable cardioverter defibrillator: Electrocardiographic documentation of 101 spontaneous discharges. PACE 1991;14:280–5.
20. Klein LS, Miles WM, Zipes DP. Antitachycardia devices: Realities and promises. J Am Coll Cardiol 1991;18:1349–62.
21. Hurwitz JL, Hook BG, Callans DJ et al. Importance of abortive shock capability with electrogram storage in cardioverter-defibrillator devices. Circulation 1991;84(IV):427 A.
22. Hook BG, Callans DJ, Kleiman RB et al. Implantable cardioverter-defibrillator therapy in the absence of significant symptoms. Circulation 1993;87(VI):1897–906.
23. Block M et al. Should implantable cardioverter defibrillators store electrograms from sensing or defibrillation leads? PACE 1993;16:853 A.
24. Savaria Y. Conception et Vérification des Circuits VLSI. Montréal: Ecole Polytechnique, 1988.
25. Lascault G, Frank R, Barnay C et al. Clinical usefulness of a 'diagnostic' dual chamber pacemaker. PACE 1993;16:918 A.
26. Limousin M, Rémy M, Ripart A. Use of temporary RAM programs to diagnose and to correct unexpected behaviour in a software based DDD pacemaker. Europace 1993, Ostend. PACE 16:1142 A.
27. Ripart A, Mugica J, Barold S et al. Le stimulateur du futur. In: Mujica J, Barold S, Ripart A, editors. La Stimulation Cardiaque. Paris: Masson, 1992.
28. Mugica J, Barold, S, Ripart A. The smart pacemaker. In: Barold S, Mugica J, editors. New Perspectives in Cardiac Pacing 2. Mount Kisco, NY: Futura, 1991.

32. Automatic measure of the interface capacitor and the total cardiac impedance

FRANCISCO PÉREZ GÓMEZ, MANUEL MONTERO,
MIGUEL A. PASTOR, FRANCISCO PÉREZ-VIZCAÍNO,
MARÍA J. PÉREZ-VIZCAÍNO & PABLO GONZÁLEZ

INTRODUCTION

Cardiac impedance can be considered as an equivalent circuit composed by the capacitor created between the electrode and the endocardium or Helmholtz capacity (C_H), a parallel resistance (Warsuf phenomenon, R_F), and in series the resistance of the cardiac tissue itself that, together with the electrode resistance and the resistance of the body, constitute the total resistance (T_r (Figure 1) [1,2]. Using low-intensity stimulation, the resistances are relatively stable, and therefore we can consider the electrode impedance as a function of the frequency for a small voltage within the linear operative range of the electrodes.

In the present chapter we describe the application of the cross-correlation method to measure cardiac impedance. We consider a dynamic system (the heart) excited by pseudorandom impulses of a voltage below the stimulation threshold to obtain information related to the total cardiac impedance and its components [3,4]. The method has been advanced to the level that the cardiac impedance curve and the value of its components can be obtained automatically by a computer-assisted system in a few seconds. Preliminary studies in experimental animal work have been done.

METHODS

The basic idea is to analyze an electrical current composed of binary stimuli of very low intensity after passing through the heart. The electrical impulses enter the heart through the endocardial stimulating electrode and leave the body through the other electrode (anode) located in the thoracic subdermis.

An auxiliary resistance of a known value (5000–15 000 Ω) is placed between the correlator and the cathodic electrode to facilitate the recordings and the calculation. Each stimulus has a constant value and a constant duration (tau). We used a sequence of 63 to more than 100 tau. The imped-

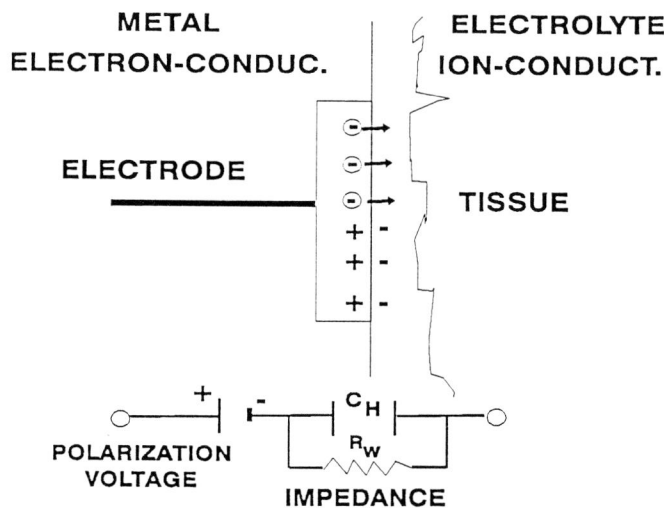

Figure 1. Capacitor created between the electrode and the tissue.

ance produced a deformation of the entering sequence so that the correlator, by comparing the entering and returning sequence, gives an $h(t)$ curve.

An artificial electrical heart model was built using a capacitor of known capacitance, a series resistance, representing the total electrode-heart-tissue resistance, and a parallel resistance. The values of these parameters were elected according to previous publications which give to the capacitor electrode/endocardium an average value of about 1 μF, to the total electrode-heart resistance a value between 500 and 600 Ω, and to the parallel resistance (Warsuf) a value of 15 000–30 000 Ω.

The cross-correlation method was used to obtain the $h(t)$ impedance curve of the heart, which adopts the shape shown in Figure 2. This shape can be modified by changing the values of the capacitor and resistances.

The determination of the values of the curve was initially done by calculating three points of the shoulder of the curve (Figure 3) [4]. Automatization of the process was finally done using a personal computer that through an analogic-digital interface performs the mathematical calculations using many points to obtain the values of T_r, R_w and H_C in a few seconds. The computer also controls an interconnexion unity capable of modifying the levels of the text signal.

The morphology of the curve, especially the shoulder and the distance to the x/y axes, are the main determinants of the impedance values. The parameters used for the calculations which better determine the values of the selected components applied to the artificial heart are those represented in Figure 4.

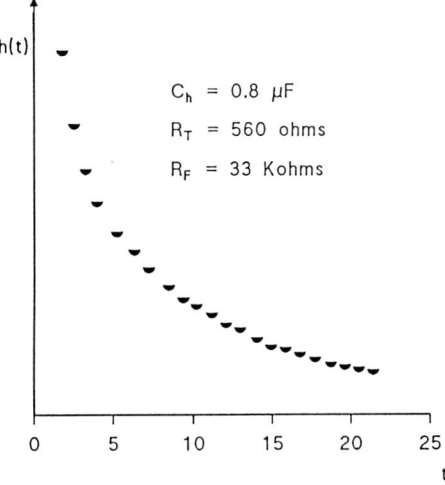

Figure 2. Cardiac impedance $h(t)$ curve obtained in a dog with a 0.8 mm tip catheter. Values of the capacitor C_H in μF, total R_t and Faraday resistances in ohms.

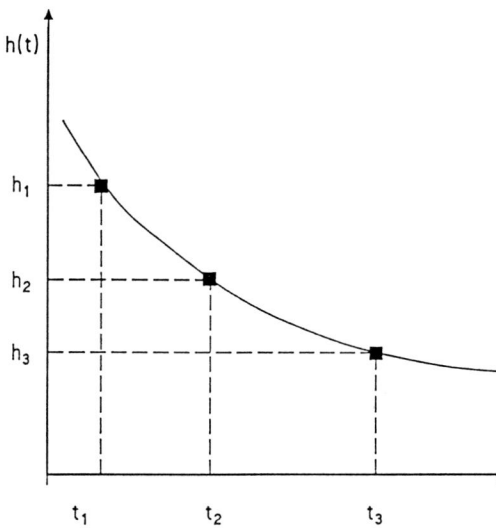

Figure 3. Cardiac impedance curve. Three points were chosen to determine the values of the curve.

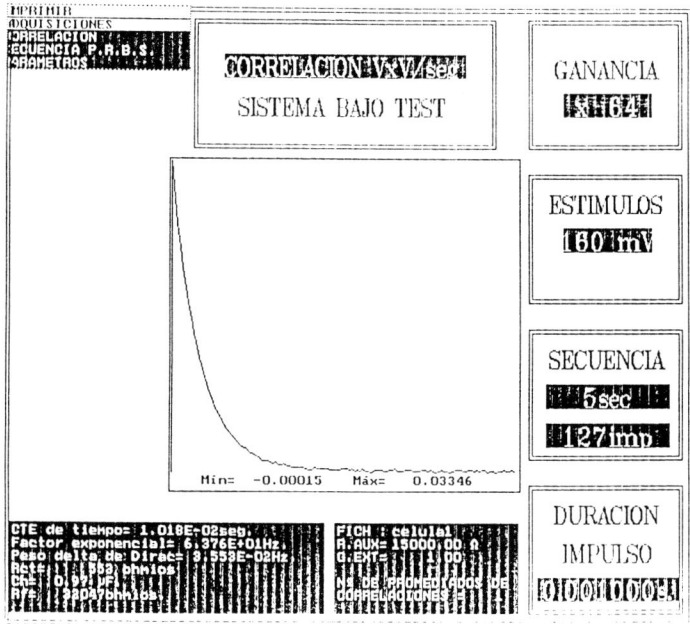

Figure 4. Typical cardiac impedance curve morphology obtained from an artificial heart model formed by a capacitor of 1 μF, a series resistance of 550 Ω, and a parallel resistance of 32 000 Ω. The values obtained were 0.97 μF, 553 Ω and 32 047 Ω, respectively.

Determination in animals

The laboratory work was accompanied by experimental animal work in dogs and lately in pigs. An electrocatheter was introduced through the femoral vein and passed to the right ventricle. The active part of the correlator was connected to the external end of the catheter and the returning side to a subcutaneous metallic plaque. Both the correlator and the monitor were grounded. An external pacemaker was used to stimulate the heart and determine the threshold in each position of the endocardial electrode.

Several determinations were made in each animal using electrodes with different tip sizes and modifying the electrode/endocardium contact. Synchronized electrical shocks (50–100 watts per second) were given to burn the contact area, and the threshold and the impedance curve were determined afterwards. Determinations were also made in one dog after acute myocardial infarction produced by successive ligature of both right and anterior descending coronary arteries.

RESULTS

The $h(t)$ curve of the artificial electrical heart model adopts an exponential shape (Figure 4) similar to that obtained in the dog (Figure 2). The precision of the method to determine the values of the curve was checked by changing the parameters of the artificial heart model, which in the case of Figure 4 was composed of a capacitor of 1 µF, a series resistance (T_r) of 550 Ω, and a parallel resistance (R_w) of 32 000 Ω. The calculated values were very similar to the real ones.

The level of voltage stimulus used varied from 50 to 160 mV, but the real range entering the heart was from 0.037 to 0.078 mV due to the reduction produced by the entering resistance of 15 000 Ω. With this level of energy there is no cardiac stimulation.

Influence of the electrode tip size. The value of the capacitor varied when the tip size was changed: its mean value using a small area electrode (8 mm) was 2 µF, 4.2 µF using a 15 mm flat electrode, and 4.8 µF using an old electrode with a large and rounded contact tip.

Influence of coronary ligation and endocardial burning. The shape of the curve changed markedly after successive ligation of the coronary arteries. After electrical endocardial shock, the threshold rose rapidly to more than 15 volts. The capacitor remained at about 2–2.5 µF and the T_r about 200 Ω.

Correlation between impedance parameters and stimulation threshold. Preliminary data were obtained from three pigs using three different catheters and variable electrode/endocardium contact. The data are not comparable since the electrode tips varied. Figure 5 shows the preliminary data of determinations with a 0.9 mm electrode tip. When the capacitance value increased (good contact) in the low threshold range, the threshold decreased, but the correlation was not significant. When the threshold was greater than 2.5 V, the value of the capacitor became almost constant with an average of about 1.5 µF. The correlation between the threshold and the total electrode-heart resistance was also better when the threshold was lower than 2 V, and this relation was significant (Figure 6). These results have to be confirmed in future studies. The morphology of the curve also changed.

DISCUSSION

In the present paper the cross-correlation method was applied to determine cardiac parameters. To our knowledge, this is the first time that this method, which is currently used to measure physical and industrial parameters, has been applied to measure cardiac impedance and its parameters. It can be easily incorporated into any internal cardiac device, functions with very low energy, and does not interfere with normal cardiac function.

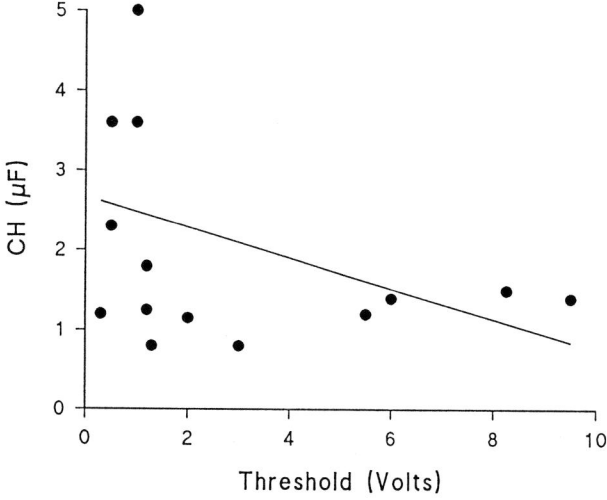

Figure 5. Correlation between stimulation threshold (volts) and the electrode-endocardium capacity (C_H). There was no significant correlation.

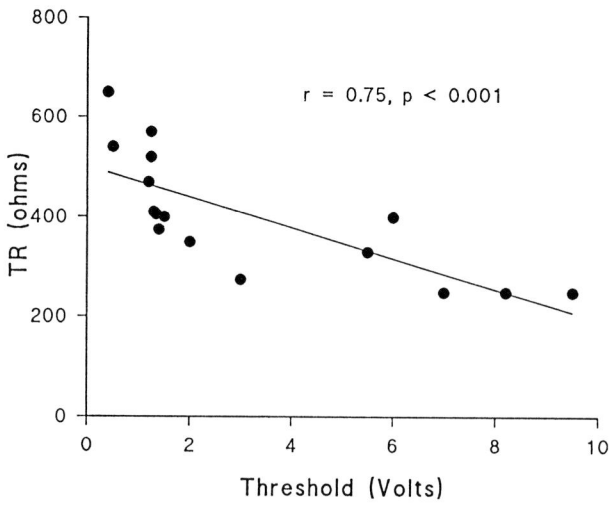

Figure 6. Correlation between the stimulation threshold (volts) and the total resistance (TR).

The $h(t)$ cardiac curve is influenced by several electrical and physiopathological conditions and consequently the value of the capacitor. The measurements obtained to date should be considered preliminary, and the real benefit of this research is still unknown. The value of the capacitor created between the stimulating electrode and the endocardium shows a clear opposite correlation with the size of the electrode, as was to be expected.

The values of the threshold, especially when they are low, indicating good contact, showed a significant correlation with the values of total electrode/cardiac resistances, whereas a nonsignificant correlation could be found with the values of the capacitor. When the contact is not good and the threshold is greater than 2 V, it seems that the capacitor and the total resistance remain unchanged.

The possibilities of employing the method in cardiac diagnosis and therapy are still unknown; advances in the design and incorporation of the automatic recording and measurement method will allow us to study these possibilities more intensively.

REFERENCES

1. Mindt W, Schaldach M. Advances in pacemaker technology. Heidelberg: Springer-Verlag, 1975:297.
2. Irnich W. Advances in pacemaker technology. Heidelberg: Springer-Verlag, 1975:241.
3. Montero M, Pérez Gómez F. Adaptative system for high performance pacemakers. Proceedings of the IV Mediterranean Conference on Medicine and Biological Engineering, MECOMBE '86. Seville, Spain, Sept 9–12, 1986.
4. Pérez Gómez F, Montero M. New method to measure cardiac impedance and its components: Preliminary results and possible clinical applications. New Trends in Arrhythmias. Proceedings 8th IC. Marileva, Italy, January, 1988.

33. Critical analysis of the different algorithms designed to protect the paced patient against atrial tachyarrhythmias in dual chamber pacing

PHILIPPE RITTER, S. CAZEAU, Y. KOJOUKHAROV,
L. HENRY, H. PODEUR, A. LAZARUS & J. MUGICA

INTRODUCTION

The introduction of microprocessors in cardiac pacing has allowed the implementation of new functions, some of them designed to improve the patient's hemodynamic status and others for safety reasons. The best example concerns the management of pacemaker-mediated tachycardias, i.e. endless-loop tachycardias (ELTs) and tachycardias induced by atrial tachyarrhythmias (AAs). Solutions for preventing and terminating ELTs are satisfactory and allow the programming of short postventricular atrial refractory periods (PVARP).

Nowadays, the management of AAs that can induce pacemaker-mediated tachycardias is of major importance for all manufacturers. Furthermore, the need for such functions is linked to extensive indications for dual chamber pacing in the bradytachy syndrome. The risk that the pacemaker will be faced with these arrhythmias is thus enhanced. Before dealing with the various algorithms available, we will review the different pacemaker behaviors induced by AAs in dual chamber pacing.

FACTORS INFLUENCING THE DETECTION OF PATHOLOGICAL ATRIAL RHYTHMS: CONSEQUENCES FOR THE BEHAVIOR OF DUAL CHAMBER PACEMAKERS

Two conditions are required for increasing the ventricular rate in the event of an AA episode. First, the sensing level must be correct for the detection of tachyarrhythmias, i.e. the amplitude of endocardial pathological A waves must be superior to the programmed sensing threshold. However, the amplitude of pathological A waves may decrease significantly in comparison with that of sinus A waves, so that the detection of pathological rhythms may be ineffective even if the detection setting is the highest available. This situation occurs frequently in the case of atrial fibrillation. Second, the capability of the pacemaker to analyze the on-going atrial rate depends on the relationship between the pathological atrial rate and the programmed refractory periods. These two parameters influence pacemaker behavior during an AA episode in DDD(R)/VDD(R).

If the amplitude of the atrial signals is lower than the programmed sensing threshold, the pacemaker is 'blind' in the atrium, and the pacing mode is DVI. Without atrioventricular (AV) block, spontaneous QRS complexes inhibit the pacemaker if the rate is higher than the basic rate or the on-going escape rate (rate-smoothing, rate-responsiveness). With AV block, AV sequential pacing occurs at the escape rate; atrial pacing is useless and wastes energy. However, in this situation, the patient is protected as the pacemaker does not accelerate the ventricular rate. Some authors have used this observation to justify the programming of atrial sensing with the detection of sinus A waves and non-detection of pathological A waves. But then two problems arise: (1) the lack of specificity in the case of sinus tachycardia, i.e. the amplitude of endocardial sinus A waves often decreases during exercise so that there is a risk for undersensing the sinus rate with no ventricular rate acceleration in this physiological situation; (2) the inability of the pacemaker to diagnose the AA episode even in the case of proper sensing of the pathological A waves. In this situation, the AV association is dependent on the on-going atrial rate, the programmed upper rate limit, and the maximal atrial detection rate (60000/AV Delay + PVARP).

With AV block, if every A wave falls outside the refractory periods, for an atrial rate between the basic rate and the upper rate limit, the AV association is 1:1. Conversely, if the atrial rate is higher than the programmed URL but lower than the maximal atrial rate detection, the AV association is Wenckebach, with progressive lengthening of AVD until an A wave falls into PVARP, neither initiating AVD nor delivering ventricular pacing.

If the atrial rate is higher than the maximal atrial detection rate, two types of AV associations can be observed: (1) if the atrial rate is lower than twice (or n times) the maximal atrial detection rate, the AV association is 2:1 (or n:1); (2) if the atrial rate is twice (or n times) higher than the maximal atrial detection rate, the AV association is Wenckebach. Last but not least, if the A waves are randomly sensed, the ECG interpretation becomes rather difficult, and ventricular pacing is irregular.

Without AV block, spontaneous QRS complexes may inhibit the pacemaker, and the behavior is difficult to analyze.

Thus, depending on the refractory periods and programmed rates, the pacemaker can or cannot analyze the atrial rate, increase the ventricular rate, and diagnose the AAs.

PROTECTION FUNCTIONS AGAINST AAs

Simple rules for protection against AAs

If advanced functions are not available, the protection possibilities are very limited and frequently unsatisfactory.
The DVI mode. In the absence of spontaneous ventricular events, pacing is AV sequential at the basic rate. With AV block, as the atrial rate accelerates, no ventricular rate acceleration is provided, and atrial pacing still persists, thus causing energy waste and also arrhythmogenicity. This pacing mode must not be used.
The DDI mode. The behavior is similar to DVI, but atrial sensing inhibits atrial pacing. The behavior is VVI except at the basic rate: AV sequential pacing if no atrial or ventricular events are sensed. The ventricular rate cannot accelerate during exercise, and in the event of AV block, the atria and ventricles are dissociated. The DDI indication is frequent AAs with preserved AV conduction.
The DDIR mode (with a DDDR device) reduces the side-effects of DDI by providing rate acceleration during exercise. The ideal indication of this pacing mode is the bradytachy syndrome with major chronotropic incompetence and preserved AV conduction.
If DDIR is not available, there are two remaining possibilities:

1. The DDD mode with a low URL, which allows ventricular rate acceleration on sinus rhythm during exercise and limits ventricular rate acceleration during AAs. However, the induced Wenckebach AV association is frequently ill-tolerated, especially during exercise.
2. Some DDDR devices allow the programming of two different URLs: a rate-responsive one (RR URL) and a P tracking one (P URL) (Siemens Synchrony I and II). If the indication for pacing is the bradytachy syndrome, programming a RR URL higher than P URL is logical. On sinus rhythm, AV synchrony is ensured up to P URL. Beyond, the AV association is Wenckebach, with limitation of the ventricular pause when an A wave falls into PVARP because the rate-responsiveness shortens the atrial escape interval. However, atrial pacing may occur when the atrium is still in a refractory or in the vulnerable period. This situation is potentially arrhythmogenic although no study has proved this hypothesis. When the RR rate is higher than the sinus rate, AV sequential pacing is ensured up to RR URL. When an AA is sensed by the pacemaker, the ventricular rate is allowed to increase up to P URL (which should be programmed low, close to 100 bpm). During exercise, the sensor accelerates the ventricular rate, and the pacing mode is VVIR between P URL and RR URL.

The VVI(R) mode is the last possibility to protect the patient, but he or she can no longer benefit from a dual chamber mode. This mode must be used in permanent AA whatever the type of pacemaker implanted.

In all these situations, the protection is satisfactory, but the pacing mode is not optimal, and the pacemaker cannot provide any information about the occurrence of AAs for retrospective diagnosis.

The specific protection functions against AAs

The ideal pacemaker provides an effective protection algorithm and stores the pathological events for retrospective diagnosis. This implies a perfect detection of AAs. Every solution brings answers to this problem, but new adverse effects occur. Furthermore, the understanding of ECG tracings becomes rather complicated when the functioning of the device is not well known by the physician. A logical classification is difficult to establish since every system is specific.

The first system to be proposed was the Siemens DDD 674 (which is no longer available), also used by the Biotronik Physios 01 (so-called dual-demand function). The device provides a retriggerable atrial refractory period in the event of a sensed A event within the atrial refractory period. The induced pacing mode is thus DVI with AV sequential pacing at the basic rate. No ventricular rate acceleration is induced, and pacing the atrium is of no use and besides wastes energy. The DVI mode is induced on short runs of pacemaker atrial complexes (PACs), and the pacemaker cannot store this information.

The second system available, the fallback, is more sophisticated. This system is found in the following pacemakers: CPI [925 model (no longer available), and Vigor (still in the evaluation process)], Telectronics [Quadra (no longer available) and Ela Medical (Chorus I, and RM)]. The fallback is based upon the comparison between the on-going atrial rate and the URL. When the atrial rate is higher than the URL, the AV association is Wenckebach. This implies the programming of a high maximal atrial detection rate (60000/AVD + PVARP). This objective is achieved by programming an automatic AVD function (when available) and a short PVARP. These programming rules (short total atrial refractory period) can be used only if reliable protection against ELTs is available. If Wenckebach AV association is impossible, the pacemaker cannot initiate fallback. If the pacemaker's programmed settings allow Wenckebach operation, and when the number of ventricular paced cycles in Wenckebach is higher than the programmed value, the VDI mode is initiated: VVI pacing with continuation of atrial rate analysis. In most pacemakers, the fallback rate is progressively decreased to a 'fallback rate', programmable or not. When AA resumes (atrial rate is below the URL), a 1:1 AV association is restored. Vigor and Chorus devices store the number of fallback initiations in their statistics, allowing retrospective diagnosis. With these pacemakers, a number of ventricular cycles in Wenckebach and fallback rate are programmable. In addition, with the Vigor system, the ventricular rate decrease is programmable. With the Quadra, the atrial rate initiating fallback, the ventricular rate at which fallback is started, and the fallback rate are all programmable.

In this concept, the discrimination between sinus rate and pathological atrial rate is based upon the comparison between the on-going atrial rate and the URL, and the duration of high atrial rates. The URL must be programmed above the maximal sinus rate that the patient can achieve during maximal exercise. If the URL is programmed lower, the system initiates fallback on sinus rhythm during strenuous exercise. In this case, the information stored in the statistics can lead to erroneous AA diagnosis. The second limitation of this system is that the ventricular rate is accelerated prior to fallback onset. This behavior may explain the sensation of palpitations.

The fallback mode provided by Sorin Physiocor 400 and Swing DRl (still under evaluation) is slightly different, but the principle remains the same. When the atrial rate goes beyond the URL, mode switching to VDI occurs immediately without Wenckebach AV association, and the ventricular rate remains just below the URL for 1000 cycles before it decreases to a nonprogrammable fallback rate. With the Swing DR1 model, and in the DDDR mode, sensor information is taken into account. When the sensor does not detect any gravimetry variation, the number of ventricular cycles with a rate close to the URL is decreased to 250, and the fallback rate is the sensor-driven rate. When exercise is sensed the number of ventricular cycles close to the URL is extended As a matter of fact, Wenckebach does not exist, and thus the hemodynamic tolerance is improved. On the other hand, the ventricular rate is accelerated prior to fallback.

A better system would avoid ventricular rate acceleration and improve the sensing capabilities of fast atrial rates The Ela Medical Chorus II 6234/44 model provides an improved fallback concept. A normal sinus event is defined as an atrial event outside the absolute atrial refractory period and outside the WARAD (window of atrial rate acceleration detection). A PAC is defined as a sensed atrial event outside the absolute atrial refractory period and during the WARAD. The WARAD starts after an atrial event and lasts 75% (nominal value) of the average of the 8 previous sinus cycles. Thus, an atrial event sensed during the WARAD has a prematurity equal or superior to 25%. When an atrial event is sensed as a PAC, the device does not trigger any AV delay but only resets the atrial escape interval (AEI). The WARAD value cannot be longer than 562 ms. This AEI is then equal to the WARAD value; in addition, at the end of the AEI, the device paces the atrium and the ventricle with a 31-ms AV interval. This functioning shortens the ventricular EI and optimizes atrial sensing for this cycle. If a spontaneous atrial event is sensed during this reset AEI, an atrial arrhythmia is suspected. For 30 s, the pacemaker limits the URL to 120 bpm (or less if the URL is less than 120 bpm), the AV association depends on the relative values of the URL and the atrial rate, and the AV interval duration is 31 ms in order to optimize atrial sensing. If an AA episode occurs, F function starts, i.e. the 'VDI' pacing mode is induced with deceleration of the ventricular pacing rate to 70 bpm. When the matrial rate decreases below 120 bpm, the 1:1 AV association is re-established.

Consequently, PVARP is divided into two parts. The first one lasts 125 ms and is an absolute atrial refractory period. The second one is a relative refractory period, but the priority is given to the WARAD period. Consequently, in sinus rhythm, the total atrial refractory period is equal to the sum programmed AVD plus programmed PVARP, but in the event of AAs, it becomes equal to 31 ms AVD plus 125 ms (156 ms). The diagnosis of all pathological atrial rates up to 385 bpm is thus possible. In addition, the number of fallback operations is stored in the events counter, and the atrial intervals are classified in programmable implantable Holter histograms. The specificity and sensitivity of the system are improved. However, in the event of frequent PACs when the sinus rate accelerates at exercise onset, fallback may be initiated at a moment when 1:1 AV synchronisation is highly desirable. Fortunately, the atrial prematurity value is programmable, and in our experience, this problem could always be solved.

Fallback always induces an automatic mode switching after a certain degree of ventricular rate acceleration. Another example of AMS from DDDR to VVIR is proposed by the Telectronics Meta DDDR 1250 model. Some information comes from the minute ventilation sensor, as the PVARP value is dependent on the programmed value and the metabolic indicated rate (MIR) calculated by the software. The calculation of MIR depends on the rate-response slope, the basic rate, the URL, and the measurement of the trans-thoracic impedance correlated to minute ventilation variations. The result is a progressive reduction of the PVARP from the basic rate to the URL. The sensor information only influences the PVARP duration and not the initiation of AMS. AMS occurs when a single A wave falls into PVARP after a 100-ms absolute refractory period. Thereafter, the atrial channel is refractory until the end of the atrial escape interval with mode switching to VDIR with a rate equal to the MIR. Consequently, a retrograde A wave or isolated PACs can induce AMS. This is the reason why the new version of the Meta DDDR device [1254 model (still under evaluation)] will improve the algorithm operation. Two conditions must be met before AMS: a counter of 5 or 11 short atrial intervals (programmable parameter) must be fulfilled, and the on-going atrial rate must be higher than 150, 175, or 200 bpm (programmable parameter) before the mode switching occurs. Three long atrial intervals or a 1-s pause in the atrium restores the DDDR pacing mode. The specificity should be increased, and the sensitivity should remain satisfactory. However, short runs of PACs would initiate AMS with alternant VVIR and DDDR periods.

Another way to protect the patient against AAs is to lower the URL in DDD mode. Intermedics Cosmos I (no longer available) and Relay devices use such a concept. In the Cosmos I model, when the atrial rate goes beyond the URL, the DDD mode is preserved, the Wenckebach AV association is induced, and the URL is lowered. When the atrial rate is below the programmed URL, 1:1 AV synchrony is restored. This algorithm has the same drawbacks as the standard fallback.

With the Relay model, the information given by the sensor is used by the soltware. When the sensor does not indicate exercise, a new URL equal to the basic rate plus 35 bpm is proposed (CVTL: conditional ventricular tracking limit). In the event of AAs, the ventricular rate is limited by the CVTL. This protection is effective at rest, but as soon as the patient exercises and when the sensor indicates an acceleration of the sensor-driven rate greater than 20 bpm, the protection is disabled, and the ventricular rate is allowed to accelerate up to the URL. In addition, if the sinus rate is higher than the CVTL at rest or at the onset of exercise or during recovery after exercise, AV dissociation occurs when AV synchrony should be maintained.

In the Quintec DDD 931 (no longer available) and Harmony devices (Vitatron), the concept is again different. After PVARP, a 100-ms period analyzes the occurrence of A waves. If A waves occur during this period for 5 consecutive ventricular cycles, the pacemaker is allowed to maintain AV synchrony in the Wenckebach mode with a 70-ms shortening of PVARP to improve the Wenckebach behavior. If an A wave occurs during this period for fewer than 5 consecutive cycles, the URL is decreased. The efficacy of this system is satisfactory, but runs of PACs may induce frequent decrements in URL and even lower the mean ventricular rate if the runs occur when the sinus rate is close to the URL.

The Ruby device compares the on-going atrial rate with the PSR (physiological sinus rate), with a maximal variation of 2 bpm from beat to beat. If the atrial rate goes above the URL and if the PSR ranges from the URL to the URL minus 15 bpm, a Wenckebach mode is initiated with a mean maximal ventricular rate equal to URL × 1.25. If the PSR is not within this rate range when the atrial rate goes beyond the URL, this atrial rate is considered pathological, and a n:1 AV association is initiated with a maximal ventricular rate equal to the basic rate × 1.5 (minimum 100 bpm). The protection initiation is counted in the pacemaker statistics. In this example, the protection function is induced by short runs of PACs.

The Diamond device offers an optional function, mode switching. In the DDDR mode, if sinus arrest occurs, the atrial escape interval is equal to the on-going sinus rate minus 15 bpm, with a subsequent decrease in the ventricular rate to the sensor-driven rate (according to the flywheel function) if this sensor rate is below the atrial rate minus 15 bpm. If not, the escape rate is the sensor-driven rate (in the DDD mode, the escape rate is the LRL). If the atrial rate goes above the on-going sinus or the sensor-driven rate plus 15 bpm for one cycle, the pacing mode is immediately switched to DDIR with an escape rate calculated according to the same modalities as described above (the short atrial interval triggering the mode switching must be shorter than 600 ms). The DDIR mode is maintained as long as the atrial rate is above the sensor-driven rate plus 15 bpm or the URL. When the AA resumes, the DDDR mode is restored. If the short atrial cycle that triggered the mode switching is isolated, 1:1 AV association is restored at the escape cycle length provided that the interval between the PAC and the atrial pacing spike is greater than 325 ms. This algorithm is also original because it combines an atrial rate analysis, sensor data [the sensor is a dual-sensor system (QT and activity)], and an automatic mode switching. The number of times the mode switched is stored in the pacemaker statistics. The limitation of this system is a possible AV dissociation at the onset of strenuous exercise when the sinus rate accelerates from the basic rate, especially if PACs occur at that particular time.

CONCLUSIONS

All manufacturers propose a protection function against AAs in their most recent pacemakers. When all the conditions for optimal AA detection are gathered, this option is effective. However, every solution has its own limitations, and AV dissociation or easy initiation of this protection during short runs of PACs may occur.

For optimal operation, atrial events falling into PVARP must be taken into account, as well as the atrial prematurity value (or abrupt changes in the atrial rate) and sensor(s) data. The initiation of the protection algorithm should be counted in the pacemaker statistics. These functions will be improved in the near future. A modern pacemaker should provide precise information about all AA and VV intervals stored in the Holter function memory.

34. Mode switching in DDDR pacing

RICHARD SUTTON

INTRODUCTION

Mode switching is a recent introduction to dual chamber pacing; its basis is disablement of the atrial tracking ventricular pacing response inherent in all DDD and VDD pacing systems in the face of atrial tachyarrhythmias. The switch is from DDD/VDD to DDI/DVI/VVI. It is provided in DDDR pacemakers whose rate-adaptive feature allows the pacing rate to remain appropriate despite the cessation of atrial tracking. It is necessary to appreciate that mode switching is a passive means of handling atrial tachyarrhythmias and in itself does nothing to prevent or abbreviate them. Despite this disadvantage, mode switching from DDDR to DDIR/VVIR can minimise or eliminate patient symptoms due to atrial tachyarrhythmias. It is an automatic means of achieving what Castallanet et al. [1] conceived as the pacing mode of choice in sinoatrial node disease in 1984.

INDICATIONS

Mode switching is selected in patients who have or are anticipated to have atrial tachyarrhythmias. These are therefore mainly sick sinus syndrome patients. It may be anticipated that all future models of DDDR pacemakers will include this feature. The other group of patients for whom mode switching is particularly pertinent are those who have undergone atrioventricular (AV) nodal ablation. They require permanent pacing and in the past have been paced in VVIR mode. However, many of them show normal atrial activity for much of the time. They can, with the benefit of mode switching, be offered physiological pacing with the ability to mode switch and avoid symptoms during an atrial tachyarrhythmia.

MECHANISMS

Manufacturers have adopted different approaches to achieve mode switching. The DDDR timing mechanisms have recently been documented [2,3].

BIOTRONIK Co. has marketed two dual chamber pacing systems with a feature known as dual demand. This is brought into operation when atrial events are sensed in the atrial refractory period. These are allowed to reset the atrial refractory period, effectively mode switching the device to DVI from DDD. This protects the patient against rapid ventricular stimulation rates during atrial tachyarrhythmias. When sensing reveals that atrial events in the atrial refractory period have ceased, the mode is switched back to DDD.

Cardiac Pacemakers Inc. (CPI) term their mode switching 'atrial tachycardia response' in their Vigor-DR pacemaker. DDDR switches to VVIR when the atrial rate exceeds the upper rate limit. Two features of this response are programmable. (1) Duration of tachycardia: this allows selection of the number of ventricular stimuli (in VVIR) at the upper rate before the rate decreases towards the lower rate. (2) Fallback: the time taken for the rate decline can be selected. Mode switching occurs after 8 A-A intervals above the upper rate limit; during these 8 beats 'normal' upper rate behaviour occurs (artificial Wenckebach). During the period known as atrial tachycardia duration, 8 detected A-A intervals must remain shorter than the upper rate limit. If this criterion is satisfied, the fallback phase commences. Mode switching back to DDDR occurs any time 8 A-A intervals are longer than the upper rate limit interval. CPI also provides a rate-smoothing option which reduces abrupt swings in rate that may occur with atrial tachyarrhythmias and mode switching.

ELA Medical SA has recently introduced a DDDR device which has available two mode commutations, DDDR to VVIR and DDD to VVIR. The operation of the algorithm is similar for both. When the atrial rate is sustained for a programmed number of cycles above the upper rate limit and pseudo-Wenckebach upper rate behaviour is in operation, the pacemaker will switch mode to VVIR. Switching back occurs when the atrial rate (monitored throughout) falls below the upper rate limit for a programmable number of sensed events.

This company also offers another type of mode switching in their Chorus II DDD device. This does not address the problem of atrial tachyarrhythmias but aims to maintain the AAI mode of pacing in a patient without overt AV block. This DDD/AMC, or automatic mode conversion, functions during normal AV conduction by monitoring the AV interval at different rates so as to maintain a 'physiological' interval whilst avoiding pacing the ventricles as far as possible. This could be described as a type of reverse AV interval hysteresis. In AV block, ventricular pacing supervenes appropriately (DDD mode). When any of the three following criteria apply: ventricular activity is sensed before the end of the AV delay, atrial sensing rather than atrial pacing occurs, or there are 100 ventricular paced beats. The device switches back to AAI mode by first lengthening the AV delay by 31 ms to encourage spontaneous AV conduction. After 16 consecutive cycles with sensed ventricular activity, the AAI mode is adopted. Use of DDD/AMC implies that some other special functions of this device are automatically activated (retro P protection and fallback with rate smoothing at 31 ms). The maximum AV time allowed is 350 ms (A and V pacing). This mode has found particular use in carotid sinus syndrome patients where it is desirable to avoid ventricular pacing except when necessary during carotid sinus attacks.

Intermedics Inc. in its Relay DDDR pacemaker has a programmable conditional ventricular tracking limit (CVTL) as its means of handling atrial tachyarrhythmias in VVIR mode. The sensor provides rate limitation depending on its input. The CVTL at rest is 35 ppm higher than the lower rate. When the sensor rate is more than 20 ppm above the lower rate, the CVTL is disabled. This allows tracking during exercise up to the upper rate limit. When the sensor rate falls to less than 20 ppm above the lower rate, the CVTL is re-enabled.

Medtronic's Elite II DDDR unit does not as such include a mode switching feature. The next generation device THERA™ DR and VDR now under clinical validation offers mode switching from DDDR to DDIR and VDD to VVIR. When an atrial tachyarrhythmia is detected, smooth sensor-determined mode and rate transition are achieved. When the atrial rate falls below the 'normal' rate (about 10 ppm below the upper rate), the ventricular rate is increased slowly towards the atrial rate. At the meeting point the mode is switched back to the higher mode. Upon a sudden cessation of an atrial tachyarrhythmia, the first three cycles are paced DDIR, after which the DDDR mode is resumed. If the device is basically VDD, VVIR switches back to VDD after three atrial detections below the upper rate.

Siemens Pacesetter AB Synchrony II DDDR unit also does not provide mode switching. However, Synchrony III will offer a mode switching feature, the details of which have not yet been released.

Sorin Biomedica's SWING DR1 DDDR pacemaker has mode switching from DDDR/VDDR/DDD to VVIR/VVI. In the rate-adaptive modes, an atrial rate above the upper rate initiates a period of ventricular pacing at the upper rate. This is approximately 250 beats (1000 beats in non-rate-adaptive modes) and allows for an emotionally driven sinus tachycardia above the upper rate without significant accelerometer input. Then the relationship between atrial rate and physical activity from the sensor is checked. If activity is present, the VVIR mode at an appropriate rate is continued (Figure 1), but if activity is not present (Figure 2), the ventricular rate declines towards the lower rate (77 ppm). Switch back to the dual chamber mode occurs when the atrial rate falls below the upper rate for three consecutive cycles. This is achieved via one cycle which has a prolonged atrial refractory period (ARP) relative to the programmed value or 400 ms (whichever is the longer).

Telectronics Inc. were the first to introduce mode switching in their Meta

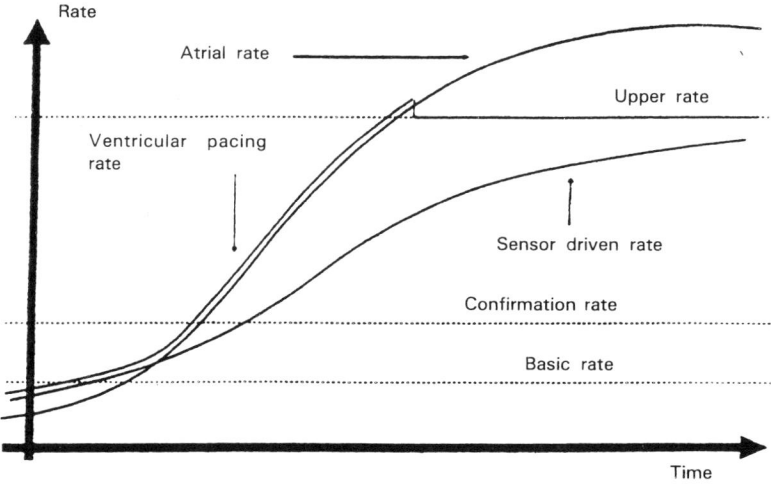

Figure 1. Sorin – swing DR1 DDDR pacemaker. Shows the behaviour of ventricular rate when the atrial rate exceeds the upper rate limit but the sensor rate is high. (Reproduced from Physician's manual with permission).

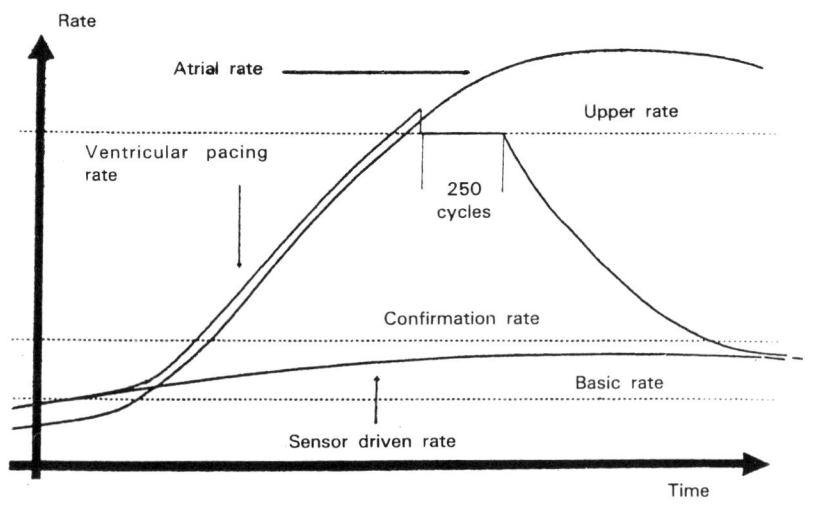

Figure 2. Sorin – swing DR1 DDDR pacemaker. Shows the behaviour of ventricular rate when the atrial rate is above the upper rate but the sensor rate is below the confirmation rate. (Reproduced from Physician's manual with permission).

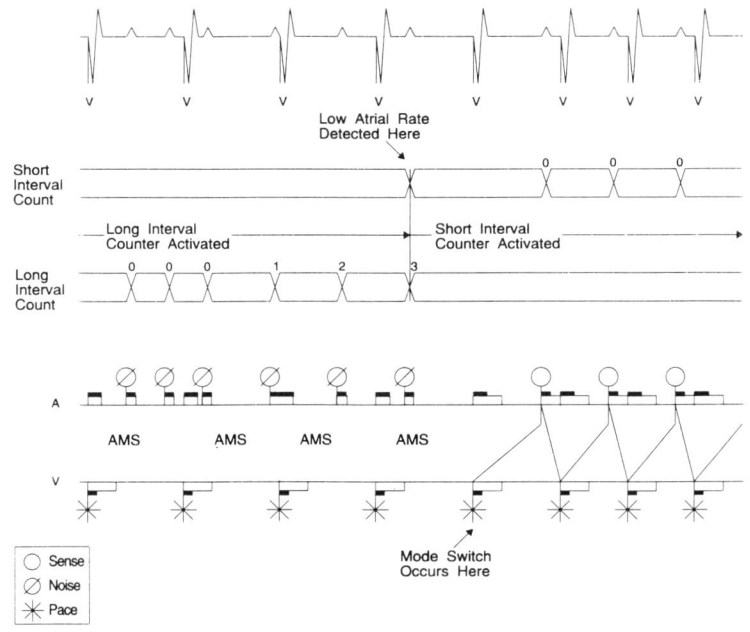

Figure 3. Telectronics meta DDDR 1254 pacemaker. Shows a mode-switch from VDIR to DDDR when the detected atrial rate falls below the upper rate. (Reproduced from Physician's manual with permission).

DDDR 1250. The DDDR mode switched to VVIR when the P-P interval was less than the total atrial refractory period, implying mode switching on the first event of this kind. In practice, this engendered too frequent mode switching, which occurred even with atrial premature complexes. Thus, the second generation unit has adopted a more sophisticated approach. For atrial tachyarrhythmia, recognition rates of 150, 175, and 200 ppm can be selected, and there is a choice of 5 or 11 beats above the chosen rate. Mode switching back to DDDR is brought about when the appropriate counter detects that the atrial rate is lower than the upper rate (Figure 3).

The rate-response behaviour of the device is the result of the influence of the metabolic indicated rate on shortening the total atrial refractory period up to the programmed upper rate. If the atrial rate exceeds the upper rate, this is judged to be non-physiological, and mode switching DDDR to VVIR occurs (Figure 4).

Vitatron Medical BV has introduced a multisensor DDDR pacemaker called Diamond. This device has adaptive mode switching which is a unique feature taking advantage of the rate of change of the atrial rate and a comparison between the atrial rate and sensor rate. The most appropriate

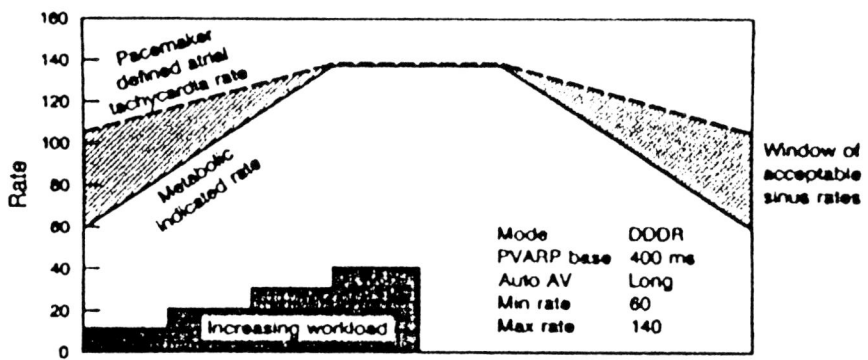

Figure 4. Telectronics meta DDDR 1254 pacemaker. Shows the influence of the Metabolic indicated rate on the mode-switching behaviour in relation to the upper rate. (Reproduced from Physician's manual with permission).

mode of pacing is selected beat-by-beat on this basis. During atrial tachyarrhythmias with an atrial rate above the upper rate, the DDIR mode is used. Physiological atrial rates are distinguished from pathological ones by employing a band of permissible atrial rates. The physiological atrial rate within this band may be paced or sensed, but it may not change more than 2 bpm without being considered pathological. The upper edge of the band is called the upper rate and is determined by the programmable maximum tracking rate. The lower edge of the band is the dynamic lower rate, which is determined by the programmable lower rate limit, and may additionally be reduced by night rate drop during sleep. In the event of a sudden fall in atrial rate, the flywheel effect is employed, a feature common to many of this company's earlier rate-adaptive pacemakers. During atrial tachyarrhythmias, mode switching occurs to DDIR or DDI (if programmed to DDD); following this, the flywheel feature is applied to reduce the pacing rate to the lower rate.

Table 1. Programmable options in mode switching as interpreted by Vitatron.

	Fixed	Automatic
Atrial tracking	Atrial rate < maximum tracking rate	Atrial rate < dynamic upper rate
Wenckebach	Atrial rate gradually > maximum tracking rate	Atrial rate gradually > maximum tracking rate
Switch to DDIR	Atrial rate abruptly > maximum tracking rate	Atrial rate > dynamic upper rate and dynamic upper rate > maximum tracking rate

The Diamond device approaches the theoretical problem of mode oscillation being precipitated by premature atrial complexes (PAC) by not tracking a single PAC. Ventricular pacing following such an event is either controlled by the flywheel or by the sensor. These permit a maximum rate change of ≤30 bpm. If necessary, an atrial synchronisation stimulus will be given so that AV synchrony can be maintained. Mode switching in the Diamond can be programmed to fixed, in which case it behaves as in Vitatron's Ruby DDD device, or to automatic (Table 1) which allows more flexibility.

AIMS OF MODE SWITCHING

The aims of mode-switching can be summarised:

1. Appropriate ventricular rate in atrial tachyarrhythmia
2. Avoidance of or limitation of F wave detection resulting in rapid and irregular ventricular pacing
3. Avoidance of prolongation of atrial tachyarrhythmia by pacing
4. Smooth transitions between pacing modes

To these ends, mode switching can be said to perform well provided that a certain number of rapid atrial beats (>1) are required for the identification of the arrhythmia. Furthermore, it may be necessary in some devices, to programme rate smoothing in addition to mode switching to achieve optimally smooth mode transitions. It remains to be seen in practice whether VVIR is superior to DDIR as the switch mode. Theoretically, there should be no difference as in DDIR atrial stimuli will not capture and therefore not perpetuate or reinitiate atrial tachyarrhythmias.

PROBLEMS OF MODE SWITCHING

The problems of mode-switching are:

1. Detection of atrial arrhythmias
2. Distinction of pathological atrial rhythm from sinus tachycardia
3. Mode oscillations
4. Passive pacemaker behaviour which offers symptomatic rather than therapeutic benefit
5. Pacemaker behaviour requires telemetric ECG analysis in order to interpret function

Mode switching algorithms can be confused by variations in F wave amplitude and slew rate, which can lead to a failure to meet mode switching criteria or mode oscillations. A rapid sinus rhythm at rest, for example in heart failure, might trigger inappropriate and physiologically negative mode switching.

Mode oscillations could occur if the criteria for switching are not sufficiently stringent.

The concept of mode switching is essentially passive, providing symptomatic benefit to the patient. It is important to recall that atrial tachyarrhythmias under these conditions can still carry with them the dangers of heart failure, systemic embolism and death [4,5]. In the future, additional therapeutic approaches are expected which may include both anti-tachycardia pacing and atrial defibrillation.

Lastly, pacemaker behaviour is now so complex that the appraisal of its function by 12-lead ECG or by Holter monitoring is inadequate, and telemetric ECGs from the device are required in order to facilitate the interpretation of function.

In conclusion, mode switching is a feature of DDDR and DDD pacemakers which has important symptomatic benefits and is anticipated soon to be universal amongst manufacturers.

REFERENCES

1. Castallanet M, Florio J, Messenger J. DDI: a new mode for cardiac pacing. Clin Prog Pacing Electrophysiol 1984;2:255–60.
2. Stroobandt R, Willems R, Vandenbulcke F, Sinnaeve A. DDDR pacemakers: a framework for the understanding of atrial and ventricular based device timing. Eur J Cardiac Pacing Electrophysiol 1992;2:151–7.
3. Hayes DL, Ketelson A, Levine PA, Markowitz HT, Sanders R, Schaney G. Understanding timing systems of current DDDR pacemakers. Eur J Cardiac Pacing Electrophysiol 1993;3:70–86.
4. Rosenqvist M, Brandt J, Schuller H. Long-term pacing in sinus node disease: Effects of stimulation mode on cardiovascular morbidity and mortality. Am Heart J 1988;116:16–22.
5. Santini M, Alexidou G, Ansalone G, Cacciatore G, Cini R, Turitto G. Relation of prognosis in sick sinus syndrome to age, conduction defects, and modes of permanent cardiac pacing. Am J Cardiol 1990;65:729–35.

PART THREE

Defibrillators

35. Indication for ICD implantation and selection of patients: present and future

LUC JORDAENS

HISTORICAL BACKGROUND

When Michael Mirowski started his clinical investigations after the development of the implantable defibrillator, he certainly dreamed about a future in which preventive implantation would be an acceptable tool for high-risk patients. However, he was very strict and applied rigid criteria to the selection of patients: they had to have survived two cardiac arrests clearly due to ventricular tachyarrhythmias. These criteria were soon made less rigid, and suffering one cardiac arrest due to ventricular fibrillation (VF) or one episode with hypotensive ventricular tachycardia (VT) was enough to be included in the first investigation, performed with the 'AID' (Intec^R, Pittsburg) [1]. It was clear that this would not remain the only indication, and patients who experienced recurrent ventricular tachycardia and remained inducible despite conventional anti-arrhythmic therapy were considered suitable. As a matter of fact, these were the criteria that were readopted in Belgium when it was accepted that the implantable cardioverter defibrillator (ICD) should be reimbursed for a few centers [2]. The only recent amendment is that previously failing drug therapy is no longer required. It was very surprising to see that Michael Mirowski also required emotional maturity and stability of patients who were scheduled for an ICD implantation. This remains a very important step when considering an ICD implantation today and will be discussed later on.

Naturally, by applying these rigid criteria a very good survival (or a very low mortality) from arrhythmic death was observed by Michael Mirowski in that first clinical series. Therefore, ICD therapy became a cornerstone of anti-arrhythmic therapy.

PATIENT SELECTION: FLEXIBILITY, DREAMS AND REALITY

Helmut Klein proposed the criteria shown in Table 1 in 1987, and they remain very acceptable after all these years. The only remark is that today

Table 1. Indications for the ICD.

1. VF or cardiac arrest >6 weeks after acute myocardial infarction
2. Rapid VT with contraindication for surgery
   - EF < 20%
   - polymorphic, multiple VT
3. Predictable surgical failure
4. Prevention of cardiac arrest in patients awaiting cardiac transplant
5. Prevention of acceleration in slow VT and with antitachycardia pacing

EF = ejection fraction; VF = ventricular fibrillation; VT = ventricular tachycardia.
After H. Klein, 1987.

we no longer require a 6-week interval if a patient has survived a stable VT late after myocardial infarction. The 'bridge to transplant' option is also from a socioeconomic point of view acceptable, and is in our experience extremely helpful for patients on the waiting list for a heart transplant [3].

If you consider these rather flexible criteria, it becomes evident that the cardiologist's decision as to who should be treated with an ICD remains very important (Table 2). Therefore, a systematic approach as proposed by Hauer to utilise the available resources in an optimal way is useful [4]. However, from the moment it became possible to terminate VT by pacing alone, without giving shocks, and without the need for an additional pacemaker and as it became clear that the non-thoracotomy approach was acceptable to the large majority of patients, the number of suitable patients increased. This is clearly reflected in the number of devices that have been implanted, e.g. as in our center during those early years (Figure 1). We are now even approaching the stage at which a device can be left in the pectoral site. Furthermore, with the modern devices it is possible to record what happened before a shock occurred so that we can be certain that shocks are really delivered for VT or fibrillation.

However, in these first few years of implantable defibrillators, there have been a few drawbacks. First, dysfunction exists. Defibrillators can become prematurely depleted or can show technical defects.

Second, patients often suffer from living with such a huge device, and it is not only the size of the device that is troublesome, but also the fact that it can deliver shocks. The patients are not cured by an ICD. The psychologist of our cardiac rehabilitation center compared ICD recipients with patients who were recovering from infarction. Incapacity, among other variables, was felt more by patients with a defibrillator. These patients had mainly been treated with investigational devices in the era of thoracotomy, but still, doubt may be entertained about the success of the ICD. Therefore, the initial suggestion of Mirowski that a patient should be very stable and very mature remains true.

Furthermore, it is clear that the excellent survival curve from the initial database is not as good as originally thought. More arrhythmic death than

Table 2. Factors influencing the decision to use ICDs.

Medical factors
  Disease-related
    Pathology
    Arrhythmia
  Patient-related
    Psychological profile
    Professional/social factors
  Physician-related
    Training
    Skills
    Scientific orientation
  Hospital-related
    Referral pattern
    Equipment

Socioeconomic factors
  Ethical considerations
  Resources
  Insurance
  Health care system governmental restrictions
  Incentives

Technical factors
  Device-related
    Investigational
    Complexity
    Non-thoracotomy option
    Size
    Availability of follow-up equipment

sudden death occurred, and the cardiac survival is not that high among these selected patients. Furthermore, if we analyze the series compiled by the Medtronic Transvene^R and the CPI Endotak^R investigators as to how many patients received shocks during these studies, then the idea of receiving a defibrillator gains negative connotations. A large majority of patients nowadays receive shocks in the first year after implantation, in contrast to the early studies [5]. This can lead to an overestimation of the benefit of an ICD.

CARDIAC ARREST

In Belgium only 7.5% of patients who have been resuscitated after cardiac arrest are long-term survivors. This study was conducted by some of the larger Flemish hospitals [6]. The hope that the proportion of survivors would increase over time seems not to be fulfilled in the actual data, at least in those from the emergency department. Ghent is a city of 250 000 people and has one central telephone number for the ambulance system. All cardiac

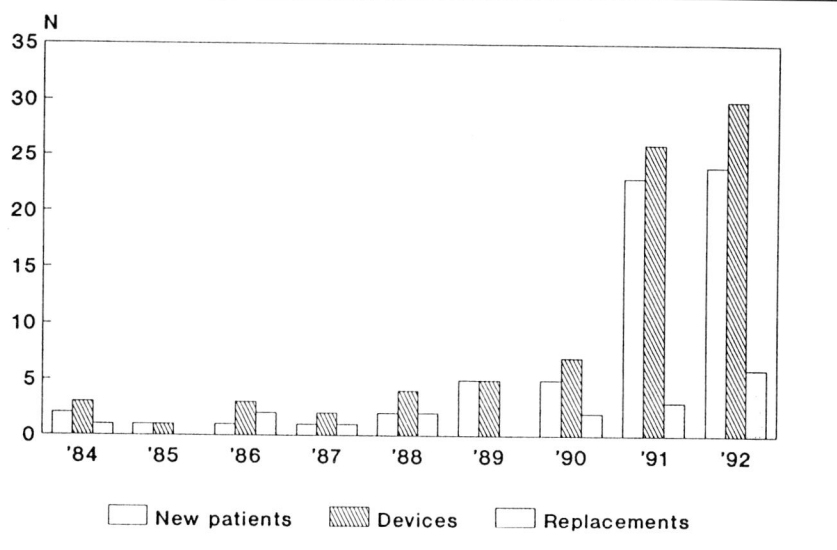

Figure 1. Number of ICD implantations in Ghent over the last 9 years.

arrests trigger the departure of a normal ambulance with resuscitation equipment. Some 125 cardiac arrests happened throughout the year in 1991 and also in 1992 (Figure 2). There were each year about 50 patients with tachycardia or fibrillation on arrival of the rescue team. Considering the survival rate in 1992, only 12 of those patients were discharged from a hospital. Most patients come from the group with VT/VF. So, this remains disappointing, as a significant proportion of these patients are not in good health. They suffer neurological sequelae, and they should not be treated with a defibrillator or even with other means of therapy. Furthermore, some of these patients have other cardiac disease (e.g. Wolff–Parkinson–White syndrome or an acute myocardial infarction) and do not require a defibrillator. The importance of ischaemia is often underscored in patients in whom cardiac arrest occurs. This should be treated very aggressively [7].

VENTRICULAR TACHYCARDIA

The second large subgroup considered nowadays for the implantation of a defibrillator are patients with VT without cardiac arrest. In our center, 43% of the total number of VT/VF studies arises because of VT, and as a matter of fact, VT also constitutes the etiology of 42% of the total number of ICDs in our department. So, the large majority of patients with VT are managed in another way than with a defibrillator [8,9]. We still are doing VT studies to suppress inducibility, and enough data support this approach. After the

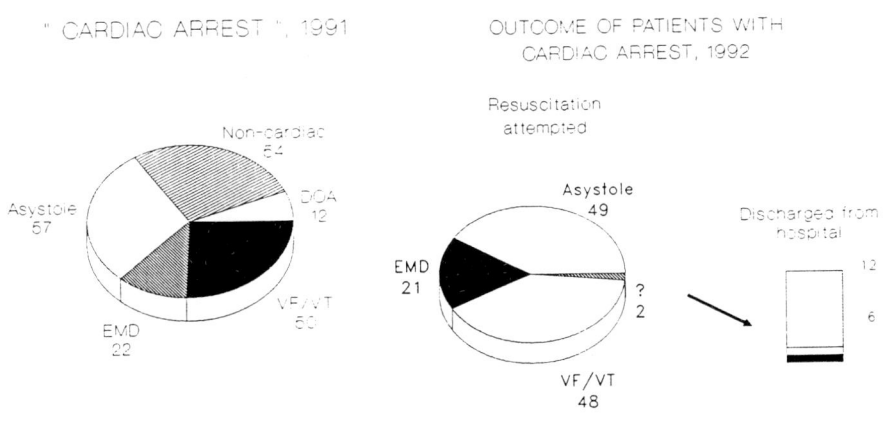

Figure 2. Cardiac arrests in Ghent during 1991 and 1992. On the left, the number of subjects 'dead on arrival' (DOA) is also included. On the right, the proportion of survivors in 1992 is shown as a bar. EMD = electromechanical dissociation. Data: Emergency Dpt., UZ, Ghent.

baseline study we usually prescribe sotalol (the ESVEM trial also identified sotalol as the better antiarrhythmic drug for ventricular tachyarrhythmias) [10]. The non-inducible patients receive sotalol, while the inducible ones receive sotalol and an ICD. Other drugs are used if side effects or proarrhythmia occurs. Over time we have seen some serious recurrences or side effects from long-term therapy with sotalol. Therefore, even this straightforward approach is not always beneficial. However, it saves time in the hospital and shortens the hospital stay, and that is also important.

Therefore, for VT a prospective study is needed to analyze how many patients really benefit from the ICD (if they are not survivors of cardiac arrest). One such effort is the SAMI trial that will start recruitment very soon and was mainly conceived by Karl-Heinz Kuck.

FUTURE INDICATIONS

So, in general, good studies are needed to understand the full implications of this therapy [11]. We can compare an ICD with a drug, or we can compare several programmable features in an ICD. We can now treat by implantation all definite indications, but it is clear that, as resources are not increasing, we will need very straightforward answers to the question who really needs an ICD, and who needs not. The health care system is now being reformed in many European countries, and in the USA there will be increasing pressure from the government in the next few years.

Therefore, in the last part of this chapter I would like to speculate on

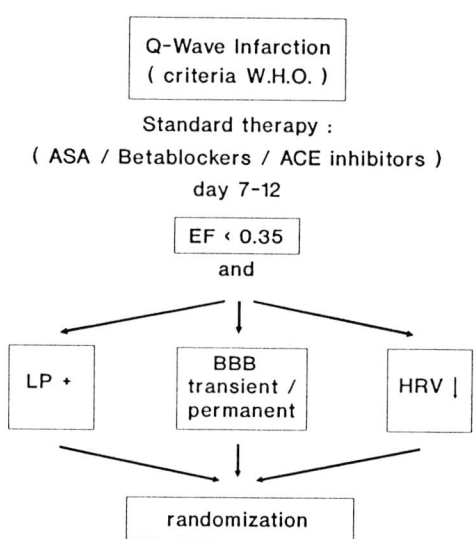

Figure 3. Flow chart of the intervention branch of the MIRRACLE'S study. ACE = angiotensin converting enzyme; ASA = aspirin; BBB = bundle branch block; EF = ejection fraction; HRV = heart rate variability; LP = late potentials.

possible future indications. Some groups of patients surviving a myocardial infarction with a very high risk for subsequent sudden death can be defined. For example, if late potentials are combined with a very poor LVEF, a very high positive predictive value for sudden death is found [12]. Selecting such a group for study could lead to the development of meaningful preventive therapy for sudden death with an ICD.

Some studies of high-risk patients have been conceived, mainly in the USA; they were summarized a few years ago (e.g. the CABG patch and the MADIT study) [13]. It must be pointed out that all those subjects underwent full thoracotomy; this will increase the risk for serious complications. Furthermore, the benefit cannot be extrapolated, as non-thoracotomy-requiring devices clearly give rise to fewer problems. A pilot study is being started called 'MIRRACLE'S' [myocardial infarction risk recognition and conversion of life-threatening events (into survival)], and one of the two branches will analyse intervention. It will study the feasibility and the safety of ICD implantation in very high-risk patients after myocardial infarction.

The flow chart for inclusion is presented in Figure 3. The study will try to answer some important questions, such as whether it is safe to implant an ICD so early after infarction. One can imagine that ischaemia, perforation, sensing problems and arrhythmic storms can arise if an ICD is implanted too early after myocardial infarction.

CONCLUSIONS

The actual indications for ICD implantation remain the following: the survivor of a cardiac arrest with a good quality of life and the patient with symptomatic VT due to organic (progressive) heart disease, who has been properly studied to exclude other ways of treatment. The patient who has survived myocardial infarction and who has a particular risk pattern could become an accepted indication. I would like to add that some patients with congestive heart failure who are not immediately candidates for heart transplantation could also be good candidates for ICD implantation, as a bridge to transplantation. Perhaps the medical therapy for congestive heart failure will improve greatly in the early 1990s [14].

REFERENCES

1. Mirowski M. The automatic implantable cardioverter-defibrillator: an overview. J Am Coll Cardiol 1985;6:461-6.
2. Jordaens L, Waleffe A, Derom F, Rodriguez LM, Clement DL, Kulbertus H. First experience with the implantable cardioverter-defibrillator: 90 patient-months of follow-up. Acta Clin Belg 1988;43:209-18.
3. Tchou PJ, Kadri N, Anderson J, Caceres JA, Jazayeri M, Akhtar M. Automatic implantable cardioverter defibrillators and survival of patients with left ventricular dysfunction and malignant ventricular arrhythmias. Ann Int Med 1988;109:529-34.
4. Hauer R. Studies examine cost effectiveness and efficacy of AICD therapy for high-risk patients. AICD Advances, CPI 1991:8-9.
5. Jordaens L, Trouerbach JW, Vertongen P, Herregodts L, Poelaert J, Van Nooten G. Experience of cardioverters-defibrillators inserted without thoracotomy: evaluation of transvenously inserted intracardiac leads alone or with a subcutaneous axillary patch. Br Heart J 1993;69:14-9.
6. Mullie A, Verstringe P, Buylaert W et al. Predictive value of Glasgow coma score for awakening after out-of-hospital cardiac arrest. Cerebral Resuscitation Study Group of the Belgian Society for Intensive Care. Lancet 1988;1:137-40.
7. Every NR, Fahrenbruch CE, Hallstrom AP, Weaver WD, Cobb LA. Influence of coronary bypass surgery on subsequent outcome of patients resuscitated from out of hospital cardiac arrest. J Am Coll Cardiol 1992;19:1435-9.
8. Jordaens L, Palmer A, Clement DL. Low-dose oral sotalol for monomorphic ventricular tachycardia: effects during programmed electrical stimulation and follow-up. Eur Heart J 1989;10:218-26.
9. Jordaens L, Vertongen P, Provenier F. Radiofrequency ablation of incessant ventricular tachycardia to prevent multiple defibrillator shocks. Int J Cardiol 1992;37:117-20.
10. ESVEM Investigators. The ESVEM trial. Electrophysiologic study versus electrocardiographic monitoring for selection of antiarrhytmic therapy of ventricular tachyarrhythmias. Circulation 1989;79:1354-60.
11. Bigger JT Jr. Prophylactic use of implantable cardioverter defibrillators: medical, technical, economic considerations. PACE 1991;14:376-80.
12. Jordaens L, Schoenfeld P, Block P et al. Risk stratification after infarction: final results of a multicenter prospective study (abstract). Circulation 1991;84:II-238.

13. Nisam S, Thomas A, Mower M, Hauser R. Identifying patients for prophylactic automatic implantable cardioverter defibrillator therapy: status of perspective studies. Am Heart J 1991;122:607–12.
14. Pfeffer MA, Braunwald E, Moyé LA et al. Effect of captopril on mortality and morbidity in patients with left ventricular dysfunction after myocardial infarction. N Engl J Med 1992;327:669–77.

36. The optimum tilt for defibrillation

W. IRNICH

INTRODUCTION

Since the early 1960s and the work of Peleska [1], it has been known that pure capacitor discharges may cause cardiac arrhythmias and reduce the efficiency of defibrillation. At that time the discharge pulse was limited by a resonant L-C circuit which reduced the discharge to 5–10 ms by simultaneously limiting the amplitude to tolerable, non-damaging amplitudes. The reduced efficiency was attributed to refibrillating effects which could be overcome by truncation of the decaying pulse [2]. Though there is no theory available so far to explain it, two aspects have found general acceptance:

1. A capacitor discharge for defibrillation should be truncated, otherwise the tail could refibrillate the heart.
2. Biphasic pulses are preferable due to their reduced propensity to produce refibrillation [3].

However, questions remain open which are not only of theoretical but also of eminent clinical importance:

1. Assuming it is correct that a capacitor discharge for defibrillation should be truncated to avoid refibrillation, which degree of truncation is necessary?
2. Is this degree of truncation, or the so-called 'tilt', independent of pulse duration?
3. If the pulse duration and the intensity of a defibrillation pulse are programmable, which combination is optimal?
4. Do current ICDs operate with or without refibrillating tilts?
5. Are optimally truncated monophasic pulses still inferior to biphasic pulses?

It is the intention of this chapter to give answers to the above posed questions. The reader should study the following text to judge whether the present concept and practice of ICD implantation need revision.

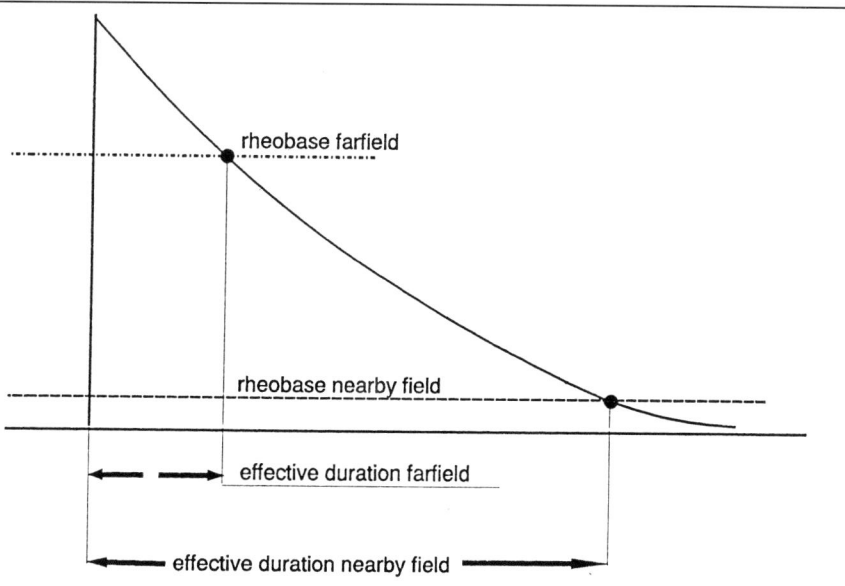

Figure 1. Application of Lapicque's rheobase principle to exponential pulses: if the declining pulse crosses the rheobase line, it is no longer effective. The effective duration of a pulse is much smaller for regions far away from the electrodes (farfield) than that very close to it. Long pulses will, thus, have regionally and temporally different effects on cell membranes, possibly causing circus movements.

THEORY

The following theory is based upon the hypothesis that defibrillation obeys the Fundamental Law of Electrostimulation [4] which is presented by a hyperbola and is characterized by Lapicque's terms of rheobase and chronaxie. The essential message of the rheobase is that an intensity below a threshold value, called the rheobase, no longer has a stimulating effect. Applied to defibrillation, the rheobase message is modified, in that an electric field spread over the whole heart is no longer capable of defibrillating all sites simultaneously. This means that for exponentially decaying capacitor discharges, if the electric field is below the rheobase, then the most distant regions of the heart are no longer electrically affected, while the closest regions, in contrast, may be stimulated much longer (see Figure 1). This regional and temporal irregularity forms the basis upon which renewed fibrillation by circus movements can be reinitiated.

Assuming the above hypothesis to be true, as supported by sufficient evidence, the problem of the correct truncation of a defibrillation pulse can be treated mathematically by the application of the Weiss 'formule fondamental' to an exponentially decaying pulse combined with the boundary condition that the intensity at the end of the pulse is equal to the rheobase, thus:

$$\int^\tau E(t)\, dt = E_0 \int^\tau e^{-t/RC}\, dt$$

$$= RCE_0(1 - e^{\tau/RC}) \geqslant E_{\text{rheo}}(t_c + \tau) \tag{1}$$

with E = electrical field strength, τ = pulse duration, E_0 = initial field strength due to the capacitor discharge, RC = product of lead resistance and discharge capacitor, E_{rheo} = rheobase field strength, t_c = chronaxie time.

Introducing the boundary condition that requires:

$$E_0 \cdot e^{-\tau/RC} = E_{\text{rheo}}. \tag{2}$$

Equation (1) can be rearranged to

$$E_{\text{rheo}} \cdot RC(e^{\tau/RC} - 1) \geqslant E_{\text{rheo}}(t_c + \tau) \tag{3}$$

The solution is independent of the rheobase field strength and can be formulated simply by normalizing the pulse duration τ and RC to chronaxie t_c:

$$e^{X/V} - 1 \geqslant 1/V + X/V \tag{4}$$

with $X = \tau/t_c$ and $V = RC/t_c$.

Equation (4) represents a transcendental function which can be solved by a simple iteration method. The solution is depicted in Figure 2.

Similarly, the energy needed for defibrillation can be expressed in a normalized form. The calculation to determine whether there is a minimum yields: The energy is minimal if the pulse duration is:

$$RC = 0.8 t_c \quad \text{and} \quad \tau = t_c \tag{5}$$

The tilt T (the change in capacitor voltage ΔU related to initial voltage) can be expressed similarly by the normalized values X and V yielding:

$$T = 1 - e^{-X/V} \tag{6}$$

Equation (6) can be evaluated by looking for the corresponding pairs of values in Figure 2 and inserting them in Equation (6). The solution is depicted in Figure 3.

DISCUSSION

According to the above theory, there is a correlation between the three parameters: pulse duration, chronaxie, and RC product of the discharge circuit. For a given RC, V can be determined if the chronaxie is known. Earlier calculations [4] led us to believe that the chronaxie for defibrillation is close to 2 ms, which is typical for stimulation with large area electrodes (such as used with external stimulation). Under this assumption, the curve

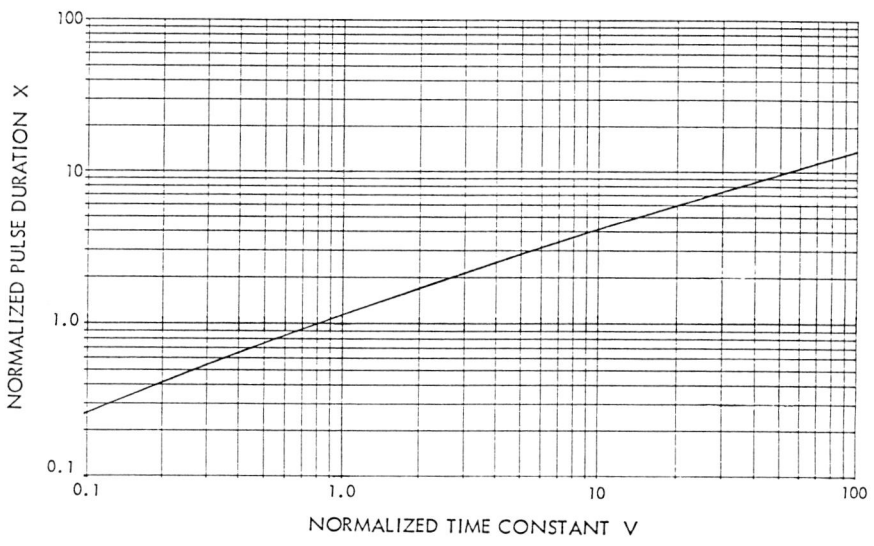

Figure 2. The normalized pulse duration $X = t/t_c$ as a function of the normalized time constant $V = RC/t_c$ (t_c = chronaxie). The curve indicates which time constant of a capacitor discharge corresponds to which pulse duration of a rectangular pulse.

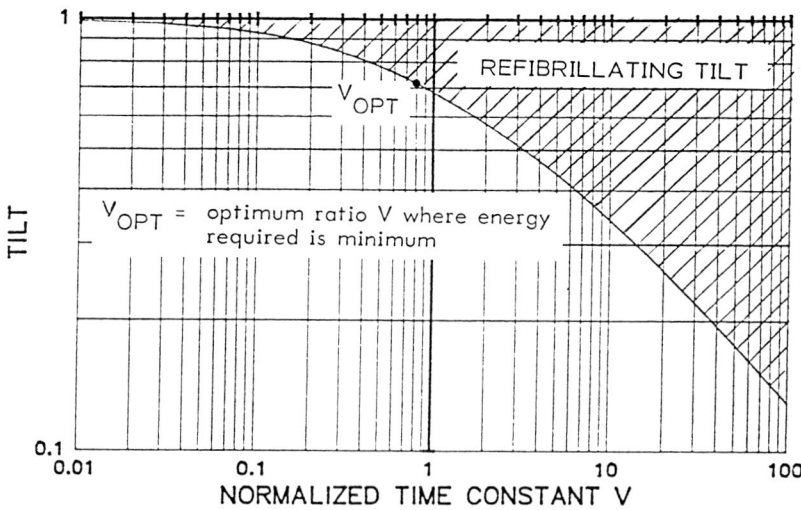

Figure 3. The tilt ($\Delta U/U$) as a function of the normalized time constant $V = RC/t_c$: The greater the tilt or the decrease in capacitor voltage, the smaller the time constant.

in Figure 3 allows for the determination of whether today's defibrillators with monophasic pulses operate adequately or not. All tilt values above the curve indicate that the voltage decrease of the discharging capacitor is too great, hence giving rise to refibrillation. For today's ICDs the capacitance of the capacitor is approximately 150 μF. Thus, together with a load of 50 Ω, a V-value of 3.75 requires a tilt of no more than 47.3%, whereas current ICDs operate at 75%. A tilt of 75% would only be adequate if V is below 1 ($RC < t_c$) or the capacitor has 40 μF or less. The best performance of a monophasic ICD would be achieved if V is 0.8 with the parameters $C = 32$ μF, $\tau = 2$ ms, and tilt = 71%. Our calculated values are very close to what was found by Kroll [5] recently. As the minimum energy for defibrillation is only 30% or less of that at 10–12 ms, we are of the firm opinion that this optimized system will operate with even lower energies than any biphasic system.

The answers to our introductory questions are:
1. The degree of truncation is dependent upon the product of the discharge capacitance of the ICD and the electrode resistance. This product related to the chronaxie, called V, determines the tilt according to Figure 3.
2. If the capacitance-resistance product RC is given, the corresponding pulse duration can be derived from Figure 2. Figure 3, then, expresses that each pulse duration needs a speclfic tilt to guarantee refibrillation-free performance. Both figures demonstrate a rather complicated tilt-pulse duration relationship.
3. The optimal defibrillation pulse is given with a 2 ms pulse duration and a 32 μF output capacitance (a R of 50 Ω and chronaxie with 2 ms assumed).
4. Nearly all of today's monophasic ICDs operate with tilts above the curve in Figure 3, indicating that they possess refibrillating capabilities.
5. It is our conviction that optimized defibrillation pulses with 2 ms pulse duration and 32 μF output capacitance (for 50 Ω load) are superior to any other pulse including biphasic pulses.

REFERENCES

1. Peleska B. Cardiac arrhythmias following condenser discharges led through an inductance: comparison with effects of pure condenser discharges. Circ Res 1965;16:11–8.
2. Schuder JC, Stoeckle H, West JA, Keskar PY. Transthoracic ventricular defibrillation in the dog with truncated and untruncated exponential stimuli. IEEE Trans Biomed Eng 1971;18:410–5.
3. Schuder JC, Gold JH, Stoeckle H, Roberts SA, McDaniel WC, Moellinger DW. Defibrillation in tne calf with bidirectional trapezoidal wave shocks applied via chronically implanted epicardial electrodes. Trans Am Soc Artif Intern Organs 1981;27:467–70.
4. Irnich W. The fundamental law of electrostimulation and its application to defibrillation. PACE 1990;13:1423–47.
5. Kroll M. A minimal model of the monophasic defibrillation pulse. PACE 1993;16:769–77.

37. Cerebrovasomotor reactivity predicts tolerance to tiered therapy with implantable cardioverter-defibrillators

IGOR SINGER & HARVEY EDMONDS, JR.

INTRODUCTION

Third-generation implantable cardioverter-defibrillators (ICDs) provide tiered therapy for ventricular tachycardia (VT) and ventricular fibrillation (VF). Tiered therapy is designed to provide an effective, rapid, and graded response for VT, so that slow VT may be terminated by antitachycardia pacing (ATP), rapid VT by cardioversion and hypotensive VT, or VF by a defibrillation shock. This philosophy, though generally sound, does not at present take into account the hemodynamic consequences of ventricular dysrhythmias nor assess the end-organ perfusion. The design of more 'intelligent' devices depends on the ability to assess the hemodynamic consequences of arrhythmias and end-organ perfusion.

Previous studies have shown that the transient cessation of blood flow which occurs during VF is associated with a temporary cessation of cerebral blood flow and, if prolonged beyond a critical time, may be followed by ischemic delta wave slowing on the transcranial EEG (QEEG), which may persist for a variable length of time [1,2]. Transcranial blood flow may be measured by noninvasive techniques, such as transcranial Doppler ultrasonography (TCD), see below. QEEG and TCD may be used together because of a close relationship among impairments of regional cerebrocortical blood flow, metabolic activity, spontaneous electrical activity, and neurologic/cognitive function [3].

QEEG analysis relies on an adaptive statistical approach [4]. The usually large interpatient variability in QEEG indices is minimized by the use of a moving window average and examining only intrapatient changes, i.e., using each patient as his own control. The logarithmic transformation of the QEEG measures to achieve Gaussian distributions then permits the familiar parametric statistical comparison of current values to those from a previously established, individualized, reference self-norm. The technique is adaptive because a new self-norm can be quickly established to adjust for major changes due to hyperventilation or sedative administration. The choice of the specific EEG descriptors is based on the loss of high-frequency activity or the development of excessive slow wave (low-frequency) activity, which are the accepted hallmarks of cerebrocortical ischemia [5].

The purpose of the present study was to: (1) assess the effects of transient cerebral hypoperfusion on cerebrocortical function with QEEG monitoring, (2) correlate QEEG changes with TCD flow changes, and (3) assess the potential usefulness of TCD and QEEG for the evaluation of cerebral perfusion and function during ICD testing and programming.

METHODS

EEG monitoring

A conventional 19-channel EEG is obtained using a nylon helmet (Electro-Cap International, Eaton, OH) with electrodes positioned according to the international 10–20 electrode placement system [6]. The electrodes are filled with a conductive gel to maintain impedances below $5\,k\Omega$ throughout the surgical procedure. An upper facial electromyogram and electro-oculogram are recorded to aid in artifact rejection. The amplifiers of the Spectrum 32 signal analyzer (Cadwell Laboratories, Kennewick, WA) have a bandpass of 0.5–70 Hz (3 dB roll-off) and a 60 Hz notch filter. Analog EEG signals are sampled at 200 Hz and digitized in sequential segments (epochs) of 2.56 s at 12-bit resolution and stored on an optical disk. The frequency content of Hamming-filtered, digitized signals from each of 8 derived bipolar channels (F7–T3, F8–T4, T3–T5, T4–T6, C3–Cz, C4–Cz, P3–01, P4–02) is determined using a fast Fourier transformation. The absolute power in picowatts (pW) is calculated for very low (0.5–1.5), low (1.5–3.5), low-moderate (3.5–7.5), high-moderate (7.5–12.5), high (12.5–25), very high (25–40), and total (1.5–25 Hz) bandwidths. The relative power is also calculated as the power in each band expressed as a percentage of total power.

CIMON QEEG Analysis

CIMON/DSA software (Cadwell Laboratories) provides unique quantitative measures of EEG change through the establishment of a high-quality baseline reference (self-norm). This baseline must accurately reflect the electrographic status of the patient's cerebrocortical function prior to testing. The self-norm is composed of 24 EEG epochs which have been determined automatically to be free from high amplitude, movement, and muscle artifacts (see below). Each of the numeric descriptors obtained from this norm is log transformed ($\log x$ for absolute power measures, $\log x/1 - x$ for relative power measures) [7] and statistically compared with like values from a moving window. The window is composed of 5 artifact-free, equally weighted epochs of 2.5 s and lags 25 s behind real time.

The CIMON display relies on boxes representing 8 bipolar derivations superimposed on a video schematic representation of the patient's head viewed from above. Within each box, the most recent moving window average is displayed as a color-coded horizontal bar. Successive moving window averages are created by adding the most recently acquired average and deleting the oldest one. The upward scrolling display has the appearance of stacks of poker chips, with each chip representing a single moving window average of 10 epochs. Each box also contains a digitized segment of unprocessed EEG waveform from the most current epoch and an indication of the mean frequency for each successive moving window average (Figure 1).

CIMON automatic artifact rejection is based on excessively high total power values (>250 pW). In addition, the unprocessed waveforms from the 19-channel EEG display, upper facial electromyogram, electro-oculogram, and ECG were examined on an adjacent video monitor for signs of contamination that may have escaped the automated artifact rejection system.

QEEG detection of cerebral dysfunction

Cerebral dysfunction was defined statistically as a >3 standard deviation change in any one of three criteria: loss of high-frequency (alpha + beta) power, gain of low-frequency (delta) activity, loss of total power. Using this statistical approach, the probability was less than 1 in 100 that detected changes in the current moving window sample mean could have been obtained from the same population as the reference self-norm.

TCD characterization of altered cerebral perfusion

The middle cerebral blood flow velocity was measured continuously via a 2 MHz ultrasonic probe held in place over the temporal region with an elastic headband [8]. The frequency composition of the Doppler shift was calculated and displayed on an Eden Medical Electronics TC2–64B pulsed wave Doppler ultrasonograph. The flow velocity profile was continuously recorded on videotape. The analog signal representing the upper edge of the profile envelope as well as that for systemic arterial pressure was also recorded as an additional channel on the QEEG analyzer. This permitted direct comparison among changes in cardiac performance, systemic and cerebral perfusion and associated EEG activity.

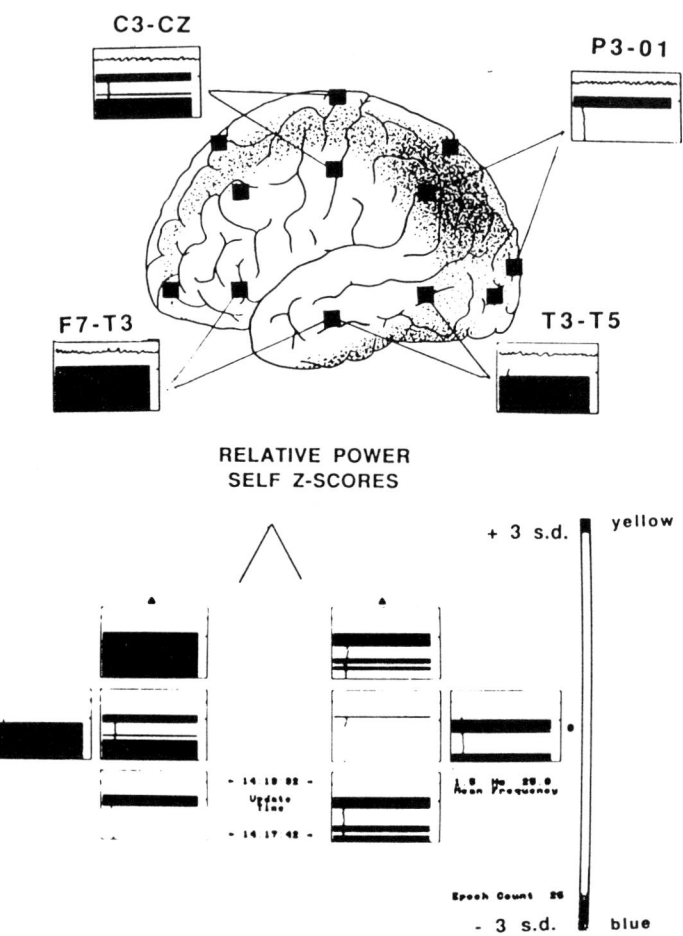

Figure 1. Topographical distribution corresponding to the various areas of the brain (above) and a schematic representation of the information displayed by the computer (below). Display: nose up, left and right frontal, parietotemporal, and occipital regions. Each region is represented by a separate 'box' of scrolling data. See text for discussion.

Patient population

Fifteen conscious patients with implanted third generation ICDs (Ventritex™ V-100, Sunnyvale, CA [8 patients] and Guardian ATP™ 4210 & 4211, Telectronics, Englewood, CO [7 patients]) underwent postoperative evaluation of their implanted ICDs in the electrophysiology laboratory. VT induction was accomplished by programmed ventricular stimulation, using the implanted EP capability and noninvasive programmed stimulation (Ventritex™ and Guardian ATP™ 4211) and via invasive programmed stimulation (Guardian ATP™ 4210). Continuous intra-arterial blood pressure, arterial saturation, electrocardiographic, QEEG, and TCD monitoring were obtained for all patients. Ventricular tachyarrhythmias were induced multiple times in each patient to test the termination of the tachyarrythmias by the device. The tiered therapy consisting of ATP, cardioversion, and defibrillation, in ascending order of treatment aggressivity, was used to terminate ventricular tachyarrythmias. If the cycle length of the tachyarrhythmia was ≤250 ms, defibrillation therapy alone was used, otherwise attempts at ATP and cardioversion preceded defibrillation. In all patients, the therapy was specifically designed to terminate VT by ATP initially, if at all possible. The programmed parameters most successful in accomplishing this task were determined by preoperative and intraoperative EP testing.

RESULTS

Cerebrovasomotor response (CVR) was determined from the time course of blood flow velocity changes after successful VT or VF reversion (CVR = number of beats to maximal velocity increase). Concomitant changes in QEEG were also analyzed independently of the TCD results. Delta wave changes, or conversely alpha loss post-hypotensive episodes (HTEs) which are associated with cerebral ischemia, were analyzed for each patient.

A total of 91 HTEs were observed in 15 patients, which ranged from 2 to 97 s. In 66 HTEs ≤ 15 s, the immediate CVR was 2 beats, i.e. the time required for the TCD to return to the baseline peak velocity. However, in 25 HTEs > 15 s, a delayed CVR response was noted, which averaged 20 beats. The percent increase in the CVR was significantly longer ($p < 0.01$) for the delayed vs. immediate CVR ($58 \pm 35\%$ vs. $35 \pm 24\%$).

Loss of alpha power (i.e. increase in delta power) occurred in 25 HTEs > 15 s, but not in HTEs ≤ 15 s, consistent with transient cerebral ischemia. Cerebral ischemia did not persist for more than 30 s.

An example of a transient cerebral ischemia due to VT is shown in Figure 2, and during VF in Figure 3. A corresponding example of typical TCD changes resulting from hypoperfusion during rapid VT is demonstrated in Figure 4. An example of CVR responses (immediate vs. delayed) is shown in Figure 5.

When the individual results are plotted, a clear separation with minimal overlap is noted between patients with immediate and those with delayed CVR responses (Figure 6).

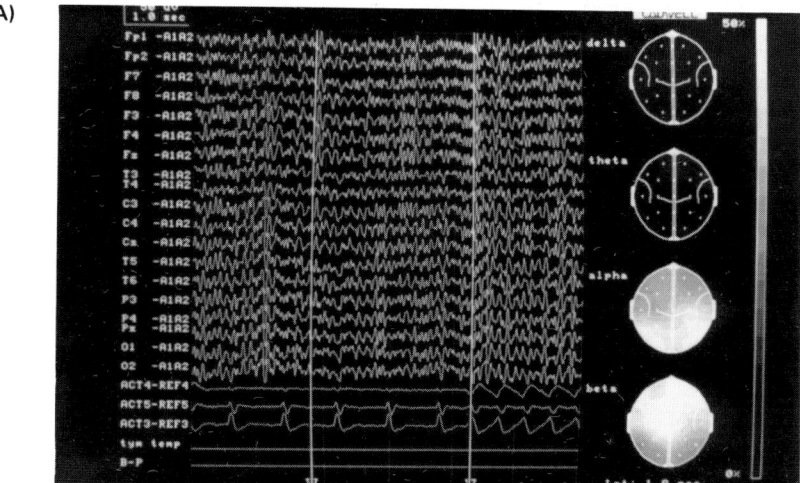

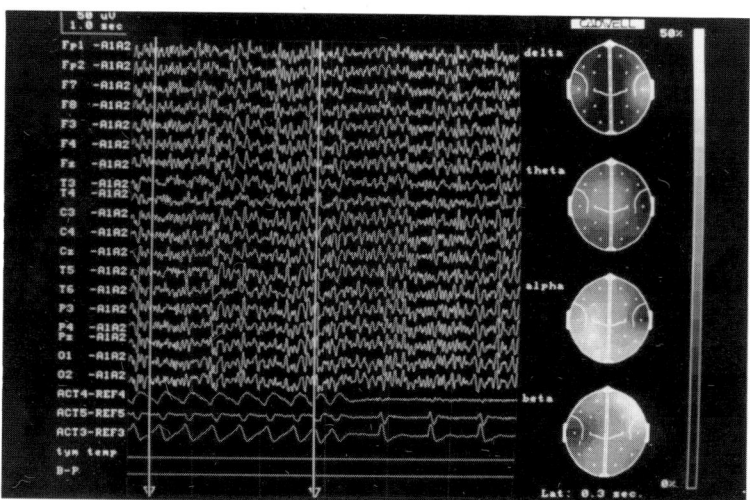

Figure 2. QEEG during an episode of VT. (A) Pre-VT induction: note that all the activity is confined to the beta and alpha regions. (B) During VT, activity shifts to theta and delta regions. (Left, analog recordings, right, schematized recordings, with head viewed from above, nose in front, occiput behind).

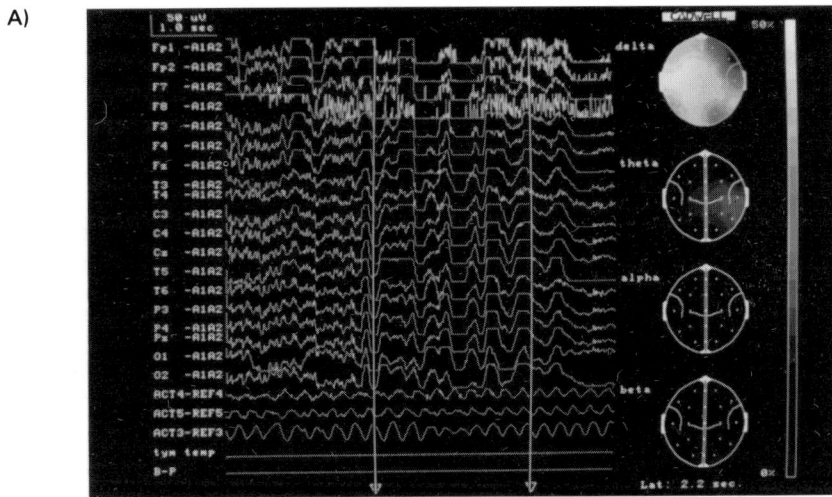

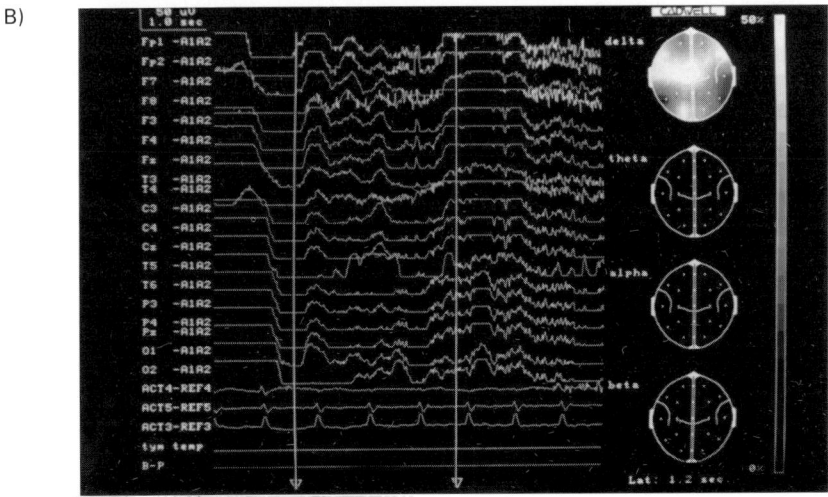

Figure 3. QEEG during an episode of VF. (A) Note a profound shift of activity to the delta region due to cerebral ischemia and (B) defibrillation: note persistence of delta slowing post-defibrillation.

DISCUSSION

More than a decade ago, Rodbard proposed that the arteriolar endothelium controlled the tone of the surrounding vascular smooth muscle by releasing vasodilator substances in response to increases in shear stress [9]. Later, this proposition was experimentally confirmed through the use of a vascular shunt [10]. Upon shunt opening, the vessel diameter initially decreased due to a

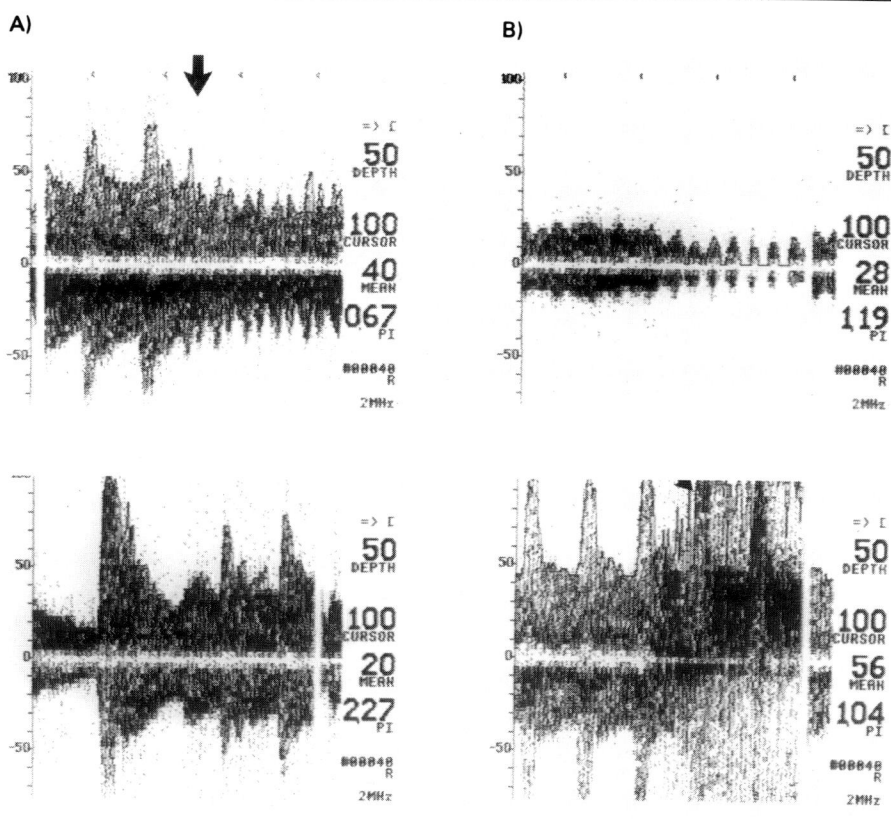

Figure 4. TCD changes during rapid VT. (A) At the onset of VT, note a profound fall in the perfusion (arrow); (B) VF, note a complete loss of perfusion; (C) return of normal perfusion on restoration of sinus rhythm by defibrillation; and (D) hyperemia following restoration of normal perfusion.

drop in intravascular pressure. However, within 10–15 s, the artery began to dilate, reaching a new plateau within 1 min. An initial moderate transient flow velocity increase occurred due to the decreased vessel diameter. In contrast, the delayed, large, sustained velocity increase seemed due to the endothelium-mediated decrease in arteriolar resistance.

The present observation extends these experimental findings from the canine gracilis muscle to the human cerebrovasculature. The brief immediate hyperemic response seen following short hypotensive episodes reflects the consequence of a sudden drop in cerebral perfusion pressure. The more sustained and larger period of hyperemia occurring after longer hypotensive episodes thus seems due to the endothelial release of endogenous vasodilators in response to continuing increases in the arterial wall shear stress. This flow-

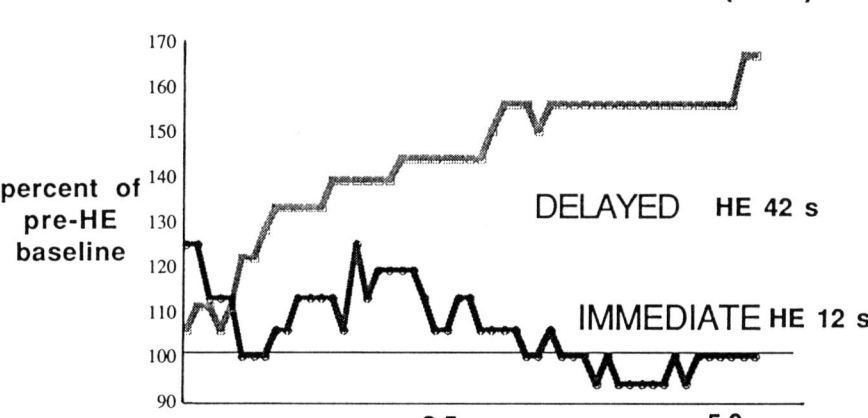

Figure 5. Differences in CVR responses for a patient with a short episode of VT (12 s) with an immediate return of CVR to the baseline, and a patient with a prolonged episode of hypotension lasting 42 s exhibiting a delayed response. HE = hypotensive episode.

induced dilation also seems to play an important part in the establishment of collateral flow [11]. Using combined QEEG/TCD monitoring, characterization of the normal pattern of vascular and neuronal reactivity may identify those patients deficient in the production and/or release of the potent vasodilators nitric oxide and the aspirin-sensitive prostacyclin [12]. These individuals seem to be at increased risk for the development of cerebral dysfunction.

Third generation ICDs use tiered therapy to terminate VT or VF. The method used for therapy stratification is most often based on the tachyarrhythmia rate (cycle length) and arrhythmia episode duration. However, the tachycardia rate (cycle length) may have dissimilar consequences in patients, depending on the status of the left ventricular function, presence or absence of cardiac ischemia, state of the extracranial and intracranial circulation, posture at the time of the arrhythmia occurrence, compensatory vasoreactive reflexes, and duration of the arrhythmia. A hemodynamic sensor may be used to evaluate perfusion during tachyarrythmias. The question as to which specific parameter should be used to evaluate end-organ perfusion is still largely unanswered, however. Perhaps the most sensitive indicator of perfusion is the brain. Since cognitive, sensory-motor and vasoregulatory reflexes are centrally controlled, it is logical to conclude that adequacy of cerebrovascular perfusion is of vital importance. Even brief episodes of cerebral hypoperfusion (>15 s), as demonstrated by this study, may result

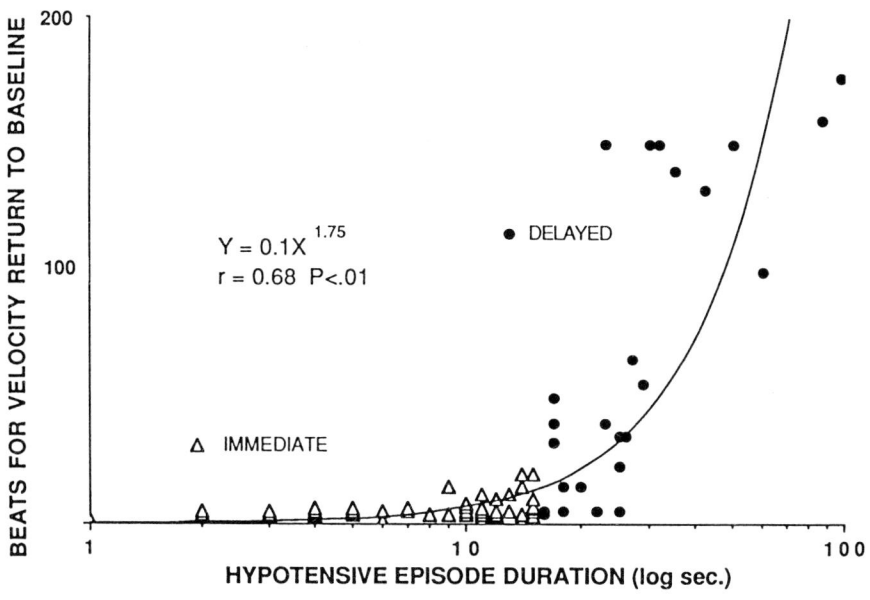

Figure 6. Data for immediate and delayed responses. Number of beats for TCD velocity to return to baseline is plotted on the y-axis and HTE duration on the x-axis (log sec.). Note that there is a clear separation with minimal overlap, indicating that CVR may discriminate the patients with a likelihood of tolerating programmed ICD therapy from patients who do not.

in profound cerebral ischemia. The consequences of ischemia may be a loss of perception or motor control or complete loss of consciousness.

Cerebral perfusion appears to be an important indicator of overall perfusion. A hemodynamic sensor for the future 'intelligent' devices, needs to be validated against some reliable measure of perfusion. TCD and QEEG parameters of cerebral perfusion may provide the absolute or a relative standard.

It is interesting to speculate what the effects of upright posture might be on these parameters. It is reasonable to expect that the observed changes in TCD and QEEG would be exaggerated in the upright posture.

Future generations of ICDs are likely to combine therapies for supraventricular tachyarrythmias with therapies for VT/VF and incorporate atrial ATP and cardioversion. Stratification of therapies based on the hemodynamic consequences of tachycardia may further enhance treatment sequencing under these circumstances. Other parameters of cerebral function may further refine and augment these techniques, e.g. evoked sensory or evoked auditory testing.

We conclude, therefore, that TCD and QEEG techniques are powerful and sensitive techniques to measure cerebral perfusion. These techniques may be used as the standard against which to test hemodynamic sensors for future ICDs.

REFERENCES

1. Nuwer MR. Quantitative EEG:I. Techniques and problems of frequency analysis and topographic mapping. J Clin Neurophysiol 1988;5:1–43.
2. Singer I, van der Laken J, Edmonds HL Jr, Slater AD, Austin E. Is defibrillation threshold testing safe? PACE 1992;14(11):1899–904.
3. Sundt TM Jr, Sharbrough FW, Piepgras DC. The significance of cerebral blood flow measurements during carotid endarterectomy. In: Bergan JJ, Yao JST, editors. Cerebrovascular Insufficiency. New York: Grune & Stratton, 1983:287–307.
4. John ER, Prichep LS, Chabot RJ et al. Monitoring brain function during cardiovascular surgery: hypoperfusion vs. microembolism as the major cause of neurological damage during cardiopulmonary bypass. In: Refsum H, Sulg IA, Rasmussen K, editors. Heart & Brain, Brain & Heart. Berlin: Springer-Verlag, 1989:405–21.
5. Niedermeyer E. Cerebrovascular disorders and EEG. In: Niedermeyer E, Lopes de Silva F, editors. Electroencephalography 2nd ed. Baltimore: Urban and Schwarzenberg, 1987:275–300.
6. Blom JL, Anneveldt M. An electrode cap tested. Electroenceph Clin Neurophysiol 1982;54:591–4.
7. John ER, Ahn H, Prichep L et al. Developmental equations for the electroencephalogram. Science 1980;210:1255–8.
8. von Reutern G-M, Hetzel A, Birnbaum D et al. Transcranial Doppler ultrasonography during cardiopulmonary bypass in patients with severe carotid stenosis or occlusion. Stroke 1988;19:674–80.
9. Rodbard S. Vascular caliber. Cardiology 1975;60:40–9.
10. Smiesko V, Khayutin MK, Kozik J et al. Flow-induced dilation of the dog gracilis muscle artery. Physiol Bohemoslov 1987;36:289–300.
11. Koller A, Kaley G. Endothelium regulates skeletal muscle microcirculation by a blood flow velocity-sensing mechanism. Am J Physiol 1990;258:916–20.
12. Smiesko V, Johnson PC. The arterial lumen is controlled by flow-related shear stress. News Physiol Sci 1993;8:34–8.

38. Clinical utility of telemetered electrograms in pacemakers and ICDs

ROLAND STROOBANDT, FILIEP VANDENBULCKE, ROGER WILLEMS & ALFONS SINNAEVE

INTRODUCTION

Bidirectional communication enables two pieces of equipment to communicate i.e. to transmit and receive information from one another. Applied to cardiac pacing, bidirectional communication is a further development of the earlier programmable devices. The same technology which permits the pulse generator to communicate with the programmer at the time of a program change also provides the means for interrogation of the pulse generator at any other time. Therefore, all present-day pacemakers have a double communication link, one for programming and another one for telemetry.

The programming link is a two-way communication established between the programmer and the implanted pulse generator. This programming link not only enables a rapid adjustment of a multiplicity of basic parameters and a selection of the stimulation mode, but also is an integral part of a quality control system. It assures the appropriate response to a programmed command while minimizing the possibility of inadvertent or phantom programming. In its simplest form, the programming link permits the pulse generator to indicate that it has received and implemented a recognizable programming code. Recent pacemakers also have a memory into which coded data can be entered and can be read later on from the pulse generator by the programmer. These data may include lead model, medication taken by the patient, indication for pacemaker implant, etc.

The purpose of telemetry in general is to make measurements at some distance and to transmit the resulting data via a telecommunication channel to the recording apparatus. The telemetry link in cardiac pacing systems allows the transfer of coded commands from the programmer to the implanted device. If a command is accepted, the pulse generator may start a new measurement or may recall results from its memory and transmit them back to the programmer.

TELEMETRY IN PACEMAKERS

The pacing system is essentially an interaction between three components: the pulse generator, the lead(s), and the patient. Therefore, a telemetry system should communicate in a way that provides information about the device and lead(s) and the way the device is programmed to deal with the patient's underlying rhythm. It may be important to recognize from the outset that not all that is printed out from a programmer is telemetered [1]. A clear distinction has to be made between programmed and measured data. Programmed data indicates how the pacemaker is supposed to perform, while measured data actually indicates how the pacemaker is performing at that time [2]. *Measured data* may give precise information about pacemaker stimulation parameters, lead impedance, and battery status. Knowing the *programmed settings* is essential before assessing any change of a parameter. It allows one to determine whether or not the pacing system is functioning in accordance with its programmed specifications and greatly facilitates the interpretation of any pacemaker electrogram [3]. Both the programmed and measured data should always be recorded on initial interrogation and filed. *Telemetry of Holter functions and event counters* provides information about the interplay between the heart and the pacemaker. It indicates the percent of time the pacemaker was either pacing or inhibited (see Chapter 29).

CLINICAL UTILITY OF TELEMETERED ELECTROGRAMS AND EVENT MARKERS IN PACEMAKERS

Since the introduction of dual chamber rate-responsive devices, the interpretation of pacemaker electrograms has become very complex. A particularly useful aid to ECG analysis is offered by the ability to telemeter intracardiac electrograms and annotated ECG channels [4]. The ECG interpretation channel provides detailed information regarding the occurrence of pacing and sensed events, refractory and alert periods. When superimposed on a surface ECG, it clearly indicates which ECG events are being sensed properly and which start a timing cycle. It allows the evaluation of normal pacemaker function and may free the user of the need to memorize characteristic features unique to a specific pacemaker model (Figure 1). It also facilitates rhythm interpretation [5] when the pacemaker is operating at its upper rate limit (Figure 2). The telemetered electrogram may also be valuable for the analysis of atrial arrhythmias which are difficult to interpret from the standard ECG.

During spontaneous episodes of pacemaker-mediated tachycardias, the surface ECG may not always be sufficiently accurate to localize the P wave. Telemetry of the atrial electrogram permits the identification of the P wave [6,7]. Telemetry of the atrial electrogram during VVI pacing at a rate which is faster than the intrinsic atrial rate offers the possibility to evaluate the potential for pacemaker-mediated tachycardia in patients equipped with a-trial tracking pacemakers. The persistence of retrograde conduction can be

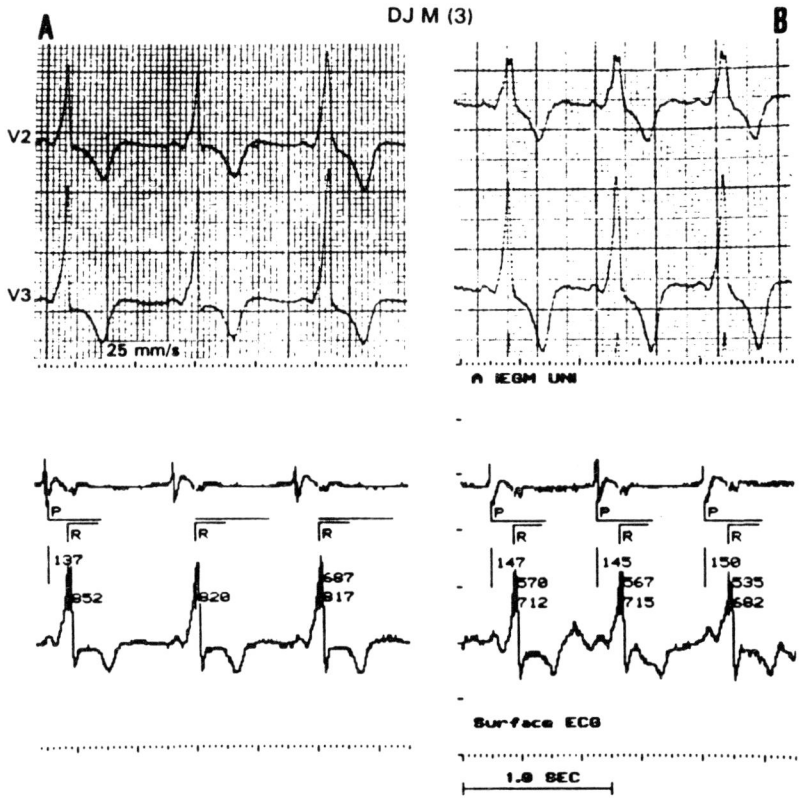

Figure 1. Top tracings are surface ECG leads V2 and V3. Bottom tracings are a printout of the surface ECG lead and a telemetered intra-atrial electrogram (A IEGM). The patient has a complete AV block, and sinus P waves are conducted over an infero-posterior located accessory pathway. As the accessory pathway blocks at higher sinus rates, a DDDR pacemaker was implanted and programmed at a lower rate of 45 ppm and an AV delay of 200 ms. (A) Although the pacemaker is completely inhibited during sinus rhythm, the telemetered atrial electrogram and the event markers indicate a malsensing of the second and third P wave. Hence, the pacemaker interprets the second and third R wave as a PVC as it is not preceded by a P wave and consequently prolongs its PVARP to 480 ms. (B) After programming the pacemaker to a higher sensitivity, the P waves are adequately sensed.

recognized and quantified (Figure 3). It allows precise measurement of the ventriculo-atrial interval (VAI), i.e. the interval from the ventricular stimulus to the retrograde P wave. This is a particularly convenient method to guide the programming of the duration of the atrial refractory period (ARI or PVARP), which will prevent recognition of retrograde P waves and prevent future episodes of pacemaker-mediated tachycardias [8]. Moreover, it allows us to maximize the upper rate limit, by selecting the shortest total atrial

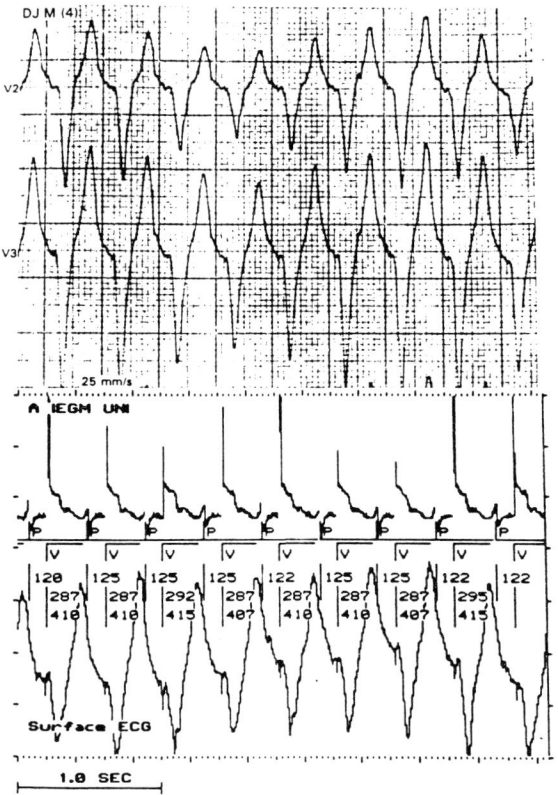

Figure 2. Upper rate behavior of DDD pacemaker. Top tracings are surface ECG leads V2 and V3. Bottom tracings are a printout surface ECG lead and a telemetered intra-atrial electrogram (A IEGM). The patient is equipped with a DDD pacemaker programmed to an upper rate limit of 150 ppm. During an exercise test the pacemaker is operating near its upper rate limit. The total atrial refractory period (TARI) equals or nearly equals the upper rate interval (URI). The sensing of the intra-atrial P wave is marked by a 'P', and the ventricular output stimulus is indicated by a 'V'. The P to V interval, the V to P interval and the V to V interval is given in ms. Telemetry of the atrial electrogram permits easy identification of the P waves that are difficult to discern on the surface ECG.

refractory interval (TARI), being the sum of the atrioventricular interval (AVI) and the postventricular atrial refractory period (ARI or PVARP) [9,10].

Myopotentials may cause myoinhibition and result in unexpected pauses. Also, myotracking may occur by sensing myopotentials on the atrial channel which then may trigger a ventricular output. Telemetry of these signals is possible and may help to adjust the sensitivity setting of the pacemaker to eliminate oversensing.

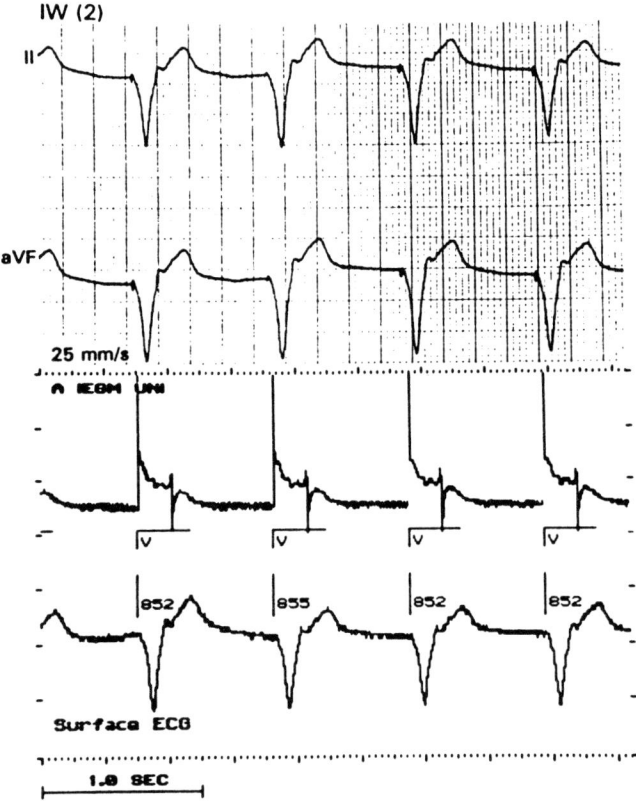

Figure 3. Evaluation of retrograde conduction in a patient equipped with a DDD pacemaker. The pacemaker is temporarily programmed in the VVI mode. Surface ECG leads D2 and AVF are shown in the top tracing. The bottom tracing depicts a printout of a surface ECG lead and the telemetered intra-atrial electrogram (A IEGM) at a chart speed of 25 mm/s. The event markers indicate ventricular paced events (V). V to V intervals are provided in ms. Retrograde VA conduction occurs at 200 ms after the ventricular pacing stimulus.

Event markers and telemetry of the intracardiac electrogram may also be a helpful adjunct in detecting electromagnetic interference caused by voltage transients from loose set screws or by physical interaction between functional and abandoned leads, make-break artifacts of a partial conductor fracture, or other spurious signals [11,12].

Lead problems can readily be identified by interrogation of the lead impedance telemetry. If lead fracture occurs, a massive rise in lead impedance will be observed. Complementary information can be obtained by event marker telemetry which will show a properly timed pacing stimulus when none is visible on the conventional ECG (Figure 4). The diagnostic capabili-

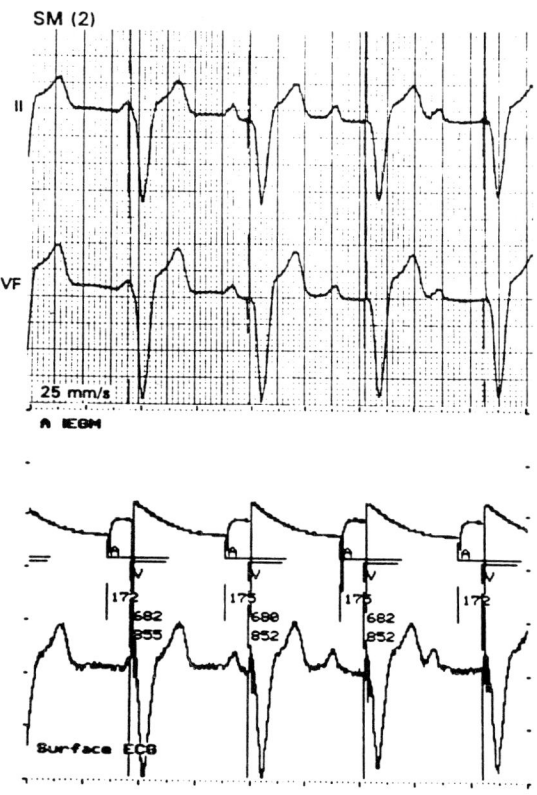

Figure 4. Lead fracture. Surface ECG leads D2 and AVF, printout of a surface ECG lead, and annotated telemetered intra-atrial electrogram (A IEGM). The patient is equipped with a DDD pacemaker programmed at a lower rate of 70 ppm, an upper rate of 120 ppm, and an AV interval of 175 ms. The surface ECG lead shows a P wave which is not tracked and which is dissociated from the ventricular paced rhythm. Telemetry of the atrial electrogram demonstrates the presence of atrial stimuli which are not visible on the surface ECG. The most likely explanation for the loss of atrial capture is either fracture of the atrial lead or a loose connection screw. Measured data indicated a massive rise in atrial lead impedance (>1990 ohms). At exploration, an internal fracture of the atrial lead was confirmed.

ties may often complement one another. Therefore, both the ECG and the annotated ECG channel must be looked at to be sure that they correspond appropriately.

VALUE OF STORED DATA IN ICDs

The introduction of third-generation ICD devices which offer a hierarchy of therapies ranging from antitachycardia pacing, low- and high-energy car-

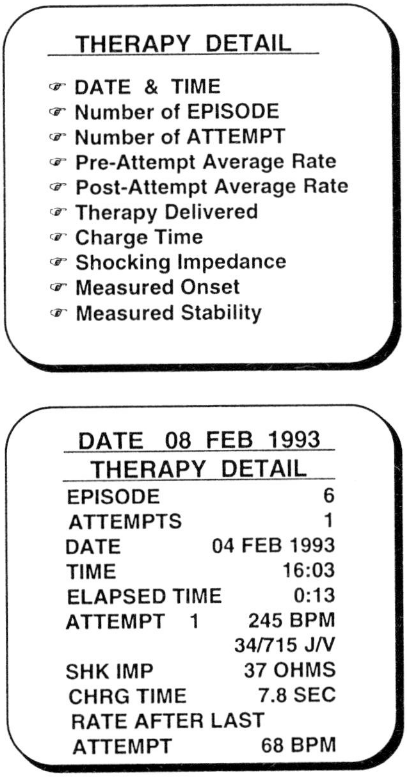

THERAPY DETAIL

- ☞ DATE & TIME
- ☞ Number of EPISODE
- ☞ Number of ATTEMPT
- ☞ Pre-Attempt Average Rate
- ☞ Post-Attempt Average Rate
- ☞ Therapy Delivered
- ☞ Charge Time
- ☞ Shocking Impedance
- ☞ Measured Onset
- ☞ Measured Stability

DATE 08 FEB 1993
THERAPY DETAIL

EPISODE	6
ATTEMPTS	1
DATE	04 FEB 1993
TIME	16:03
ELAPSED TIME	0:13
ATTEMPT 1	245 BPM
	34/715 J/V
SHK IMP	37 OHMS
CHRG TIME	7.8 SEC
RATE AFTER LAST ATTEMPT	68 BPM

Figure 5. Example of a therapy detail telemetered by an ICD (CPI Ventak P2).

dioversion, and bradycardia pacing has expanded the patient selection criteria for implantation of an ICD. In contrast to the implantation criteria of the early ICDs, in which virtually all patients had to have sustained a cardiac arrest [13], the recipients of third-generation ICDs may have fewer symptomatic ventricular tachyarrhythmias and experience less hemodynamic compromise before device response [14]. Therefore, the presence and severity of symptoms preceding device response may become a very unreliable indicator of the presence of sustained ventricular arrhythmias. The inability to document the rhythm leading to device intervention was a persistent limitation in the early generations of ICDs. A major advance in the latest generation of ICDs is the incorporation of sophisticated telemetry capabilities [15]. This diagnostic feature may provide information concerning the therapy delivered, the number and types of detection, and the rate of the tachycardia. The therapy history allows the physician to assess the effectiveness of the therapy delivered for a detected arrhythmia (Figure 5). The number of episodes indicate the number of detected arrhythmias, while the number of attempts is defined as the number of treatments within an episode. Date and time

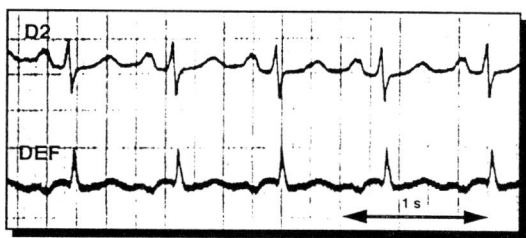

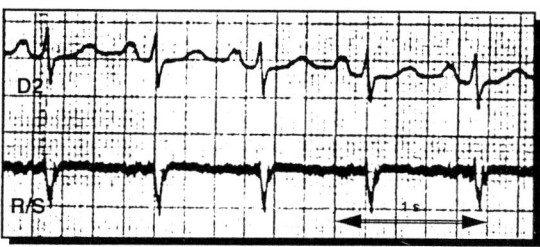

Figure 6. Real-time telemetered electrogram simultaneously recorded with surface ECG lead D2. The top panel shows the real-time electrogram from the shocking electrodes (DEF), being the proximal and distal coil of an endocardial single lead system (CPI Endotak-C). P waves are clearly visible. The lower panel depicts the real-time electrogram from the rate-sensing, bipolar detection electrodes (R/S).

indications are very helpful in correlating symptoms with events. Information stored concerning sudden onset ratios and measured stability of the tachycardia may supply important information to enhance the detection criteria for tachyarrhythmias.

Real-time electrograms may be available from both the rate sensing leads and the shocking leads (Figure 6). The electrogram recorded between the shocking leads is superior in quality compared with the electrograms obtained from the rate-sensing leads because they are more spread apart and cover larger areas of myocardium. Therefore, they appear much like a cross between a surface ECG and an intracardiac electrogram. As electrograms

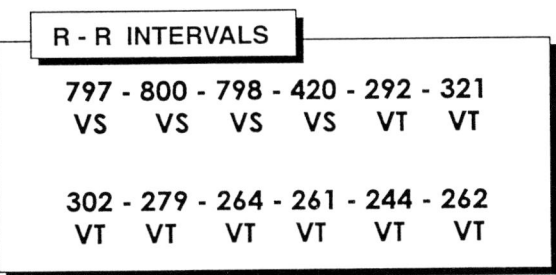

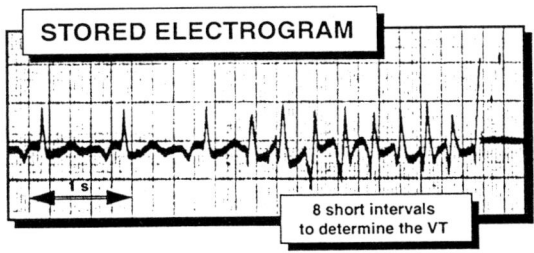

Figure 7. Onset of ventricular tachycardia. The top panel shows the annotated R-R intervals of a detected ventricular tachyarrhythmia. VS = ventricular sensing during sinus rhythm; VT = sensing in the ventricular tachycardia zone. The lower panel shows the stored electrogram. The onset of the detected tachycardia is determined by 8 short intervals at a frequency above the rate cutoff. As the electrograms are stored from the shocking electrodes, the transition from sinus rhythm to tachycardia can clearly be diagnosed.

obtained by shocking leads are easier to interpret, they should be used preferentially for storage.

The new devices not only store R-R intervals but can also store and telemeter electrograms at the onset of tachyarrhythmia episodes (Figure 7), as well as electrograms pre- (Figure 8) and post-therapy (Figure 9). This can provide reconstruction of the events leading to device activation, together with a correlation of symptoms with events.

Pre-attempt and post-attempt average rates provide information about the heart rate before and after treatment. Marked cycle length variability prior to device therapy with a rate of less than 220/min suggests a diagnosis of

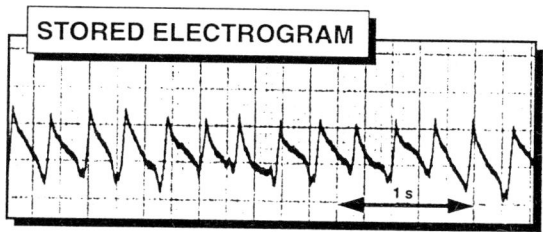

Figure 8. Pre-treatment. (Top) Annotated R-R intervals during the detection of the arrhythmia and subsequent charging of the capacitors. VT = detection in the ventricular tachycardia zone; Chrg = charging the capacitors. (lower) Stored electrogram during ventricular tachycardia.

atrial fibrillation, while a regular tachycardia with an abrupt onset most likely represents a recurrence of VT [16].

Annotated R-R intervals show what the device is really sensing and how it classifies the different rhythms within predefined rate zones such as brady- and tachy zones, zones of normal sinus rhythm, and ventricular fibrillation. It further demonstrates the delivery of pacing pulses by the device (either as bradycardia backup pacing or as antitachycardia pacing) and the charging of its capacitors. Stored electrograms may also allow the recognition of the delivery of inappropriate shocks and the induction of new arrhythmias by the device.

Information retrieved by stored electrograms will enhance the understanding of the mechanisms responsible for the initiation of arrhythmias. Furthermore, it will certainly lead to the improvement of the algorithms for

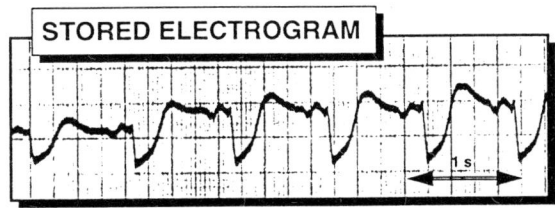

Figure 9. Post-shock redetection. (top) Annotated R-R intervals post-shock. VS = ventricular sensing during sinus rhythm; VP = ventricular pacing (post-shock pacing). (lower) Stored electrogram after the delivery of a 34 J shock. Clearly visible P waves indicate sinus rhythm. Changes in QRS complex morphology due to lesion potentials are usually observed in the acute post-shock period.

arrhythmia detection and may help to reduce the frequency of recurrent responses for non-VT rhythms.

REFERENCES

1. Furman S. Telemetry. In: Furman S, Hayes DL, Holmes DR Jr, editors. A Practice of Cardiac Pacing. Mount Kisco: Futura, 1993:605–33.
2. Castellanet M, Garza J, Shaner SP, Messenger JC. Telemetry of programmed and measured data in pacing system evaluation and follow-up. J Electrophysiol 1987;1:360–75.
3. Luceri RM, Catellanos A, Thurer R. Telemetry of intracardiac electrograms: Applications in spontaneous and induced arrhythmias. J Electrophysiol 1987;1:417–24.
4. Duffin EG Jr. The marker channel: A telemetric diagnostic aid. PACE 1984;7:1165–9.
5. Stroobandt R, Willems R, Sinnaeve A. Dual chamber rate responsive (DDDR) pacing: ventricular versus atrial timing. In: Andries E, Brugada P, Stroobandt R, editors. How to

face 'the faces' of cardiac pacing. Kluwer Academic Publishers, Dordrecht, The Netherlands: 1992:127-37.
6. Levine PA, Sholder J, Duncan JL. Clinical benefit of telemetered electrograms in assessment of DDD function. PACE 1984;7:1170-7.
7. Clarke M, Allen A. Use of telemetered electrograms in the assessment of normal pacemaker function. J Electrophysiol 1987;1:388-95.
8. Marco DD, Gallacher D. Noninvasive measurement of retrograde conduction times in pacemaker patients. PACE 1988;11:1673-7.
9. Stroobandt R, Willems R, Holvoet G, Backers J, Sinnaeve A. Prediction of Wenckebach behavior and block response in DDD pacemakers. PACE 1986;9:1040-6.
10. Stroobandt R, Willems R, Vandenbulcke F, Sinnaeve A. DDDR pacemakers: A framework for the understanding of atrial and ventricular based device timing. Eur J CPE 1992;2:151-7.
11. Levine P. The complementary role of electrogram, event marker, and measured data telemetry in the assessment of pacing system function. J Electrophysiol 1987;1:404-16.
12. Sarmiento JJ. Clinical utility of telemetered intracardiac electrograms in diagnosing a design dependent lead malfunction. PACE 1990;13:188-95.
13. Mirowski M, Reid PR, Mower MM et al. Termination of malignant ventricular arrhythmias with an implanted automatic defibrillator in human beings. N Eng J Med 1980;303:322-4.
14. Hook B, Callans DJ, Kleiman RB et al. Implantable cardioverter-defibrillator therapy in the absence of significant symptoms: Rhythm diagnosis and management aided by stored electrogram analysis. Circulation 1993;87:1897-906.
15. Newman D, Dorian P, Downar E et al. Use of telemetry functions in the assessment of implanted antitachycardia device efficacy. Am J Cardiol 1992;70:616-21.
16. Marchlinski FE, Gottlieb CD, Sarter B et al. ICD storage: Value in arrhythmia management. PACE 1993;16:527-34.

39. High patient acceptance for implantable cardioverter/defibrillator (ICD): quality of life and patient acceptance

BERNDT LÜDERITZ, WERNER JUNG & MATTHIAS MANZ

INTRODUCTION

The primary treatment of ventricular tachycardia (VT) and/or ventricular fibrillation (VF) intends to influence the outcome of the underlying cardiac disease. Symptomatic therapy is subdivided into drug therapy, electrotherapeutic tools [e.g. antitachycardia pacing, implantable cardioverter-defibrillator therapy (ICD), catheter ablation], antiarrhythmic surgery and cardiac transplantation [1-9]. Since the implantable automatic defibrillator as ICD or later on as ICD + ATP (antitachycardia pacemaker) was clinically introduced, there has been an increasing number of patients receiving these implants as a means of preventing sudden arrhythmic deaths. The clinical experience today has suggested that the device can significantly reduce mortality in malignant ventricular arrhythmia patients who meet the selection criteria for implantation [10]. The implantation of an ICD via sternotomy with epicardial or with non-thoracotomy leads is a major procedure. Patients are faced with psychological and social adjustments. Their lifestyle is further complicated by their psychological and social adjustments and the dependence on an implantable device which would 'save' them should they experience recurrences of life-threatening ventricular arrhythmias [11].

PATIENTS AND METHODS

Up to August 1992, at the Bonn University Hospital, 112 patients presented with drug-refractory ventricular tachyarrhythmias in whom implantation of the cardioverter-defibrillator was deemed necessary: 138 ICD systems (including 26 replacements) were implanted, 66 AICD (automatic implantable cardioverter/defibrillator; CPI Inc., St. Paul, MN), 32 PCD (pacer cardioverter/defibrillator; Medtronic Inc., Minneapolis, MN), 10 Res-Q (Intermedics

Table 1. Details of ventricular tachyarrhythmia: implantable cardioverter-defibrillator patient group studied.

ICD-ATP	
Patients:	57 (m: 50, f: 7)
Age:	59 ± 13 years
Diagnosis:	
– CAD	40
– CMP	11
– Myocarditis	1
– ARVD	2
– Idiopathathic VF	3
Treatment:	
– PCD	32
– Res-Q	10
– PRX	13
– Cadence	2
Transvenous approach:	38
Shocks:	13 ± 10
ATP	39 ± 16
Months:	20 ± 17

CAD = coronary artery disease; CMP = congestive cardiomyopathy; ARVD = arrhythmogenic right ventricular dysplasia; VF = ventricular fibrillation; PCD = pacer cardioverter/defibrillator; ATP = antitachycardia pacing.

Inc., Freeport, TX), 13 PRX and 15 Ventak P 2 (CPI) and 2 Cadence (Ventritex Inc., Sunnyvale, CA). Thus, 57 of the 112 patients received a third generation ICD-ATP device.

The study population included all these patients with multiprogrammable ICD devices. The underlying heart disease was coronary artery disease in 40 patients, idiopathic dilated cardiomyopathy in 11, myocarditis in 1, arrhythmogenic right ventricular dysplasia in 2, and primary electrical disease in 3. The mean left ventricular ejection fraction as assessed by contrast ventriculography was 36 ± 11% (Table 1). There was no perioperative mortality.

The patient acceptance for ICD-ATP concerned:

- Perception about device
- Perception about discharge
- Integration into body image
- Lifestyle alterations
- Patient and family perceptions
- Home-going concerns
- Complications

All patients underwent psychological assessment 12 ± 2 months after defibrillator implantation. Their state of anxiety was evaluated 1, 3, 6 and 12 months post-ICD-ATP device implantation. A specifically designed questionnaire including the following 8 questions was addressed to the patients by their physician [12,13].

1. Do you feel more comfortable and at ease since the implantation of the ICD, as compared with before you had the added protection?
2. Are you constantly aware of the device or just at particular times?
3. How long did it take you to get used to the ICD device?
4. When it becomes necessary to replace the battery:
   - Would you be willing to have another electrophysiologic (EP) study to determine if the device is still necessary?
   - Would you insist on a battery replacement without EP study?
5. What is your greatest concern about the ICD?
6. Knowing what you know, was it worthwhile having the electrotherapeutical tool implanted?
7. Has the ICD allowed you to return to a full active life?
8. Would you advise another patient to undergo ICD implantation if necessary?

RESULTS

Complete results could be obtained from all 57 patients (Table 2). A total of 47 patients felt more comfortable with the ICD system, 32 were constantly aware of the device, and 24 patients got used to it within less than 2 months. Concerning battery replacement, only 27 of 57 patients requested an electrophysiologic study.

Twenty patients stated fear of ICD discharges, 12 patients revealed physical discomfort due to the device, limited quality of life occurred in 8 patients. Fifty-five patients answered that it was worthwhile having an ICD device implanted, 30 (53%) had returned to active life, and 56 (98%) would advise another patient to undergo implantation if necessary. Thus, the acceptance for ICD was very high.

For differentiation of the anxiety and social impact, see Table 3. Pain during ICD discharge occurred in 27 patients and limited physical activity in 40; and as far as anxiety is concerned, the fear of ICD shock was present in only 20 patients and fear of device failure in only 16. Forty-two patients experienced no decreased sexual activity; in 15 patients the answer to this question was 'yes' (Table 3). A return to an active lifestyle was possible for 35, to work only in 7, to hobby (sports) in 39, and to unemployment in 32 patients.

Our results concerning the state of anxiety available in a cohort of 42 patients are shown in Table 4. No change occurred after the 1st, 3rd and 6th months in 50% of the patients. A slight and moderate decrease in their state of anxiety was present in 4 and 13 patients, respectively, after the 1st month;

Table 2. Answers to the questionnaire (57 patients).

Do you feel more comfortable with the ICD?	
yes: 47	no: 10
Are you constantly aware of the device?	or just at particular times?
yes: 32	yes: 25
How long did it take you to get used to the ICD?	
<2 months: 24	>2 months: 33
Battery replacement – EPS requested?	
yes: 27	no: 30
What is your greatest concern?	
– Fear of the ICD discharge	20
– Physical discomfort due to the device	12
– Limited quality of life (job, sport, social activity)	8
– None	17
Was is worthwhile having an ICD device implanted?	
yes: 55	no: 2
Has the ICD allowed you to return to active life?	
yes: 30	no: 27
Would you advise another patient to undergo ICD implantation if necessary?	
yes: 56	no: 1

Table 3. Results of questionnaire concerning anxiety and social impact ($n = 57$).

Anxiety	Yes	No
Pain during ICD discharge	27	30
Limited physical activity	40	17
Fear of ICD shock	20	37
Fear of device failure	16	41
Decreased sexual activity	15	42
Social impact		
Return to active lifestyle	35	22
Return to work	7	50
Hobby (sport)	39	18
Unemployment	32	25

Table 4. State of anxiety (n = 42 patients) over time.

	Month 1	Month 3	Month 6	Month 12
No change	21	21	21	
Slight decrease	4			42
Moderate decrease	13		7	
Marked decrease		14		
Moderate increase	4	7		
Marked increase			7	
Strong increase			7	

a marked decrease was observed in the patients after 3 months, a marked and strong increase in 8 patients each after half a year. However, the most interesting result seems the (slight) decrease in all patients after 12 months, i.e. the decrease in the state of anxiety in all patients 1 year after ICD implantation.

DISCUSSION

As part of this retrospective study by means of specific questioning of patients, a high acceptance rate was formulated for the automatic ICD. Over half the patients resumed an active lifestyle and almost all patients (98%) would advise other patients, where indicated, in favour of an ICD-ATP system. Disappointing is the extent of the incapacity to work, which amounts to 56% of patients. This figure appears to be relatively high compared with the USA, where the majority of patients return to their original profession following ICD implantation [14]. The low level of a return to work in this country might well be explained by the specific social system.

Naturally, in this study, the limited period of 12 months overall must be taken into account. It is quite possible that the details during an additional period of time would alter both from the positive as well as from the negative aspect. Whilst the complications of the system might increase, further psychological and social stabilization could be expected, as individual observations of our patients have already demonstrated.

Over the 1-year period of observation, it appears to be important that a reduction in the state of anxiety occurred amongst all patients, even though this was only slight. Our findings are in agreement with the results obtained by other authors [13].

Analyses of the anxiety as a condition or as a trait show that the state of anxiety, but not the trait of anxiety, is clearly reduced after ICD implantation. The studies by Vlay et al. indicate that the patients suffering from malignant ventricular tachyarrhythmia sent for defibrillator treatment, were more prone to a higher degree of anxiety than normal people or patients with some other disorder. This finding appears to be understandable in view of the clear syndrome of malignant ventricular tachyarrhythmia, which is generally due to a severe organic heart disease.

Subsequently, even after ICD implantation, anxiety is retained as a characteristic, even though the anxiety condition or the readiness to be anxious decreases [13]. Similar results are reported by Obel et al. in a small group of six patients [15]. By comparison, the state of a possible malaise where the electronic system is concerned remains unchanged. The number of ICD interventions probably affects the attitude of the patient towards the device. The number of ICD electroshocks was higher during the initial 6 months than in the subsequent period.

Even though the overall acceptance of the ICD is positive, it must be pointed out that the anxiety and critical awareness amongst patients is high and that the relevant effect, like the so-called type A and type B attitude, is still unclear in the long term [13].

A comparison between ICD patients and those following a heart transplant may be of interest with regard to satisfaction and quality of life as indicators of treatment success. Bunzel et al. [16] evaluated the details given by 47 patients following heart transplants with regard to their physical, psychological, spiritual, professional, sexual and financial situation, as well as to leisure activities, partnership and family. On average, the patients reported a noticeable improvement in the quality of life and their satisfaction, apart from their financial situation. Significant differences between the expressed condition and the satisfaction were observed in the sectors of the spiritual, professional and financial situation as well as in the partnership and family, whereby satisfaction with what had already been achieved was noticeably higher than the change in the particular sector. The basic positive evaluation, which mainly concerned the physical capacity, also included the psychosomatic and emotional situation [16].

A study of Angermann et al. in long-term survivors of orthotopic heart transplantation showed that the subjective quality of life is similar to that of healthy individuals of the same age group. Thus, survival is certainly not the only indicator of success; aspects of quality of life must also be included in the cost effectiveness and/or cost benefit considerations in those patients [17].

Our study aimed to take into account that not just the ICD, but also the accompanying antiarrhythmic treatment may have affected the psychosomatic care and treatment of awareness and the condition of anxiety. In this multifactor relationship, which includes the interaction of a variety of variables, treatment with anxiolytic drugs will also have to be investigated. Prior to the start of treatment, patients and their relatives were informed by the physician of the possible psychological and social changes that can result from an ICD implantation. It also appears important to us to carry out additional, accompanying, systematic psychological studies on the innovative treatment method of the ICD so as to clarify the importance of the individual influencing factors.

Limitations of the study

Since the quality of life may change over time, one limitation of this study is that the questionnaire was addressed to the patients at a specific time only and was not repeated during follow-up. Furthermore, to improve the importance of this study, a control group including patients suffering from malignant ventricular tachyarrhythmias may be desirable. However, at the present time, it seems to be unethical and unjustifiable to withhold a treatment modality which has been proven to be safe and effective in patients at a high risk for sudden cardiac death.

CONCLUSION

Patients who have survived sudden cardiac death often experience subsequent anxiety, feel a loss of control and helpless; common problems that decrease over time after ICD implantation, including emotional lability, depression, fear and hyperarousal with night wakefulness. Helpful treatment interventions include education, individual and family counseling, and relaxation techniques [18].

The actual activation of the devices during sexual activity is a rare occurrence. Even so, descriptions indicate that the sensation of an ICD discharge is quite mild and not painful. All patients were mildly disturbed by the seemingly large size of the device but nonetheless accepted it. In general the acceptance for the ICD as a tool for the management of life-threatening ventricular tachyarrhythmias is very high [19]. Besides the survival aspect, the quality of life and patient acceptance of ICD-ATP are important criteria of defibrillator therapy.

REFERENCES

1. Kelly PA, Cannom DS, Garan H et al. The automatic implantable cardioverter/defibrillator. Efficacy, complications and survival in patients with malignant ventricular arrhythmias. J Am Coll Cardiol 1988; 11:1278–86.
2. Morady F. A perspective on the role of catheter ablation in the management of tachyarrhythmias. PACE 1988;11:98–102.
3. Parsonnet V. Antitachyarrhythmia devices. PACE 1988;11:5–6.
4. Saksena S. Nonpharmacologic therapy for tachyarrhythmias: The tower of Babel revisited? PACE 1988;11:93–7.
5. Saksena S, Hussain SM, Gielchinsky I. Surgical ablation of tachyarrhythmias: Reflections for the third decade. PACE 1988;11:103–8.
6. Steinbeck G, Haberl R, Kemkes BM. Heart transplantation in drug-resistant recurrent ventricular tachycardia and electrophysiology. In: Belhassen B, Feldman S, Copperman Y, editors. Proceedings of the VIIth World Symposium on Cardiac Pacing and Electrophysiology, 1987;509–12.

7. Troup PJ. Lessons learned from the automatic implantable cardioverter/defibrillator: Past, present and future. J Am Coll Cardiol 1988;11:1287–9.
8. Wilber DJ, Garan H, Finkelstein D et al. Out-of-hospital cardiac arrest. Use of electrophysiologic testing in the prediction of long-term outcome. N Engl J Med 1988;1:19–24.
9. Winkle RA. Nonpharmacologic therapy of tachycardias: The role of implanted devices. PACE 1988;11:109–13.
10. Winkle RA, Mead R, Ruder MA et al. Ten years experience with implantable defibrillators. Circulation 1991;84(Suppl II):426.
11. Tchou PJ, Piasecki E, Gutmann M et al. Psychological support and psychiatric management of patients with automatic implantable cardioverter/defibrillators. Int J Psychiatry Med 1989;19:393–407.
12. Pycha C, Calabrese JR, Gulledge AD, Maloney JD. Patient and spouse acceptance and adaptation to implantable cardioverter/defibrillators. Cleveland Clin J Med 1990;57:5:441–4.
13. Vlay SC, Olson LC, Fricchione GL, Friedman R. Anxiety and anger in patients with ventricular tachyarrhythmias. Responses after automatic internal cardioverter defibrillator implantation. PACE 1989;12:366–73.
14. Kalbfleisch KR, Lehmann MH, Steinmann RT et al. Reemployment following implantation of the automatic cardioverter/defibrillator. Am J Cardiol 1989;64:199–202.
15. Obel IWP, Lasersohn B, Dateling F. General and psychological aspects of defibrillator implantation. In: Kappenberger LJ, Lindemans FW, editors. Practical Aspects of Staged Therapy Defibrillators. Mount Kisco, NY: Futura, 1992;65–8.
16. Bunzel B, Wollenek G, Grundböck A et al. Quality of life and satisfaction after cardiac transplantation: An indicator of results of treatment. Herz 1991;16:257–66.
17. Angermann CE, Bullinger M, Spes CH et al. Quality of life in long-term survivors of orthotopic heart transplantation. Z Kardiol 1992;81:411–7.
18. Pycha C, Gulledge AD, Hutzler J et al. Psychological responses to the implantable defibrillator: Preliminary observations. Psychosomatics 1986;27:841–5.
19. Lüderitz B, Jung W, Manz M. Patient acceptance for implantable cardioverter/defibrillator (ICD). New Trends Arrhyth 1992;VII:631–40.

40. Cardiac pacing and electrophysiology: how much technology do we need?

R.W.F. CAMPBELL

INTRODUCTION

Technology is fashionable, and like it or not, cardiologists are slaves to fashion. Scientifically respected researchers vie with each other to be the first to use a new device. Only much later, and usually when a new model is on the horizon, is critical scrutiny brought to bear. Is our obsession with high technology appropriate? Is high technology really needed'?

CARDIAC PACING

For decades, simple VVI pacing systems have saved lives and improved the quality of life for thousands of patients, yet the days of VVI pacing seem numbered. Rate-adaptive pacing systems and, for those with relatively stable atrial electrophysiology, dual chamber pacing systems are displacing VVI pacemakers to such an extent that the indications for simple VVI pacing seem few. In a controversial policy document, the British Pacing and Electrophysiology Group recommended sophisticated pacemaker technology for the vast majority of clinical situations [1]. Subsequent correspondence and research focused principally upon the additional costs that would be incurred by abandoning simple VVI pacing [2,3].

Cost is certainly an issue, but it must be examined in the context of benefit. Sophisticated pacemaker technology is unlikely to save any more lives than simple VVI pacing. The issue is not one of mortality but rather of morbidity and quality of life. These factors are notoriously difficult to measure, and clinical research is still in its infancy when faced with the challenge of determining differences in these types of outcomes [4]. Nonetheless, in almost every comparative study of simple VVI pacing versus more sophisticated pacing, a putative benefit of this sophisticated technology is claimed [5,6]. For many physicians, however, the case is still far from proven. Many are still sceptical of the results of quality of life assessments, and others, quite rightly, are reluctant to change their practice on the basis of what may be marginal improvements in a measured haemodynamic index such as cardiac output, end-diastolic pressure, etc.

On the other hand, the dramatic success of VVI pacing with its life-saving potential should be re-evaluated. The benefits of pacing are beyond question for well-defined and easily defined clinical situations. The basic technology has been refined, and the challenge is to make the treatment even better for our patients. The dramatic benefits of technological progress as applied to even simple VVI pacing should not be overlooked. Generators are but a fraction of their size of a decade ago, simplifying their implantation and significantly reducing the risk of their extrusion [7]. Lithium battery technology has dramatically increased the longevity of pacemakers, so that replacements are less frequent and the associated morbidity is reduced [8]. Electronic and encapsulation technology has become more reliable, making sudden failures and modifications a rarity, and outpatient surveillance need not be so intense.

Pacemaker costs vary from country to country. Sophisticated pacemakers are expensive, but the additional cost of, for instance, rate-responsive dual chamber pacing (DDDR) versus simple VVI pacing is the financial equivalent of a can of soft drink daily over the life of the generator. Set in these terms rather than the total capital costs, the price of sophisticated technology not only seems but is affordable.

Were we ourselves to require pacemaker implantation, few would opt for simple VVI pacing except under the most unusual circumstances. We, however, would not purchase complex and potentially unreliable technology redundant to our clinical need. We would not choose an improper technology which might place us in jeopardy. The field of cardiac pacing has been one of the greatest success stories in medicine. We should not jeopardise the track record of success by the whimsical endorsement of new technology. Cardiologists and physicians should be firmly in control of what is desirable for their patients and should clearly establish for technologists the future directions and the clinical challenges to be addressed.

ANTITACHYCARDIA PACING

Antitachycardia pacemakers are a technological tour de force. These implantable units on detecting a tachyarrhythmia can deliver a remarkably varied selection of preprogrammed tachycardia-terminating pacing sequences [9,10]. As early work established that when used on their own, these units were not appropriate for the management of ventricular tachycardia (VT) as they could provoke ventricular fibrillation (VF) in an appreciable proportion of patients, antitachycardia pacing concentrated on the termination of supraventricular tachycardias. The pacemaker systems are relatively simple to implant, but their programming and tailoring for individual patients is complex and demands great skill, patience and experience.

Antitachycardia pacemakers were developed at a time of decreasing satisfaction with antiarrhythmic drug management of arrhythmias, and for a time they seemed likely to have considerable clinical impact. The advent of radio-frequency ablation which is applicable to the majority of types of narrow QRS tachycardias has dramatically changed the situation [11]. Whilst intellectually satisfying and technologically brilliant, the role of antitachycardia pacemakers for the management of supraventricular tachycardias has all but disappeared. The technology, however, has not been abandoned. Antitachycardia pacing is emerging as an important component of the implantable cardioverter-defibrillator (ICD) in which it can safely offer an anti-VT action with backup defibrillator shocks should VF be precipitated [12,13].

IMPLANTABLE CARDIOVERTER-DEFIBRILLATOR

The most expensive and most technologically complex implantable device is the ICD. There can be no question that this device can save life [14]. It represents a remarkable development, and its clinical introduction has silenced its many initial critics [15]. It has been enthusiastically endorsed in those countries where its cost can be met. In other countries, its use is governed not so much by clinical indications as by financial resource. The systems are expensive in capital expenditure and are expensive to maintain. The function of the ICD is to save life, and set against this, perhaps any expense is justifiable. The incorporation of antitachycardia pacing and anti-bradycardia pacing into ICDs has significantly improved their clinical performance [12,13], although this has yet further increased their technical sophistication. The technical development of ICDs is still at an early stage. There is much to improve, and as with pacemakers, it can be confidently expected that ICD technology development in the next 10 years will be dramatic.

The expense, sophistication and disadvantages of ICDs are acceptable to those patients in whom the units offer benefit. It remains that a high proportion of patients in whom ICDs are implanted receive neither shocks nor pacing sequences [15,16]. Identifying optimal candidates for ICDs is important, but the current techniques are unreliable. Too often, ICDs are recommended for patients 'just in case' they have another (or a first) arrhythmic event. Patients need ICD technology, and patients need that technology to be refined. There is every reason to expect that this will be achieved. It depends largely upon an appreciation of current knowledge and improved production processes. The greatest stumbling block is not technical but clinical. Too little is known about the risk stratification and natural history of cardiovascular disease. Only with that knowledge can sophisticated technology be appropriately applied and achieve acceptable cost-benefit targets.

REFERENCES

1. Recommendations for pacemaker prescription for symptomatic bradycardia. Report of a working party of the British Pacing and Electrophysiology Group. Br Heart J 1991;66:185–91.
2. de Belder MA, Linker NJ, Jones S, Camm AJ, Ward DE. Cost implications of the British Pacing and Electrophysiology Group's recommendations for pacing. BMJ 1992 10;305:861–5.
3. Ray SG, Griffith MJ, Jamieson S, Bexton RS, Gold RG. Impact of the recommendations of the British Pacing and Electrophysiology Group on pacemaker prescription and on the immediate costs of pacing in the Northern Region. Br Heart J 1992;68:531–4.
4. Linde-Edelstam C, Nordlander R, Unden AL, Orth-Gomer K, Ryden L. Quality of life in patients treated with atrioventricular synchronous pacing compared to rate modulated ventricular pacing: a long-term, double-blind, crossover study. PACE Pacing Clin Electrophysiol 1992;15:1467–76.
5. Oto MA, Muderrisoglu H, Ozin MB et al. Quality of life in patients with rate responsible pacemakers: A randomized, cross-over study. PACE Pacing Clin Electrophysiol 1991;14:800–6.
6. Kruse I, Arnman K, Conradson TB et al. A comparison of the acute and long-term haemodynamic effects of ventricular inhibited and atrial synchronous ventricular inhibited pacing. Circulation 1982;65:846–55.
7. Har-Shai Y, Amikan S, Ramon Y, Kahir G, Hirshowitz B. The management of exposed cardiac pacemaker pulse generator and electrode using restricted local surgical interventions; subcapsular relocation and vertical-to-horizontal bow transposition techniques. Br J Plast Surg 1990;43:307–11.
8. Greatbatch W, Holmes CF. The lithium/iodine battery: a historical perspective. PACE Pacing Clin Electrophysiol 1992;15:2034–6.
9. Griffith MJ, Bexton RS, McComb JM. Financial audit of antitachycardia pacing for the control of recurrent supraventricular tachycardias. Br Heart J 1993;69:250–4.
10. Jung W, Mletzko R, Manz M, Luderitz B. Long-term therapy of antitachycardia pacing for supraventricular tachycardia. PACE Pacing Clin Electrophysiol 1992;15:179–87.
11. Jackman WM, Wang XZ, Friday KJ et al. Catheter ablation of accessory atrioventricular pathways (Wolff-Parkinson-White syndrome) by radiofrequency current. N Engl J Med 1991;324:1660–2.
12. Leitch JW, Gillis AM, Wyse DG et al. Reduction in defibrillator shocks with an implantable device combining antitachycardia pacing and shock therapy. J Am Coll Cardiol 1991;18:145–51.
13. Porterfield JG, Porterfield LM, Smith BA, Bray L, Voshage L, Martinez A. Conversion rates of induced versus spontaneous ventricular tachycardia by a third generation cardioverter defibrillator. The VENTAK PRx Phase I Investigators. PACE Pacing Clin Electrophysiol 1993;16:170–3.
14. Winkle RA, Mead RH, Rudar MA et al. Long-term outcome with the automatic implantable cardioverter-defibrillator. J Am Cardiol 1989;13:1353–61.
15. Campbell RWF. Life at a price—the implantable defibrillator. Br Heart J 1990;64:171–3.
16. Zilo P, Gross JN, Benedek M, Fisher JD, Furman S. Occurrence of ICD shocks and patient survival. PACE Pacing Clin Electrophysiol 1991;14:273–9.

41. Medical technology assessment and reimbursement policy of implantable devices in Belgium: possibilities and limitations for the future

ROB VAN DEN OEVER

INTRODUCTION

The Belgian health care system is based on a mixture of public and private initiatives. It is financed by social contributions proportional to income (70%) and by state subsidies (30%) in a Bismarck model of national solidarity and compulsory health insurance covering the whole of the 10 million population. The administration of the system is exclusively assigned to five recognized sickness funds, and its policy-making structure is built on an advisory and consensus mechanism between government officials, health insurers, and interest groups of providers and institutions. In order to coordinate and supervise a uniform application of insurance cover by the sickness funds a National Institute of Health and Disability Insurance (R.I.Z.I.V.) was created in 1963. Health care delivery is paid through the reimbursement of a per diem price for the hospital and of a fee-for-service for the provider. It is obvious that this output-financed health care system in Belgium has led to an increase of services offered and a generalized purchase of the latest and most expensive technology.

Because of growing concern over health care budgets, the government has to observe a maximum percentage of the GNP that can be spent, access to care for every member of the society and maintaining the quality of care. It is the responsible authority that has to guarantee sufficient means in order to achieve these goals. The total health care budget is set yearly in consensus with providers and insurers, taking into account the medicotechnical evolution, the objective needs and the real costs. The National Council of Hospitals advises the Minister of Health and Social Security on the planning, financing, or subsidizing of hospital facilities. The Medical Technical Committee proposes the reimbursement of new techniques and procedures, and the Technical Committee for Implants and Devices can propose reimbursement for medical materials agreed for marketing by the Ministry of Health. These three advisory bodies are composed of representatives of the medical schools, of the providers associations, and of the health insurers.

The process of choices in health care can thus be brought about on medical criteria, and superfluous procedures, especially diagnostic (e.g. clinical chemistry, medical imaging, endoscopy), or needless use of expensive therapies (e.g. implants, pharmaceuticals) can be avoided. It is preferred to achieve a limitation of the medical offer in health care by evaluation and planning techniques while maintaining a flexible and at least partial fee-for-service financing but within certain budgetary constraints. This substantial engagement of provider and insurer, a first step on the way to managed care, has recently led to the introduction of a new reimbursement system for implantable devices and has already proved useful in obtaining health insurance cover for the implantable cardioverter-defibrillator (ICD).

THE REIMBURSEMENT OF IMPLANTABLE DEVICES

The evolution in total numbers and expenditure for implantable devices has always been accepted as a normal expression of modern medicine and quality care. The results of medical technology such as implants in orthopedic surgery (hip, knee, spine) and cardiovascular medicine (pacemaker, heart valve) have proved to be cost-effective, and their increased use was welcomed by the health insurance through general and until recently unlimited reimbursement. Time-consuming agreement procedures and a fixed quota or budget for implants per hospital or provision center are extremely unpopular, and a rapid reimbursement with rates calculated on average selling prices of comparable products was the rule, once a marketing agreement (declaration procedure) of the Ministry of Health and a maximum retail price by the Ministry of Economic Affairs had been obtained. The obvious advantages of this system consist in a direct follow-up of medical technology and a health insurance that is able to offer the latest acquisitions to every patient, because progress in medical science is not hampered by overregulation, limited spread or non-reimbursement.

The budgetary consequences however weigh heavy, and the growth rate in expenditures for implantable devices like pacemakers – perhaps attaining a saturation point in next few years – and articular prostheses in Belgium (Table 1, Figure 1) illustrates the need for regulation of this free market model if its total health care budget share is not soon to become as important as that of the pharmaceuticals. The R.I.Z.I.V. therefore was challenged to judge implantable devices on their objective therapeutic value and their social interest and also to make choices based on criteria of quality care with respect to certain financial limits. In 1989, the Technical Committee of Implants at the R.I.Z.I.V. was set up as a multidisciplinary organ for medical technology assessment, where providers and insurers together can discuss with the health authorities, and the industry can propose new devices for reimbursement. In order to obtain both cost control and protection for the patients against unreasonable copayments, agreements on conditions and rates of reimbursement are negotiated between representatives of the medical

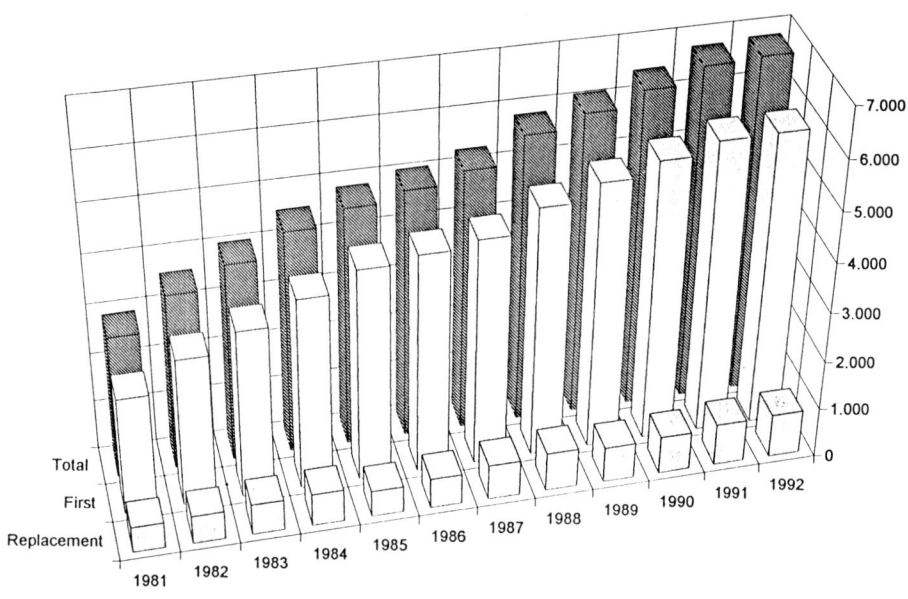

Figure 1. Pacemaker implantation in Belgium.

Table 1. Evolution of reimbursement amounts for implantable devices by health insurance in Belgium.

Year	Reimbursement (in million US $)		
	Orthopedic implant	Pacemaker	All implants
1982	4.0	6.9	14.2
1985	10.9	17.5	37.5
1989	27.3	29.8	87.3
1991	39.5	38.0	116.7
1992	49.1	43.3	143.5

schools, provider associations, and insurance companies in a flexible follow-up of medical technology.

Following the directives of the European Commission on the regulation and harmonization of national legislation on medical aids to guarantee free trade, the implantable devices are defined and classified in five categories:

 I. Active implant (e.g. pacemaker, neurostimulator)
 II. High-risk implant (e.g. heart valve, vascular prosthesis)
 III. Relative risk implant (e.g. clips, staplings)
 IV. Custom made implant (e.g. special articular prosthesis)
 V. Clinical trial implant

Devices of categories I and IV are individually accepted by the committee on a limitative list of products according to their therapeutic use and social benefit. Reimbursement is fixed on the retail price agreed by the Ministry of Economic Affairs (I) or on the manufacturing price (IV), and there is no patient share.

Products of categories II and III are reimbursed at fixed rates based on average retail prices of comparable products with a maximum 25% margin for copayment. Category II implants that exceed the reimbursement rate by more than 25% are excluded from insurance cover, but can in exceptional cases be introduced on the limitative list and financed as in category I.

The hospital pharmacist is appointed as a provider of implantable devices in relation to the health insurance and occupies an important position with financial responsibilities towards the implanting physician, the hospital administrator, the patient, and his or her health insurer. Depending on his or her purchasing policy the pharmacist, who receives a delivery fee, can avoid extra costs for the hospital and for the patient.

An innovation is category V, referring to category I devices newly introduced on the market, that in case of demonstrable medical and social benefit can obtain the committees' agreement for provisional reimbursement during an evaluation period and for a restricted number, even before official marketing is granted by the Ministry of Health. The reimbursement rate for the clinical trial implant is based on that of similar earlier-generation devices of the same production series. After the assessment period and with a positive outcome, the clinical trial model can become a category I implant reimbursed at its own retail price.

ICD REIMBURSEMENT

Specialized care provision by highly trained personnel and expensive equipment for individual indications based on pluridisciplinary medical teamwork is not covered by routine health care insurance or general reimbursement rules, but can be financed by convention between the R.I.Z.I.V. and the treatment centre. The detailed conditions for reimbursement are negotiated between the College of Medical Directors of the five sickness funds and the applying physicians under the auspices of the R.I.Z.I.V. This assessment tool permits a fine tuning on demand of the financing of new and exceptional therapies before their effectiveness is proven beyond any doubt or before widespread applicability.

Just like reimbursing drug addiction treatment programs, readaptive therapy for severe neurological pathology, and comprehensive care for diabetics with an insulin pump, the convention model was also successfully used for the defibrillator. Before the ICD was internationally accepted as effective in patients at risk of sudden death [1–3], the conditions for reimbursement

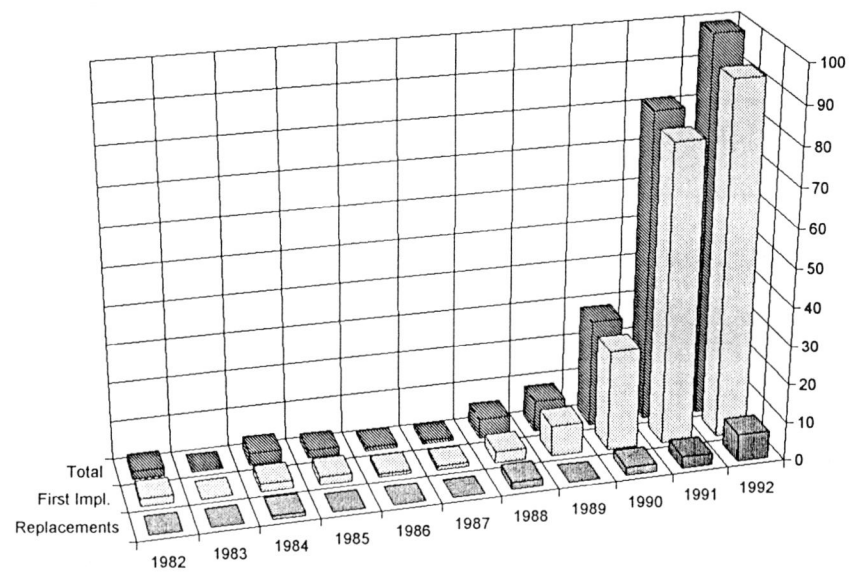

Figure 2. ICD implantation in Belgium.

were set down in 1986 as a result of constructive negotiation between health insurers and interested cardiologists.

The R.I.Z.I.V. developed a policy of reimbursement that included the individual evaluation of candidates for an ICD by the above-mentioned College of Medical Directors. Only documented ventricular fibrillation (VF) or hemodynamically unstable ventricular tachycardia (VT) not caused by acute ischemia or reversible causes, refractory to drugs, and not eligible for interventional therapy are accepted as indications.

Under drug therapy failure are included spontaneous or exercise-induced arrhythmia recurrences, remaining inducibility by electrical stimulation of ill-tolerated or rapid VT, or major side effects. The recognized implantation centres agree to perform a mutual peer review and to accept a fixed yearly reimbursed quotum of ICDs, of which every participating centre has a share according to the number of its allowed implants [4].

The ICD quotum in 1987 was set to 30 for a 2-year period in consensus with four recognized centres and has been raised since 1992 to 100/year with 15 recognized centres, which corresponds to 1 ICD per 100 000 inhabitants exclusive of replacements. Only two centres have more than 10 implantations/year, and the evolution of total ICD therapy is shown in Figure 2. Even if ICD reimbursement for a candidate matching the criteria will not be refused and the yearly quotum is rather flexible during review, the convention

Table 2. Total health care expenditure as % of GNP and average ambulatory per capita consumption of drugs at wholesale purchase price (in US $) vs. percentages of diagnoses by general practitioners and specialists with drug prescription in 1991.

	% GNP[a]	Per capita consumption	% Drug prescription
United Kingdom	6.1	85	74
The Netherlands	8.1	86	56
Spain	6.6	113	80
Belgium	7.6	136	86
USA	12.5	146	64
Italy	7.6	179	73
France	8.8	193	84

[a] 1990 figures; 1989 figures for the UK and Spain.
Source: OECD and Nefarma, Utrecht.

model thanks to the obligatory individual application for reimbursement and peer review has proven to be an effective way of managing health insurance expenditure for the ICD to the satisfaction of all parties concerned [5].

HOW TO AFFORD NEW MEDICAL TECHNOLOGY IN THE FUTURE?

The 1993 budget for health care in Belgium has been set at US $10 billion by a government concerned for years about cost containment. The accepted growth rate of 6.2% seems underestimated compared with the yearly 10% increase during the 1989–1992 period, while the revenues of the social security system do not follow this trend due to a shortfall of state subsidies and increasing unemployment.

Health authorities, hospital administrators, and providers — as in other industrialized western countries — are looking for additional means of financing through raised patient copayments and private insurance.

The acute budgetary problem in Belgian health care with still moderate expenditures and a small price per provision is caused by too many providers, facilities, and care production in a fee-for-service payment system, resulting in supplier-induced health care demand and in the overprescription of diagnostic tests and pharmaceuticals. In Table 2, the total health care expenditures as part of the GNP are compared with the rate of drug prescription and the per capita drug consumption figures, illustrating aberrant prescription together with reasonable expenditures per inhabitant due to the low drug prices in Belgium.

Demographic changes (1 in 5 Belgians will soon be over 60 years old) and the shift to more expensive procedures of a highly sophisticated and technological health care explain some of the growth in total expenses but are not the origin of the overconsumption. The reimbursed fees for specialized care are below the European average, which is why cardiac surgery and organ transplant centres in this country are attractive to foreign patients and their health insurers.

The excellent performance of the nations' health care system together with complete coverage and accessibility, and with patient copayment restricted to ambulatory and non-critical care, produce the high satisfaction score. While most Western countries are in the middle of a radical reform of their health care systems with choices between compulsory insurance covering only essential care and complementary private insurance [6], Belgium can preserve its current system provided that a more coherent policy and a financially responsible administrator are obtained.

The described reimbursement systems for implantable devices and for the ICD have to prevent future medical technology becoming a threat instead of a gain to the health care system. To do so, providers, hospitals, and health authorities have to accept joint responsibility for total health expenditures, not with respect to a rigid budget but in redefining values and consumer attitudes in practice, training, and research.

High-tech cardiac pacing and electrophysiology can lower health care costs by a better diagnosis, a more direct therapy, and the prevention of ineffective treatment or prolonged hospital admission, but correctly specified output measuring has to be our first concern.

The beneficial effects of the ICD on total cardiovascular mortality and on total survival remain to be established in comparison with alternative antiarrhythmic therapies, since past studies show several methodological pitfalls in using historical control data, different selection criteria, or hypothetical sudden death events extrapolated from 'appropriate shocks' [7–11]. Randomized trials in patients surviving cardiac arrest are being carried out and the results of these prospective cost-effectiveness analyses of ICD implantation could broaden the acceptance and the reimbursement conditions [12]. Indications for ICD therapy will probably also increase thanks to the longer generator life, lower defibrillator threshold, pacing facilities, and nonthoracotomy approach, and reimbursement of a defibrillator as an effective electronic bridge to transplantation for patients at risk [13] is already accepted in this country.

However, even if we can afford the prophylactic use of the ICD in the future, this would in spite of the considerable extra costs only mean a significant delay in death for more patients at risk of malignant arrhythmias, with a negligible impact on total mortality from cardiac disease in the population [14]. The development and diffusion of effective medical technology must not be limited, but a well-organized assessment capability in close collaboration between physicians and health authorities is essential if we want to provide delivery and insurance cover of high quality care in the future.

REFERENCES

1. Fogoros RN, Fiedler SB, Elson JJ. The automatic implantable cardioverter-defibrillator in drug-refractory ventricular tachy-arrhythmias. Ann Int Med 1987;107:635–41.
2. Tchou PJ, Kadri N, Andersen J, Caceres JA, Jazayeri M, Akthar M. Automatic implantable cardioverter defibrillator and survival of patients with left ventricular dysfunction and malignant ventricular arrhythmias. Ann Int Med 1988;109:529–34.
3. Winkle RA, Mead RH, Ruder AM et al. Longterm outcome with the automatic implantable cardioverter-defibrillator. J Am Coll Cardiol 1989;13:1353–61.
4. van den Oever R. Arrhythmia technology. The insurer's point of view. In: Andries E, Brugada P, Stroobandt R, editors. How to face 'the faces' of cardiac pacing. Dordrecht, The Netherlands: Kluwer Academic Publishers, 1992:255–65.
5. Brugada P, Van Royen M, Andries E, van den Oever R. The Belgian system to control indications for the implantable defibrillator: a model for other European countries? Eur J Med 1993;2:86–8.
6. OECD. The reform of health care: a comparative analysis of seven countries. Health Policy Studies no. 2. OECD, Paris, 1992.
7. Saksena S, Camm AJ. Implantable defibrillators for prevention of sudden death. Technology at a medical and economic crossroad. Circulation 1992;85:2316–21.
8. Saksena S. The social and economic impact of the new implantable cardioverter defibrillator technology. In: Alt E, Klein H, Griffin JC, editors. The implantable cardioverter/defibrillator. Berlin: Springer-Verlag, 1992:293–9.
9. Larsen GC, Manolis AS, Sonnenberg FA, Deskanski JR, Mark Estes NA, Pauker SG. Cost-effectiveness of the implantable cardioverter-defibrillator: Effect of improved battery life and comparison with amiodarone therapy. J Am Coll Cardiol 1992;19:1323–34.
10. O'Brien BJ, Buxton MJ, Rushby JA. Cost-effectiveness of the implantable cardioverter defibrillator: a preliminary analysis. Br Heart J 1992;68:241–5.
11. Heidbüchel H, Ector H. Cost-benefit analysis of arrhythmia technology. In: Andries E, Brugada P, Stroobandt R, editors. How to face 'the faces' of cardiac pacing. Dordrecht, The Netherlands: Kluwer Academic Publishers, 1992:241–54.
12. Hauer RNW, Wever EFD, Cryns HJGM. Automatic implantable cardioverter defibrillator: cost effectiveness. Pace 1993;16:559–63.
13. Jeevanandam V, Bielefeld MR, Auteri JS et al. The implantable defibrillator: an electronic bridge to cardiac transplantation. Circulation 1992; 86(II):276–9.
14. Kottke TE, Stanton MS, Bailey KR, Decker WW, Hammill SC. A population-based estimate of candidacy rates for the implantable cardioverter-defibrillator. Am J Cardiol 1993;71:77–81.

42. Socioeconomic aspects of implantable devices: can we afford new technology?*

KONRAD K. STEINBACH

INTRODUCTION

In the 1960s and 1970s the only task of the cardiologist was to develop new therapeutic and diagnostic procedures. In many countries in Europe at that time, the implementation of new methods into clinical practice was not impeded by a financial barrier, for two reasons: nearly unlimited financial resources for medical care were available at least in the Western countries of Europe, and less therapeutical options – and thus less expensive – became available. The situation has changed in the 1980s because less money and more expensive therapeutic modalities were available. Based on these facts, cardiologists at the present time and in the future will be obliged to implement socioeconomic aspects in their decision-making concerning diagnostic interventions and treatment.

Financial aspects influence decision-making concerning treatment at three levels: (1) no restriction, (2) shortage of financial resources, or (3) no money. The ideal, but not realistic situation is the first one. The third one allows no option for decision-making for the physician. In the middle case, the physician has to decide how much money can be used for a certain therapeutic intervention.

EPIDEMIOLOGY AND CALCULATION OF COSTS

In Europe, 900 000 patients die suddenly per year, about 90% because of an arrhythmogenic event. If 25% of the victims in whom sudden cardiac death (SCD) is the first manifestation of their disease are excluded, theoretically 600 000 patients would be candidates for an implantable cardioverter-defibrillator (ICD). If our community would accept the hypothesis that any risk of arrhythmogenic death has to be prevented, ICD implantation in all these

---

* Supported in part by Österreichische National Bank, Jubiläumsfonds 4025.

patients would be justified. The costs for this treatment would be 13 milliard ECU per year. Not only the limited financial resources for health care, but also the limited number of implanting hospitals make such a proceeding impossible. Therefore, the indications for ICD implantation have to be based on the evaluation of the individual risk [1]. There are two patient groups at risk for SCD:

1. Patients with organic heart disease but without ventricular tachycardia or fibrillation (VT/VF). The evaluation of risk in this group can use the following criteria:
   - Underlying heart disease
   - Left ventricular ejection fraction (LVEF)
   - Heart rate variability
   - Late potentials
   - Arrhythmia profile
   - Clinical symptoms

   The degree of impairment of LVEF, lack of heart rate variability, and the existence of late potentials have been documented as the most predictive parameters for the risk of SCD [2,3].
2. Patients with documented VT and survivors of SCD.

Table 1. Characteristics indicating low and high risk for SCD.

SCD risk below 10%	SCD risk above 10%
Ventricular tachycardia: Idiopathic ARVD DCM without syncope HCM without syncope	Ventricular fibrillation: Idiopathic DCM HCM
Postmyocardial infarction: VT without syncope NYHA I–II	Postmyocardial infarction: VT without syncope NYHA III–IV VF exercise-related VT with syncope exercise-related VF, VT with syncope NYHA III VF, VT with syncope, multiple MI

The question remains as to which incidence of SCD can be used as the boundary between low and high risk. A definite answer is not possible. Follow-up studies have elucidated the outcome of patients grouped according to the underlying heart disease NYHA classification and occurrence of syncope (Table 1) [4].

For the physician treating any kind of disease, the guideline for selecting a specific treatment should be that this therapeutical intervention will improve the patient's prognosis and quality of life and be psychologically acceptable. If a therapeutic intervention probably will not improve the quality of life and may even worsen it, e.g. severe heart failure, it should not be

Table 2. Socioeconomic aspects of treatment.

Return to work
Less expensive alternative treatment possible
Availability of a specific therapeutic method
No financial resources available

applied. In principle, the professional ethics of physicians preclude taking into consideration the socioeconomic aspects (Table 2) [5,6]. This means offering patients the best treatment even if it is very expensive, like an ICD. The significant criteria are a prolongation of life and improvement of the quality of life. Being able to return to work has a socioeconomic impact, and only under this aspect is it relevant for decision-making.

The physician also has to decide if another, 'less expensive' treatment in a given case is appropriate and if the costs of treatment can be reduced in this way. For this calculation not only the primary cost, e.g. the cost of the implantable cardioverter/defibrillator, but also follow-up costs have to be taken into account. From the economic point of view, in patients with ventricular tachycardia, ablation as the cheapest intervention should be first, antiarrhythmic surgery second, and ICD third choice. The costs of pharmacological treatment including expenses for regular medical check-up and hospital admission depend on the expectation of life of the patient. Thus, it is difficult to compare the costs of pharmacological and nonpharmacological interventions in patients with ventricular arrhythmias [7,8]. A comparison with other therapeutical methods has not only an economic but also a medical aspect. This is the evaluation of the benefit for the patients, the advantage, the disadvantage, and the inconvenience.

Finally, the availability of different therapeutic interventions has a socioeconomic impact. A department which treats patients with malignant ventricular arrhythmias should offer all kinds of pharmacological and nonpharmacological interventions. Only in this case can financial considerations be included in the decision-making process.

Not only the costs of a specific diagnostic and therapeutical intervention, but also the number of hospitals which can take care of patients with arrhythmias are of economic importance. The implementation of a department which is able to offer all methods of pharmacological and non-pharmacological treatment of arrhythmias is costly because of the necessary training of the staff, the expensive equipment in the laboratories and the materials (ICD, catheter). In most countries in the past, arrhythmia centers were not founded based on a regional or a national plan, but according to the activity of a cardiologist and/or local health authorities. As an example of this development, pacemaker implantation can be used. In countries like Belgium, France, and Germany, pacemaker implantation is performed in too many hospitals [9]. As a result the implantation ratio in these countries is high, probably too high. At the other end of the scale in the United

Kingdom and in Eastern and Southern countries of Europe, the number of implanting hospitals is too low. As a result, the number of pacemaker implantations does not correspond with the need.

At the present time guidelines for organizing the management of patients with malignant ventricular arrhythmias do not exist. The paper published by the Task Force of Working Groups on Cardiac Arrhythmias and Cardiac Pacing of the European Society of Cardiology presents guidelines for the use of ICDS and for the qualification of cardiologists who are involved in this treatment. This chapter does not cover organizational details [10]. In this situation it is extremely important to work out recommendations concerning the number of necessary centers per million inhabitants, staff, training criteria, and the minimal and maximal number of interventions per center [11–13].

It is impossible to compare the costs of ICD treatment with other therapeutical interventions on an international level. The reason for this is that the costs of ICD, including hospital fees and follow-up expenses, differ considerably throughout Europe. This is also true for the other therapeutical interventions. Studies dealing with the comparison of costs are retrospective, and the choice of antiarrhythmic agents in these investigations was individualized and not predesignated [14]. This can bias the comparison between pharmacological and non-pharmacological treatment.

In Austria the costs for an ICD based on a calculated lifetime of the implanted unit of between 48 and 60 months range per life-year saved between 5000 and 6000 ECU, for antiarrhythmic surgery 2000 to 4000 ECU, ablation 1200 to 1700 ECU, and drug treatment 1500 to 2100 ECU. These figures are different in other countries. In the USA, an ICD compared to pharmacological treatment reaches the break-through point after 3 years of treatment. This is mainly caused by the much higher hospital fees, which increase the costs for pharmacologically treated patients because of the more frequent rehospitalisation.

ORGANIZATION OF MANAGEMENT OF PATIENTS WITH VENTRICULAR TACHYCARDIA/FIBRILLATION IN EUROPE AT THE PRESENT TIME

Complete figures concerning the number of centers and number of interventions per year in the different countries in Europe are not available. In Table 3 the number of ICD implantations/million inhabitants for 1992 are presented. It ranges between 1.7 and 14.0. In Table 4 the relation between centers performing ICD implantation and the population in four countries is listed, and the relation between other special cardiological interventions and population is included. This list does not take into consideration the number of interventions per center. The accuracy of these figures is limited because

Table 3. ICD implantations per million inhabitants in various European countries in 1992.

Austria	6.8
Belgium	6.5
France	1.3
Germany	14
Italy	1.8
The Netherlands	1.7
Norway	7.1
Spain	1.8
Sweden	4.5
United Kingdom	2.2
Europe	1.8

Table 4. Relation between centers performing ICD implantation and population (in units per million).

	Austria	Germany	Italy	UK
Cardiac surgery	1.2	0.8	0.9	0.6
Catheter	3.8	2.5	1.4	0.8
PTCA	1.3	1.7	0.2	0.6
EPS	1.0	2.2	0.9	0.8
Pacemaker	5.6	13.1	4.7	1.1
ICD	0.6	0.2	0.3	0.1
Ablation	1.3	0.4	0.15	0.06

Table 5. Calculated figures of possible and definite ICD candidates per million inhabitants.

	Definite	Possible
Austria	32	20
USA	65	17

they have been collected through personal contact with rhythmologists in different countries and companies producing ICDs.

FUTURE PLANNING

Only a little information is available concerning the adequate number of ICD implantions per million inhabitants [15,16]. The calculated figures range between 32 and 65 definite and 17 to 20 possible candidates per million (Table 5). In reality, this figure is not achieved by far (Table 3). Based on this calculation, an amount of 6.9–13.5 million ECU per million people would be necessary to cover the costs of this treatment for definite candidates. Another prerequisite is the implementation of an adequate number of specialized centers. At the present time, the number of centers performing ICD implantation ranges between 0.1 and 0.6 per million people. This figure gives no information about the number of implantations, which differs remarkably.

Based on a survey in Austria, a figure of 212 patients with VT/VF per million/year has been calculated. Two-thirds of these patients are below the age of 70 years. Assuming that 60% of them are candidates for non-pharmacological treatment, at very least 1 specialized center/million inhabitants for treating patients with malignant arrhythmia is necessary [17]. It will be mandatory to work out recommendations for the organization of management of patients with arrhythmias. This recommendation has to include:

1. Number of centers
2. Number of patients with malignant arrhythmias/center
3. Minimal number/center of
   a) Cardioverter/defibrillator implantations
   b) Ablation
   c) Surgical interventions
4. Size and training of staff
5. Follow-up facilities
6. Documentation of data
7. Quality control

It is the task of the European Working Groups on Cardiac Pacing and Arrhythmias to take over the responsibility of planning the adequate number of centers for treating patients with malignant ventricular arrhythmias. This activity has to take into consideration the medical as well as the socioeconomic aspects mentioned in this chapter.

REFERENCES

1. Akhtar M, Avitall B, Jazayeri M et al. Role of implantable cardioverter defibrillator therapy in the management of high risk patients. Circulation 1992;85(Suppl I):131–9.
2. Farrell TG, Bashir Y, Cripps T. Risk stratification for arrhythmic events in postinfarction patients based on heart rate variability, ambulatory electrocardiographic variables and the signal-averaged electrocardiogram. J Am Coll Cardiol 1991;18:687–97.
3. Klein H, Trappe HJ, Fiegeth HG, Nisam S. Prospective studies evaluating prophylactic ICD therapy for high risk patients with coronary artery disease. PACE 1993;16:564–70.
4. Brugada P, Andries E. The rationale for prophylactic implantation of a defibrillator in 'high risk' patients. PACE 1993;16:547–51.
5. Hauer RNW, Wever EFD, Crijns HJGM. Automatic implantable cardioverter defibrillator: Cost effectiveness. PACE 1993;16:559–63.
6. Winkle RA. Early automatic implantable cardioverter-defibrillator implantation: Medical and economic considerations and inequities in health care reimbursement. J Am Coll Cardiol 1990;16:1264–6.
7. Kuppermann M, Luce BR, McGovern B. An analysis of the cost effectiveness of the

implantable cardioverter-defibrillator: Is early implantation cost-effective? J Am Coll Cardiol 1990;81:91–100.
8. O'Donoghue S, Platia E, Brooks-Robinson S, Misipireta L. Automatic implantable cardioverter-defibrillator: Is early implantation cost-effective? J Am Coll Cardiol 1990;16:1258–63.
9. Feruglio GA, Rickards AF, Steinbach K, Feldman S, Parsonnet V. Cardiac pacing in the world. A survey of the state of the art in 1986. PACE 1987;10:768.
10. Coumel PH. Guidelines for the use of implantable cardioverter defibrillator. Eur Heart J 1992;13:1304–10.
11. Steinbeck G, Meinertz T, Andresen D. Empfehlungen zur Implantation von Defibrillatoren. Z Kardiol 1991;80:475–8.
12. Lehmann MH, Saksena S. Implantable cardioverter defibrillators in cardiovascular practice: Report of the Policy Conference of the North American Society of Pacing and Electrophysiology. PACE 1991;14:969–79.
13. Dreifus LS, Fisch C, Griffin JC. Guidelines for implantation of cardiac pacemakers and antiarrhythmic devices. J Am Coll Cardiol 1991;18:1–13.
14. Kuppermann M, Luce BR, McGovern B, Podrid PJ, Bigger T, Ruskin JN. An analysis of the cost effectiveness of the implantable defibrillator. Circulation 1990;81:91–100.
15. Podczeck A, Frohner K, Kaltenbrunner W, Steinbach K. Epidemiology and decision making in patients with sustained ventricular tachycardia. Eur Heart J 1991;12(Suppl I):1793.
16. Kottke TE, Stanton MS, Bailey KR. Estimated candidacy rates for implantable cardioverter defibrillators in a defined population. J Am Coll Cardiol 1992;19:208A.
17. Bigger JT. Future studies with the implantable cardioverter defibrillator. PACE 1991;14:883–9.

Index

ablation 137, 138, 139, 411, 436
ablation of the bundle of His 139
adverse effects of VVI/VVIR pacing 236
alcohol 58
aliasing 105
amiodarone 42, 132
analog-to-digital converter 107
antiarrhythmic drugs 23, 24
antiarrhythmic treatment 42
antitachycardia pacing 387, 411
antitachycardia systems 319
atenolol 20
atrial chronotropic incompetence 230
atrial escape interval 304
atrial fibrillation 355
atrial flutter 139
atrial leads 221
atrial pacing 357
atrial rate histogram 328
atrial refractory period 358
atrial tachycardia 139
atrioventricular nodal reentrant tachycardia 138, 145
Autocorrelation methods 51
autonomic nervous system 170
AV delay 238
AV nodal pathway 138
AV block 356, 357

baroreflex sensitivity 55
bidirectional filter 112
BIOTRONIK 364

cardiac death code 44
cardioinhibitory 16, 17
cardiomyopathy 31, 33, 275

cardioversion 387
chaos 52
Chorus II 364
chronic atrial fibrillation 229
chronic AV block 230
chronotropic incompetence 228
clonidine 20
common-mode rejection ratio 99
conditional ventricular tracking limit 365
congestive heart failure 236
CPI 364

DAT mode 233
DDI mode 19
DDD pacing 275, 333
DDDR pacing 363
DDI and DDIR modes 255
DDI mode 311
defibrillator 426
delayed potential 33, 34
Diamond 367
different modes of pacing 163
disopyramide 20
dual atrium pacing 232
dynamic QT interval 73
dynamic variations of the QT interval 67

effect of age 55
effect of heart rate 56
effect of posture 56
effect of exercise 57
ELA Medical 364
electrode 169, 181, 186, 189, 190, 194, 196, 199, 200, 203, 221, 223, 347, 350, 351, 353

electrode replacement 163
electronic filtering 102
electrophysiological testing 28
Elite 306
emotion 58
ensemble averaging 103
EP 390
equipment 3
electrophysiology laboratory 3
etilefrine 20
Eur Heart 129
event counter 310
event counter telemetry 312
event histogram 312, 328
event markers in pacemakers 400

fallback 305, 358, 359, 360, 364
Fast Fourier Transformation 102
fast pathway ablation 138
finite impulse response 111
Fourier transformation 51
Frank lead system 94
frequency domain 100

heart failure 41
heart rate oscillations 64
Heart rate variability 49, 63, 79, 80, 81, 82, 83, 84, 89
heart transplant patients 230
high-degree AV block 228
high-resolution electrocardiography 93
Holter 83, 87, 88, 333, 336, 341, 360, 362, 370
HRV 49, 56, 57, 58
hypertrophic obstructive cardiomyopathy 245

ICD 41, 336, 341, 342, 377, 378, 385, 387, 388, 395, 396, 412, 413, 415, 416, 426, 429, 431, 433, 434
idiopathic atrial chronotropic incompetence 231
impedance 181, 199, 347, 350
implantable cardioverter-defibrillator (ICD) 424, 433
implantable cardioverter-defibrillator therapy (ICD) 411
implantable defibrillator 373
implantable devices 424
Implantable monitors 321
indications for pacing 161
infarction 86
Infinite impulse response 112
ischaemia 131

interatrial conduction 239
Intermedics 365
Intermedics Cosmos 312
ischaemia 131

Johnson (or Nyquist) noise 99

late potentials 93, 125, 126, 131, 135, 378
left-sided pathways 139
linear averaging 103
Lorentz plots 52

malignant vasovagal syndrome 15, 17, 20
mapping 4
Medtronic's Elite II 365
mental stress 58
Meta DDDR 365
mode switching 330, 361, 363, 364, 365, 368, 369, 370
motion artifacts 97
myocardial infarction 79, 81, 83, 84, 86, 125, 136
myocardial ischaemia 131
myopotentials 97

normal ventricular activation sequence 244
nonobstructive hypertrophic cardiomyopathy 275

oxygen saturation controlled pacing 290

pacing in chronic AV block 238
pacing in dilated cardiomyopathy 275
pacing in hypertrophic cardiomyopathy 269
pacemakers 424
pacemakers controlled by minute ventilation and body activity 294
pacemaker syndrome 236
pacemaker syndrome during atrial-based pacing 251
Pacemaker syndrome with AAIR pacing 260
pacemaker syndrome with dual chamber pacing 251
phase shift 111
physical training 57
physiological cardiac pacing 227
Poincaré plots 52
posteroseptal pathways 139
postmyocardial infarction patients 73
predictive accuracy 119
pre-pacing ECG 161
programmed stimulation 4
pseudo atrial exit block 258

pulse generator replacement 163
P wave amplitude histogram 326
P wave synchronous pacing 231

QRSD 118
T interval 63

radiofrequency 137
rate-adaptive AV delay 305
rate-adaptive pacing 161
rate-adaptive PVARP 305
rate smoothing 305
relay 365
repetitive nonreentrant VA synchrony 257, 258
repetitive nonreentrant ventriculoatrial resolution 107
retrograde SP mapping 146
reverse AV interval hysteresis 364
right-sided septal accessory pathways 139
ringing 111

SAECG 119, 133, 134, 135, 136
sampling technique 105
SCD 432
scopolamine 20
screw-in 222
screw-in electrodes 221
sensor-driven pacing 233
sensor-indicated rate counters 315
sensor-indicated rate histogram 329
sequential averaging 103
Shot (or Schottky) noise 99
sick sinus syndrome 363
Siemens Pacesetter 312, 365
signal-averaged 126
signal-averaged analysis 128
signal-averaged electrocardiogram 131
signal-averaged electrocardiography 93
signal averaging 125
sinus node disease (SND) 230, 237
skin potentials 97
slow-pathway ablation 145
slow potentials 146, 148
smoking 58

Sorin Biomedica's SWING DR1 365
spectral methods 51
spectral window filters 112
spike potentials 146
stored data in ICDs 404
stratify risk 73
sudden cardiac death 431
sudden death 42, 378
synchrony 257, 306
Synchrony II 365
Synchrony III 365
Synergyst 306
syncope 132

Telectronics 365
Telectronics Guardian 320
telemetered electrograms 399
telemetry in pacemakers 400
template 109
THERA 365
time domain 99
time domain averaging 103
time domain methods 50
time-domain SAECG 118

Upper rate behaviour 304

vasovagal syncope 15
    incidence 15
    cardioinhibitory 16, 17
    vasodepressor 16, 17, 20
VA synchrony nonreentrant arrhythmia 258
VDD mode 254
VDD pacing 209
venous oxygen saturation controlled pacing 290
ventricular chronotropic incompetence 228
ventricular fibrillation 184, 373, 387, 411
ventricular tachycardia 373, 387, 411
Ventritex Cadence 320
Vitatron Medical 367
VT 379, 390

Wolff-Parkinson-White syndrome 138